Clinical Imaging
in Non-Pulmonary Tuberculosis

Springer

Berlin
Heidelberg
New York
Barcelona
Hong Kong
London
Milan
Paris
Singapore
Tokyo

Francis E. McGuinness

Clinical Imaging in Non-Pulmonary Tuberculosis

With Contributions by
D. Hamilton and J. Al Nabulsi

With 172 Illustrations in 345 Parts

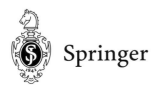 Springer

RC 311.2
M36
2000

Dr. Francis E. McGuinness
Korte Prinsengracht 87
1013 GR Amsterdam
Netherlands

Contributors
Dr. David Hamilton
Dr. Jawada Al Nabulsi
Riyadh Armed Forces Hospital
P. O. Box 7897
Riyadh 11159
Saudi Arabia

ISBN 3-540-65940-4 Springer-Verlag Berlin Heidelberg New York

Library of Congress Cataloging-in-Publication Data
McGuinnes, Francis, 1930–. Clinical imaging in non-pulmonary tuberculosis / Francis McGuinness, with contributions of David Hamilton and Jawada Al Nabulsi. p. cm. Includes bibliographical references and index. ISBN 3-540-65940-4 (hc.: alk. paper) 1. Tuberculosis – Imaging. I. Hamilton, David, Dr. II. Al Nabulsi, Jawada. III. Title. [DNLM: 1. Tuberculosis – diagnosis. 2. Diagnostic Imaging – methods. WF 220 M478c 1999]. RC311.2.M36 1999. 616.9'950754–dc21. DNLM/DLC. for Library of Congress 99-35196

This work is subject to copyright. All rights are reserved, whether the whole or part of the material is concerned, specifically the rights of translation, reprinting, reuse of illustrations, recitation, broadcasting, reproduction on microfilm or in any other way, and storage in data banks. Duplication of this publication or parts thereof is permitted only under the provisions of the German Copyright Law of September 9, 1965, in its current version, and permission for use must always be obtained from Springer-Verlag. Violations are liable for prosecution under the German Copyright Law.

The use of general descriptive names, registered names, trademarks, etc. in this publication does not imply, even in the absence of a specific statement, that such names are exempt from the relevant protective laws and regulations and therefore free for general use.

© Springer-Verlag Berlin Heidelberg 2000
Printed in Germany

Product liability: The publishers cannot guarantee the accuracy of any information about dosage and application contained in this book. In every individual case the user must check such information by consulting the relevant literature.

Cover design: Erich Kirchner, Heidelberg
Typesetting: Fotosatz-Service Köhler GmbH, 97084 Würzburg
Computer to film and binding: Universitätsdruckerei Stürtz AG, 97080 Würzburg

SPIN: 10554336   21/3135 – 5 4 3 2 1 0 – Printed on acid-free paper

To Annelies Heuker of Hoek,
who made this book possible

Acknowledgements

It is impossible to produce a text book without the help of many co-workers. In my case, most of the background work was carried out in two Saudi Arabian hospitals: The King Khaled National Guard Hospital in Jeddah and, latterly, The Armed Forces Hospital in Riyadh.

I would like to thank all those physicians and surgeons in both hospitals who have given me access to their clinical cases. My thanks in particular must go to Dr. Mona Al Shahed, whose carefully preserved film library in Riyadh is the source of many of the illustrations in the sections on bone and joint tuberculosis, and tuberculosis of the alimentary tract. Dr. Monir Madkour gave me valuable advice on the expression of tuberculosis versus brucellosis.

The co-operation of the Diagnostic Imaging Department at Riyadh was essential to my work, and I am most grateful to the head of the department, Dr. M.Y. Aabed Al Thagafi, and his staff, including Mrs. Wendy Stonehouse, Mrs. Sue Ferguson, Mrs. Sharan Fergie, Ms. Eileen Henderson and Dr. John Morgan, for their advice and co-operation. Steve Nally of the Medical Illustration Department produced the slides for the illustrations.

Other co-workers at the Armed Forces Hospital provided me with material, including Professor Price-Evans, Dr. W.M. Othman and Dr. Saleh Hamza.

The Nuclear Medicine Department, under the leadership of Dr. U.J. Miola, deserves special mention in that Dr. David Hamilton and Dr. J.J. Nabulsi wrote the chapter on isotope imaging in tuberculosis.

Even after many years in clinical practice, it is impossible to collect cases representing all the facets of tuberculosis imaging. I am therefore grateful to many colleagues from around the world for allowing me to use their previously published material. These include Dr. Ravi Ramakantan of Bombay, Dr. Shu-Hang Ng of Taiwan, Drs. Chan and J. Pang of Hong Kong, Dr. F.G. Arias of Oviedo, Spain, Dr. J. Berciano of Santander, Spain, Dr. Denath of Kuwait, Dr. Dorothy Makanjuola of King Saud University, Riyadh and Dr. Clive Levine of University of Missouri, Columbia, USA.

As there is a low incidence of AIDS in Saudi Arabia, I am particularly grateful to Dr. Nuria Bargallo of Barcelona and Dr. P. Goodman of the University of Texas, Houston for the inclusion of illustrations in Chap. 8. Dr. Brian Cremin also provided me with many excellent illustrations from his book *Childhood tuberculosis: modern imaging and clinical concepts*. Springer-Verlag and another South African colleague, Dr. Jan Lotz, were also helpful to me. I thank them all.

Contents

CHAPTER 1

Introduction

"Events during the past decade have dramatically changed the nature and magnitude of the problem of tuberculosis. Much of what many physicians learned in training about this disease is no longer true. In many respects tuberculosis has become a new entity" [1].

The return of tuberculosis as a major infectious disease in Western industrialised countries has taken doctors by surprise and found them unprepared to fight it. Globalisation is a word that is constantly applied by governments, economists and financial gurus to the transfer of money and information around the world; however, it does not only apply to politics but also to the transfer of populations and of disease. Due to new methods of rapid transport, all countries are more accessible, and this has occurred at a time of global financial and political instability. Refugees from war zones and from undemocratic regimes, as well as economic refugees, are crossing internal and international boundaries in increasing numbers. In our societies, these people represent a new group who are at particular risk of contracting tuberculosis. This risk is compounded by the world-wide epidemic of acquired immunodeficiency syndrome (AIDS), where the lowering of immunity has allowed tuberculosis a new vehicle through which to spread. This, as well as the new manifestations of tuberculosis, has led the World Health Organisation (WHO) to set up a tuberculosis programme.

Tuberculosis occurs not just in sub-Saharan Africa and the Far East, where there is a rapid increase in patient numbers, but in countries such as the former Soviet Union, where the recent collapse of financial structures leaves governments unable to carry out their anti-tuberculosis programs. The disease also occurs in eastern Europe, where post-communist democracies are struggling to keep their health services viable, and in Latin and Middle America, where natural disasters, population explosions and poor socio-economic structures are making it more and more difficult to combat disease. Finally, there is China, which is in the shadow of the Asian financial crisis and is plagued by internal economic problems, the result of flooding and the mass migration of agricultural workers to overcrowded cities.

In the West, we can no longer say that we are a fortress, safe from these problems. The time to say that we are safe is long past. Our own success has led to the development of a society with relatively high numbers of older people who are susceptible to tuberculosis and to the development of an under-class who are particularly exposed to the disease. It has also made us attractive to many economic refugees, who will cross the borders in the near future. Not only has tuberculosis changed but, during the past 20 years, the methods of investigation available to the radiologist and the physician have developed.

The purpose of this book is to increase our awareness of the many clinical patterns of non-pulmonary tuberculosis, often called the great imitator. Professor P. E. S. Palmer has said that the only thing to expect from tuberculosis is the unexpected. Many of us have a whole armoury with which to fight against tuberculosis. Others are less fortunate and fight against a combination of tuberculosis and financial constraint. Because of this, I have included accounts of some of the less sophisticated methods of investigation as well as those available in modern Western hospitals.

With the introduction of effective anti-tuberculous chemotherapy in the early 1950s, the disease declined rapidly, and public health specialists claimed a victory over it [2]. This led to a decrease in funding for the established anti-tuberculous programmes, with the closure of many centres in Europe and North America and less support for research. However, the very nature of the disease, with its slow insidiousness and ability to reactivate, meant that there was always a pool of active infection in society.

Until recently, it seemed that, in Western countries, the problem was under control, with the number of cases continuing to decline annually in Europe and North America, but the picture changed in the 1980s. The rate in the USA fell from 95 per 100,000 in 1944 to less than 10 per 100,000 but, since 1986, there has been a continuing annual rise from 9.3 per 100,000 in 1987 to 10.4 per 100,000 in 1991, when more than 26,000 new cases were reported. Since 1985, there has been an increase of 18 % per annum [3].

Globally, the situation raises even more cause for concern. Now, the WHO points to tuberculosis as having the highest mortality of all present-day infectious diseases [4].

WHO statistics estimate that, in 1990, 1.7 billion people were infected, with 20 million active cases. Annually, 8 million new cases are diagnosed, resulting in 3 million deaths [5]. Among the 8 million, 1.3 million are children, with 450,000 dying under the age of 15 years. Of these cases, 95 % are in developing countries and, among 15–59 year olds, tuberculosis accounts for 25 % of avoidable deaths [6]. The WHO also notes that reported cases of tuberculosis in some African countries doubled during the last 4 years of the 1980s [7]. In a 1995 WHO update, it was estimated that one-third of the world population is infected by *Mycobacterium tuberculosis*. The number of new active cases is still 8 million per annum. Significantly, Southeast Asia, the most densely populated area of the world, is singled out as a problem area. There are approximately 2 million cases in this area each year, with more than 500,000 deaths. Co-infection with the AIDS virus is extremely high in the region and may rise by a factor of seven in the coming decade [7].

Historically, tuberculosis was a widespread and deadly infectious disease until the introduction of effective anti-tuberculous chemotherapy. The ability of the organism to lie dormant intracellularly in a closed off nidus and to reactivate when the immunity of the host changes made it impossible to eradicate totally.

Bad socio-economic conditions, such as overcrowding, poverty and malnutrition, favour the spread of tuberculosis through the target groups. Alcoholics, diabetics and the immunocompromised have always been susceptible. To these groups are now added those infected with the AIDS virus and people addicted to intravenous (IV) drugs. Tuberculosis was epidemic during Western industrial revolutions, while European wars and refugee problems of this century supported its spread. Today, conditions in inner cities and large-scale immigrations provide suitable conditions for the dissemination of tuberculosis in both Europe and the Americas. The decision to reduce the amount of investment in anti-tuberculous measures during the last 40 years has now been shown to be a fundamental error. In recent years, there have even been shortages of anti-tuberculous drugs in North America [8]. In the developing world, the disease has been ever present, but expertise, finance and logistics to combat it have not been available. With the introduction of chemotherapy in the 1950s, an opportunity was lost. It was quickly shown that, with good supervision and patient follow-up, it was possible to cure sputum-positive cases by 18 months of triple-drug therapy. The emergence of the neurotoxic effects

of streptomycin and the gastrointestinal side effects of para-aminosalicylic acid led many patients to abandon treatment. Centres of excellence that led the fight, such as Edinburgh [9], found to their dismay that many others introduced less adequate drug therapy, without meticulous supervision, and that bacterial drug resistance emerged. The development of new anti-tuberculous drugs only postponed the inevitable, for the lack of supervision in medication led once more to patient non-compliance and drug resistance. Further closure of public health programmes and sanatoria compounded the problem.

The basis of WHO's anti-tuberculous-therapy plan is short-course chemotherapy (SCC). This is 6 months of therapy combining isoniazid, rifampicin and pyrazinamide, administered as directly observed therapy (DOTS) [10]. Local culture and politics, as well as the financing of drugs and health care workers, present major problems that, in Asia and Africa, are very difficult to overcome. The worst outcome is that a badly run programme is a potential source of further drug resistance. In the West, patient non-compliance is as high as 20 % [10]. This has led to a surge in multi-drug-resistant mycobacteria. In New York, from 1982 to 1984, 9.8% of isolates in new cases were resistant to at least one drug, while the figure for relapsed cases was 52 % [3].

Multi-drug resistance is increasing among problem groups of patients, including IV drug users, AIDS patients, alcoholics and recidivist prisoners, who are unlikely to comply with the regimes without close supervision. This means that the DOTS system will have to be introduced into Western countries as well.

If direct microscopy is negative, the diagnosis of tuberculosis by culture takes up to 6 weeks, mycobacterial resistance studies from 3 weeks to 12 weeks. New, faster methods, using polymerase chain reaction techniques are being developed but, at this time, are expensive and not generally available. The time lag associated with relying on conventional laboratory culture to isolate the bacterium facilitates the spread of tuberculosis. This is especially so in closed communities, for example: prisons, hostels, hospitals and welfare homes, and among their inmates and employees. Patients with AIDS are found in many of these institutions, and this leads to co-infection. In AIDS patients, the chance of co-existent tuberculosis is 8 % per annum, in contrast to a lifetime risk of 10 % in healthy, Mantoux-positive individuals. Although making the initial diagnosis may be difficult because of its many difficult presentations, the cure rate of tuberculosis in AIDS patients after supervised chemotherapy is comparable with that in sero-negative patients [11]. However, if the organism is multi-drug resistant, the mortality in AIDS patients is 80 % [3, 12].

The chance of the infection being extra-pulmonary in AIDS patients increases dramatically if the immunodeficiency is advanced. The resurgence of tuberculosis paints a bleak outlook for world populations. Early diagnosis is essential in limiting the devastating consequences of infection. In order to achieve this, re-education of the public, doctors and health care workers will be necessary. The disease must be included in differential diagnosis more often. Many authors have emphasised the fact that, in order to make the diagnosis, the physician must possess a high index of suspicion for the disease [13]. Since the early innovative period of diagnostic X-rays, radiologists have always been a major link in the chain leading to the diagnosis of tuberculosis. The technical advances of the last 40 years have placed many new diagnostic modalities in the radiologists' hands, and the radiograph – the basic tool – has never diminished in value. The introduction, by the WHO, of the basic radiographic unit to many centres in Asia, Africa and Latin America has been an important step forward, but it is the awareness that the disease affects all types and levels of society and all age groups that is important. Doctors must also recognise the many unexpected manifestations of tuberculosis and its wide spectrum of disease patterns. As a systemic disease, there is no organ in the body that cannot be infected, leading to a chimera of disease patterns and radiological images.

Many papers have appeared in the world radiological literature over the past decade dealing with diverse aspects of non-pulmonary tuberculosis, but there has been no general bench book dealing with the plurality of the disease since the early 1980s. This book is an attempt to bridge that gap and to illustrate, as widely as possible, the diversity of the disease as well as provide pointers to appropriate radiological investigation. Bearing in mind that highly advanced technology is spread thinly throughout the world, simple technology is also emphasised.

■ References

1. Snider DE, Roper WL (1992) The new tuberculosis. N Engl J Med 362:703–705
2. Bignall JR (1971) Tuberculosis in England and Wales in the next 20 years. Postgrad Med J 47:759–762
3. Bloom BR, Murray CJL (1992) Tuberculosis: commentary on a re-emergent killer. Science 257:1055–1063
4. Murray CJL, Styblo K, Rouillon A (1992) Disease control priorities in developing countries. Oxford University Press, New York
5. WHO (1990) The work of the World Health Organization 1988–89. WHO, Geneva
6. WHO (1990) Global estimates for health situation assessment and projections. WHO, Geneva
7. WHO (1995) World health statistics quarterly. 48 no 3/4
8. Peloquin CA (1992) Shortages of antimycobacterial drugs. N Engl J Med 5:714
9. Leitch AJ (1996) Two men and a bug: one hundred years of tuberculosis in Edinburgh. Proc R Coll Physicians Edinb 26:295–308
10. Raviglione MC, Snider DE, Kochi A (1995) Global epidemiology of tuberculosis. JAMA 273:220–226
11. Small PM (1991) Treatment of tuberculosis in patients with advanced human immunodeficiency virus infection. N Engl J Med 324:289–294
12. Snider DE Jr, Cauthen GM, Farer LS, Kelly GD, Kilburn JO, Good RC, Dooley SW (1991) Drug-resistant tuberculosis. Am Rev Respir Dis 144:732
13. Cook GC (1985) Tuberculosis: certainly not a disease of the past. Q J Med New series, 56:519–521

CHAPTER 2

Intracranial Tuberculosis

■ Histopathology of Intracranial Tuberculosis

The manifestations of tuberculosis are diverse and are reflected in imaging appearances. In interpreting the images, an understanding of the underlying histopathology of the disease is helpful. Detailed descriptions of the histopathological changes of tuberculous infection of the central nervous system are to be found in the literature [1–4]. A brief account of the major changes that influence the imaging appearances in central nervous system tuberculosis follows. Central nervous system tuberculosis is almost invariably the result of haematological spread of the infection from a focus elsewhere in the body.

Direct spread from tuberculous spinal or cranial osteomyelitis is a rarity due to the effective barrier of the dura mater. In the majority of cases, the primary source of disease is a focus of pulmonary or pulmonary – lymphatic tuberculosis. In infants and children, a primary pulmonary focus leading to local lymph-node involvement with the development of progressive primary tuberculosis is the common cause of spread of the disease to the nervous system. In older patients (from adolescence onwards), reactivation of pulmonary disease, miliary tuberculosis or spinal tuberculosis are the common causes of haematogenous dissemination to the central nervous system. Miliary tuberculosis, resulting from gastrointestinal or non-spinal bone or joint infection, is a less common cause of central nervous system involvement.

The initial response of the host to tuberculous infection is to surround the bacilli with phagocytic polymorphonucleocytes in an attempt to enclose it. Inside this focus, the organism continues to multiply. It is not until about 2 weeks after the original infection that an immune response initiates, leading to the development of the tubercles characteristic of the disease. The destruction and replacement of host tissue is more the result of the immune response than any local destruction caused by the bacillus itself. The basis of immunity to tuberculosis is a cell-mediated process. At first, virulent microbacteria are phagocytosed – but not killed – by polymorpho-

nucleocytes. T-lymphocytes stimulate the development of activated macrophages by producing an immune lymphokine. This is the result of a response of the T-cells to the immunising tuberculoprotein of *Mycobacterium tuberculosis*. The activated macrophages are able to kill the intracellular bacilli residing within themselves. Recently, it has been proposed that cytotoxic T-lymphocytes may also play an important role in destroying the mycobacterium [1].

■ Tuberculous Meningitis

The initial lesion in the central nervous system is a microscopic granuloma or Rich focus [5–8]. This lesion either develops superficially (in the parenchyma of the brain) or in the wall of an arteriole. When it ruptures into the subarachnoid space tuberculous meningitis (TBM) develops. A Rich focus developing deeper in the brain parenchyma will lead to the development of a parenchymal tuberculoma. Due to the paucity of polymorphonucleocytes, the cerebrospinal fluid (CSF) and the subarachnoid space have poor defences against the tubercle bacillus, which spreads rapidly along the meninges through the basal cisterns [9–11].

Cell-mediated immunity (CMI) leads to the development of a glutinous exudate. In the first stages, the exudate is largely confined to the basal subarachnoid areas but rapidly involves the basal cisterns, particularly the inter-peduncular and suprasellar spaces [2–4, 12]. Spread of the exudate along the periarterial spaces of the major arteries is favoured, and circumferential encasement of the common carotid, middle, anterior and posterior cerebral arteries follows, facilitating spread of the exudate to the ambient system, pre-pontine cistern and the supratentorial subarachnoid spaces [9–11, 13–16].

The exudate is an inflammatory response to the presence of both intra- and extracellular tubercle bacilli. The cell-mediated reaction from activated T-cells leads to an outpouring of lymphocytes and monocytes, which reorganise into countless, microscopic tubercles. The characteristic of these tubercles

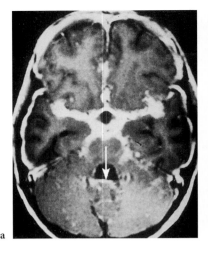
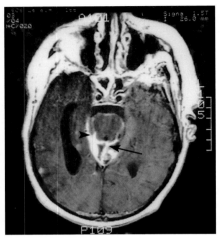

a   b

Fig. 2.1. a Axial T1-weighted, post-gadolinium scan, demonstrating intense enhancement of the basal meninges in a case of tuberculous meningitis. The *white arrow* points to borderzone disease adjacent to the fourth ventricle. **b** A similar scan at a lower level. There is enhancement of the surface of the brain stem and of exudates in the surrounding cisterns (*arrow*). On both scans, there is enhancement of the meninges over the convexities, and a number of small parenchymal granulomas. There is hydrocephalus

is an outer layer of lymphocytes and an inner core of monocytes and epithelioid cells, which fuse to form Langerhans'-type giant cells. They are spread in great numbers throughout the infected area, leading to the development of the associated exudate and, importantly, to the development of arteritis in both the larger and smaller arteries and arterioles of the basal areas. The occlusion of the vessels involved in the

process of arteritis leads to infarction of the areas of brain that they supply, particularly the basal ganglia, but also, less commonly, the large territories of the anterior and middle cerebral arteries. The common triad of imaging changes in TBM are: basal meningeal enhancement on contrast-enhanced computer tomography (CECT) and gadolinium (Gd)-enhanced magnetic resonance imaging (CEMR), hydrocephalus on computed tomography (CT) and magnetic resonance (MR), and parenchymal supratentorial and brain-stem infarctions. These are the direct result of the underlying histopathological changes. Enhance-

Fig. 2.2 a, b. Sagittal T1 and proton-density scans. There is a grape-like cluster of tuberculous granulomas obstructing the outflow of the fourth ventricle, resulting in hydrocephalus (*arrow*)

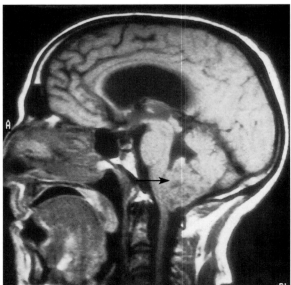
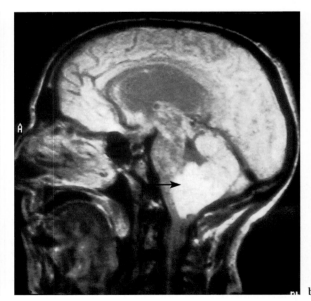

a   b

Fig. 2.3 a, b.
Extensive, bilateral, thalamic
infarction and hydrocephalus
on coronal magnetic resonance
imaging (*arrows*). Images by
courtesy of Dr. J. Lotz, Riyadh
Military Hospital, Saudi Arabia

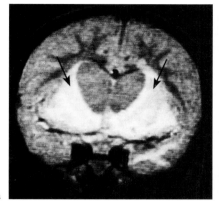
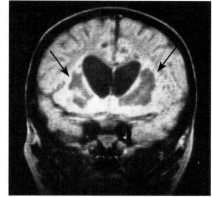

a

b

ment is due to the intense basal inflammatory exudates. Hydrocephalus is due to blockage of the CSF
pathways, and infarction is the result of closure of the
basal cerebral vessels. Basal contrast enhancement
follows the pathway of the distribution of the cerebral arteries (Fig. 2.1). Linked with the other two
elements of the triad, this enhancement is highly
suggestive of TBM but is by no means pathognomonic. Other conditions – bacillary meningitis,
fungal meningitis, other granulomatous diseases and
meningeal metastatic disease – may demonstrate a
similar picture, usually with a less intense enhancement and a narrower distribution [9 – 11, 14 – 22].

The second almost universal feature, hydrocephalus, rarely precedes the development of basal enhancement [20, 23] and, in most cases, develops simultaneously with basal meningeal exudates. The resulting
interruption of the circulation of CSF prevents its
passage over cerebral convexities to points of re-
absorption at the arachnoid granulations. Hydrocephalus develops and is characteristically of high
pressure, and the periventricular white matter is suf-
fused, to a greater or lesser extent, with hydrostatic
oedema [9, 10].

Rarely, the hydrocephalus results from obstruction of the aqueduct of Sylvius due to pressure from
a parenchymal lesion (Fig. 2.2). It is of great importance that the radiologist recognises this as, in these
cases, ventricular shunting will be necessary [1, 9, 11,
24]. The third manifestation of the triad is parenchymal brain infarction.

Arteritis, encasement by exudate, vessel spasms
and vessel occlusion lead to compromise of the arterial flow in the vessels of the Circle of Willis and their
peripheral branches. Angiographic and post-mortem
studies have demonstrated occlusion ranging from
closure of the intracranial segment of the carotid
artery to thrombosis of its major branches, leading
to large territorial infarctions. However, the smaller
perforating branches are more commonly affected
than the larger arteries, such as the medial striate and

thalamo-perforating arteries, leading to a characteristic picture of infarction in the thalamus and
caudate nucleus (Fig. 2.3) [1, 9, 10, 12, 16, 20, 25].
According to the literature, supratentorial infarction
occurs in 30 – 60 % of cases [1, 9, 10, 20, 21, 25 – 27].
Brain-stem infarction is much less common, with an
incidence of 2 – 3 %. Brain-stem infarction is particularly difficult to recognise, especially in the presence
of border-zone disease. It may be more common than
is at present assumed.

Apart from the triad of enhancement, hydrocephalus and infarction, other manifestations are
common. As TBM progresses, border-zone leptomeningeal encephalitis develops in those parts of the
brain invested with meningeal exudate [10, 26]. The
areas likely to be involved are the cortex and white
matter related to the basal exudates, the surface of
the cerebral peduncles abutting onto the interpeduncular fossa and the part of the brain stem adjacent to
the ambient system.

Recognition of these lesions is difficult, as the
bright signal seen on MR T2-weighted images in
these border zones merges with the high signal of the
leptomeningeal exudate (Fig. 2.4) [10]. Around the
third ventricle, encephalitic changes are almost invariably present post-mortem [1, 28]. On MR imaging
studies, the basal ganglia fail to show a high signal
in these areas and, more often, demonstrate the
changes of parenchymal infarction. Tuberculomas
are present in the brains of between 10 % and 50 % of
patients with TBM. This wide variation may be dependent on the duration of the disease at the time
the cases present. The lesions, both peripheral and
supratentorial, are usually less than 1 cm in diameter.
Instances of thalamic, midbrain and brain-stem tuberculomas in TBM are also well documented. The
clinical presentation and distribution of tuberculomas in TBM is different from those developing
as sporadic, parenchymal lesions and may be over-
shadowed by the other manifestations of the disease
(Fig. 2.5).

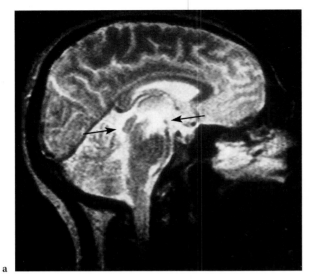

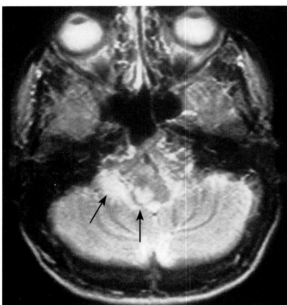

Fig. 2.4 a, b. Axial and sagittal, T2-weighted images demonstrate extensive basal exudates and border-zone disease. This encroaches on the anterior margin of the right cerebellar hemisphere (*arrows*)

High signals on MR T2-weighted studies have been demonstrated in the sheaths and substance of the cranial nerves and are usually associated with clinical deficits in cranial-nerve function. The second, third, fourth and sixth cranial nerves are often damaged as a result of their passage through the basal exudate and their long anatomical courses. The fifth and seventh nerves are affected as they leave the midbrain. Late-stage histological change in TBM, in which the combination of long-term chemotherapy

and tissue healing convert the basal exudates into dense, fibrotic tissue, is the reason for permanent loss of function in these nerves, the pattern of deficit varying from patient to patient [14, 21, 26, 29]. Severe or late-stage TBM also demonstrates the advance of leptomeningitic changes over the cerebral convexities and ependymitis in the ventricular walls.

TBM Cerebral Infarction

The vascular lesions of TBM are the result of focal arteritis affecting the carotid artery, its subdivisions and small venules [1]. These vessel-wall changes lead, eventually, to obliteration of the lumen and infarction of the area of brain supplied or drained. This process particularly affects the small arterial subdivisions (Fig. 2.6). Classically, the basal perforating arteries are involved. These changes, demonstrated by vascular studies and at post-mortem, have been well documented [1, 19, 21, 25, 26, 28].

The most frequently involved areas are the basal ganglia and, as is the case with many of the manifestations of TBM, infarction appears to be most common in the under-5 years age group. This underscores the notion that the vessels become involved in the inflammatory process as they pass through the basal exudates surrounding the Circle of Willis. The small calibre of arteries in children makes them more vulnerable and susceptible to thrombotic occlusion than the larger arteries of adults. However, even large branches of the carotid arteries may become severely affected by arteritis, leading to demonstrable narrowing on digital subtraction angiography (DSA) and magnetic resonance arteriography (MRA) and large-territorial infarctions in the areas supplied by the anterior and middle cerebral arteries (ACA and MCA, respectively), giving rise to extensive cortical and white-matter infarctions [1, 9, 10, 13, 19, 21, 25–28, 30].

At post-mortem, the incidence of infarction is around 40% [1, 28]. Most recent work involving CT studies suggests an infarction discovery rate of between 28% and 38%. MRI studies demonstrate that a high proportion of these infarctions are haemorrhagic and that this may lead to cavitation [9–11]. Much higher rates of infarction in a group of 27 children were noted by Schoeman [10].

Twenty of these patients with stage-II, or -III disease, according to the Medical Research Council classification [31], had midbrain or basal ganglia infarctions, and ten had brain-stem/parahippocampal-gyri/hypothalamus changes. Some of the changes in the latter group were due to infarction and some were due to the probable result of border-zone disease associated with ambient-system exudates. Eight of the 27 demonstrated non-communicating

Fig. 2.5.
a Post-contrast computed tomography scan demonstrates a cluster of enhancing tuberculomas in the left thalamus (*arrows*). There is hydrocephalus as well as a meningeal enhancement. b MRI of an enhancing, grape-like cluster of tuberculomas (*arrow*). Note also the ependymitis in the temporal horn of the right lateral ventricle (*arrowhead*). This was in a terminal case of tuberculous meningitis

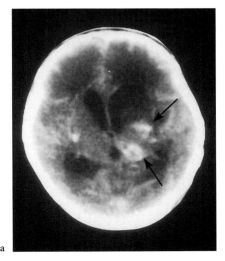

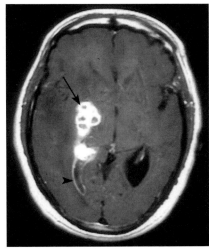

a

b

hydrocephalus, requiring surgical intervention, suggesting that the stretching of vessels may play a role in the occlusive process. The lower incidence of the demonstration of infarction by CT studies appears to be the result of a lower sensitivity of tissue differentiation when compared with MR imaging [10, 11, 21, 27, 30]. Angiographic changes in TBM include irregularities in the calibre of vessels branching from the Circle of Willis, occlusion of the medium-sized arteries at the base of the brain and early venous drainage. This, combined with a hydrocephalic pattern of vessel distribution, was described by Lehrer as the angiographic triad of TBM [32].

Although rare, the arteritis of TBM can lead to aneurysm formation, with fatal consequences, and a small number of such cases have been described [20, 21, 25, 26, 33]. One such case [33], described by Cross et al., responded to endovascular occlusion treatment and presented with life-threatening epistaxis. Rochas-Echeverri lists the angiographic findings in 24 patients examined by DSA and notes that the

Fig. 2.6. a A carotid angiogram with suprasellar thrombosis of the carotid artery (*arrow*) in a case of severe tuberculous basal meningitis. There is pronounced reflux of the contrast into the external carotid system. b A vertebral-artery angiogram with much wall irregularity in the basilar artery and the posterior fossa branches, resulting from tuberculous arteritis (*arrows*)

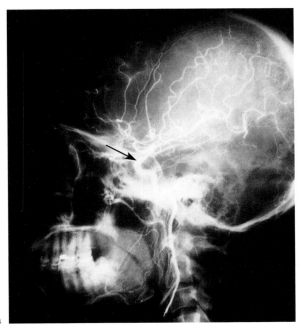

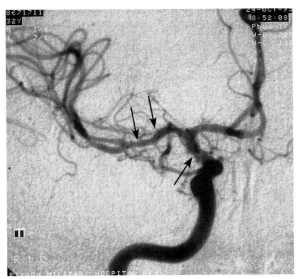

a

b

examination could not predict the clinical outcome of TBM. In this group of patients, ischaemic infarction was present in 82% of those with an abnormal DSA but also in 54% of those with a normal DSA.

In this series, the frequency of infarction in a parallel MR imaging study, 66%, was higher than in most other studies. Rochas concluded that routine DSA studies were not justified in TBM, despite the lack of morbidity resulting from the examination in his group [34].

MRA introduces the possibility of producing useful information about the distribution of arterial lesions by a non-invasive method, despite the lower quality of the images when compared with DSA [19, 21, 26]. What is certain is that, when available, Gd-enhanced MR imaging is much more sensitive in outlining cerebral infarction in TBM than contrast-enhanced CT [21, 24–26, 30].

Tuberculous Basal-Ganglia Infarctions

The areas commonly affected by infarctions are documented in the literature [1, 9–11, 13, 19, 20, 23, 25–28, 30, 34]. The preponderance of infarctions in the basal ganglia is related to the occlusion of the basal perforating arteries and their relationship to the extensive basal meningeal exudates that characterise TBM. The anatomy of these vessels and the portions of the basal ganglia they supply have been extensively studied by Takahashi et al. [35].

Using the nomenclature of Foix and Hillmand [36], Takahashi studied basal-ganglia infarctions utilising CT studies and post-mortem microangiography. Incorporating the anatomical findings of Plets [37], he described the following groups:

a. Thalamotuberal (TTA) or premammillary arteries, which originate from the posterior communicating artery (PCoA), enter the hypothalamus and thalamus.
b. Thalamoperforate arteries (TPA), which originate from the interpedunculate segment of the posterior cerebral artery (PCA), penetrate the posterior perforated substance and are distributed in the thalamus.
c. Thalamogeniculate arteries (TGA), which arise from the ambient segment of the PCA, enter the brain between the medial and lateral geniculate bodies and are distributed within the thalamus.
d. The medial posterior choroidal artery (MPChA).
e. Choroidal vessels of the lateral ventricles (Ch-VLV), which arise from the lateral posterior (LP-ChA) and anterior choroidal arteries (AchA).

This study shows that the small branches of the PCA and its ambient segment are vulnerable to the excessive basal meningeal exudate in the ambient system and the interpeduncular fossa, giving rise to infarction in both the medial and lateral basal-ganglia nuclei.

Hsieh et al. suggest the existence of a tuberculous (TB) zone and an ischaemic zone [38]. In a study of 14 TBM patients and 173 patients suffering ischaemic infarctions, Hsieh points out two different distribution patterns of infarction. The TB zone is supplied by the medial striate artery, TTA and TPA. This includes the heads of the caudate nuclei, antero-medial thalamus, the anterior limbs of the internal capsule and the genu of the internal capsule [39]. In contrast, the ischaemic zone, lenticular nuclei, postero-lateral thalamus and posterior limbs of the internal capsules are fed by the lateral striate artery, anterior choroidal artery and TGA. Although the number of cases studied by CT and described by him is small, the statistics of the study appear to be supportive of his theory. The 14 TBM patients expressing infarction were 35% of his group of patients with TBM; 75% of these infarctions were in the TB zone. Of those control patients with ischaemic infarctions, only 10% occurred within the TB zone out of a total of 441 lesions. Further study of the distribution of larger numbers of TB infarctions will be needed in the future to test this theory.

If true, the proposition will be of value in suggesting the diagnosis of TB when it is not clear from bacterial and other studies. In contrast, Rojas-Echeverri et al., in a study of 24 adults with proven TBM, found the lateral striate territory to be the most common site of infarction. All of their patients were examined by means of MR imaging, and the lower sensitivity of CT may play a role in the difference between the two studies [34, 38]. The development of cerebral infarction in TBM is a grave complication, and those patients who recover are often left with severe neurological deficits. Also, the onset of infarction greatly increases the chance of death as the outcome [9–11, 13, 22, 25, 27, 29, 31, 34, 40–42].

Parenchymal Cerebral Tuberculosis

Parenchymal cerebral tuberculous disease may be subdivided into:

1. Parenchymal tuberculomas
2. Tuberculous abscess
3. Tuberculoma en plaque

Parenchymal tuberculomas may occur sporadically in patients with detected or undetected tuberculosis in other systems or in cases of TBM. Atlas suggests a 10% incidence of tuberculomas in TBM cases [43]. Jinkins, in a study of 80 patients with in-

Fig. 2.7 a, b.
Post-contrast computed tomography scans of a young patient. As well as hydrocephalus, the scans demonstrate multiple enhancing, sub-cortical tuberculomas in the frontal and parietal regions and at the higher level beneath the convexity (*arrows*)

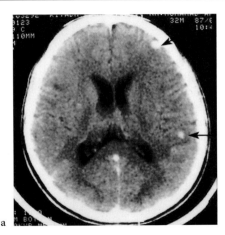 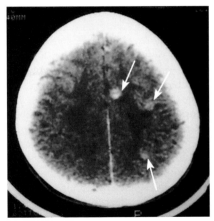

a   b

tracranial tuberculosis, found 11% with compound meningeal/parenchymal lesions and 89% with parenchymal tuberculomas [19].

In developing countries, parenchymal tuberculomas make up a large proportion of intracranial-space-occupying lesions. In patients from India, Gupta suggests that between 10% and 40% of intracranial lesions are parenchymal tuberculomas [40]. In Saudi Arabia, Jinkins found 10–15% of all mass lesions to be tuberculomas. Salgado points out an increasing incidence of cerebral tuberculoma in developed countries [44]. In children, Cremin and Jamieson found parenchymal tuberculoma formation in 10% of their cases [9, 11]. Sporadic cerebral tuberculous masses had a different clinical presentation from lesions in TBM, which were multiple in 15–20% of TBM patients.

Distribution of Tuberculomas

Tuberculomas of the central nervous system may occur at any level in the brain and spinal cord, and there are an increasing number of reports in which both areas are shown to be simultaneously affected [13, 21, 45]. These lesions are more common in the cerebral hemispheres than in the subtentorial structures. Studies suggest that subtentorial tuberculomas are more common in children than in the elderly [20, 27, 46]. Peripheral tuberculomas occur commonly in TBM but are very uncommon as sporadic lesions. However, in TBM, suprasellar, intrasellar, pineal and pre-pontine tuberculomas have been described, as have rare, intraventricular lesions. In these cases, differentiation from tumours is difficult.

Tuberculomas may be single or multiple and, when multiple, may demonstrate differing degrees of development in the same patient at the same time (Fig. 2.7). Most tuberculomas occur at the cortico-

medullary junction, suggesting origin by haematogenous spread. A small number develop from direct extension of a pial or arachnoid Rich lesion, in which case the surrounding meninges enhance on CECT or MR imaging T1-Gd studies. The origin, in a few cases, is by spreading from venous sinuses.

In the less common lesions of the basal ganglia, brain stem and cerebellum, differentiation from primary and secondary neoplasms is a problem (Fig. 2.8). Beneath the tentorium, both single and multiple lesions are described [9, 11, 19–21, 26, 40, 42, 44–52].

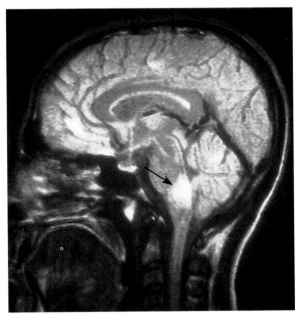

Fig. 2.8. Sagittal, post-contrast magnetic resonance imaging demonstrates an isolated tuberculoma of the brain stem. It is impossible to differentiate it, on this image, from a primary brain-stem tumour (*arrow*)

Parenchymal tuberculomas affect all age groups. In developing countries, tuberculomas show a predilection for children, but occur at any age [19, 53, 54]. In developed countries, the elderly, as well as those groups with a susceptibility, are likely to be affected; however, exceptions occur, and even infants may develop tuberculomas [41]. The onset of symptoms is insidious, and gradual elevation of intracranial pressure, focal epilepsy and focal neurological deficits are the presenting signs. Fever may be present.

Clinically, differentiation from tumour, fungus or parasitic disease is difficult, and this is also a problem radiologically. Search should be made for a focus of tuberculosis elsewhere in the body, but this is often occult. Both chest radiographs and CSF studies are commonly negative for tuberculosis.

The tuberculous cerebral mass may be present for a considerable time before clinical symptoms develop. This gives rise to very wide variations in the histology and internal structure, which in turn leads to variations in the radiological characteristics. Tuberculosis is the great mimic of other pathological entities [20, 21].

Before the advent of CT and MR imaging, most tuberculomas were diagnosed at operation or post-mortem and some by their response to anti-tubercular therapy. Surgical intervention still carries a high mortality [48] and should be reserved for cases requiring a shunt for raised intracranial pressure, those with a life-threatening mass effect and those few cases where differential diagnosis from malignancy is impossible without stereotactic brain biopsy.

Many radiologists have expressed the opinion that radiological diagnosis of parenchymal tuberculoma is always tentative. Recent developments in MR imaging T1-Gd studies have defined groups of patients, for which the probability of the diagnosis of tuberculoma is extremely high, especially in areas where tuberculosis is endemic.

CT and MR imaging studies carried out without contrast agents are likely to overlook both isodense parenchymal tuberculomas and TBM (Fig. 2.9). In cases of suspected cerebral tuberculoma, particularly in those groups presenting with raised intracranial pressure and focal fits, a careful search for an active focus of infection in other systems should be made. For this, sputum testing, gastric washings, CSF study and chest radiography, including lateral radiographs in children, are necessary. Abdominal ultrasound will demonstrate peritoneal tuberculosis if present and, in women, pelvic disease can be the source. Urine bacteriology is also necessary. However, in some cases, even after careful central nervous system radiological investigation, examination of the response

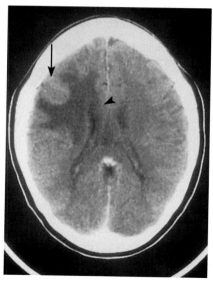

Fig. 2.9. Pre-contrast computed tomography demonstrates an isodense right-frontal, subcortical, tuberculous mass (*arrow*). There is a surrounding zone of oedema and a pressure effect on the lateral ventricle (*arrowhead*)

to anti-tuberculosis therapy will be the only way to make the diagnosis [9, 11, 19, 24, 40, 47, 52].

The radiological image is dependent on both the histology and the age of the lesion. A tuberculoma commences as an aggregation of polymorphonucleocytes, lymphocytes and macrophages but, as CMI develops, the cell population changes to include epithelioid cells, active macrophages, giant cells and a fibroid structural network. At first, there are many tubercle bacilli but, as the macrophages activate, these are mainly destroyed, and caseation develops. The brain tissue is displaced rather than destroyed, producing a surrounding zone of gliosis. Inside this, a sphere or ovoid of collagen tissue forms a capsule enclosing the caseating material. At the next stage, central necrosis occurs, producing caseation and a soft, fluid or semi-fluid core. Eventually, if treated, the lesion will either calcify or disappear totally. This is a slow process, which may take months or two or more years [19, 30]. The tuberculoma may leave no scar or, in some cases, overlying encephalomyelopathy may be visible [19–21]. The activity of the tuberculoma may be judged by the degree of contrast enhancement on follow-up CT or MR imaging studies as well as by clinical assessment of the patient. Focal seizures and neurological deficits may continue, but any resurgence of symptoms heralds reactivation, drug resistance or drug non-compliance.

The Radiology of Parenchymal Intercranial Tuberculomas

Plain films of the skull do not help in the diagnosis of symptomatic tuberculomas. In infants, widening of the suture lines often accompanies elevated intracranial pressure, but it is a non-specific finding, as is intracranial calcification in older patients with mature tuberculomas. Angiography and dynamic CECT demonstrate non-specific findings of a space-occupying lesion and, in some patients, the lack of vascularity in the lesion is helpful in differentiating it from an intracranial neoplasm.

All authorities agree that, in the early phases, granulomatous tuberculomas are slightly hypodense or isodense to the surrounding brain tissue on CT studies. On CECT, these solid lesions, which are characteristically round, oval or lobular, enhance homogeneously. When first discovered, tuberculomas are usually less than 2 cm in diameter and are often single or multiple. If multiple, the lesions are usually of different sizes. There is accompanying low-density, white-matter oedema, which in these early lesions may be intense. The resulting mass effect can cause displacement of the ventricular system.

The neurological deficit will depend on the site of the lesion and the extent of the oedema, as well as focal epilepsy; monoplegia and hemiplegia are relatively common. Changes in consciousness may result from the raised intracranial pressure. If the ventricular foramina are compromised, hydrocephalus will develop, often requiring shunting. Mesencephalic and brain-stem tuberculomas obstructing the aqueduct of Sylvius or the fourth ventricle are also a cause of hydrocephalus. As central caseation and encapsulation develop, the pattern of enhancement on CECT becomes heterogeneous centrally, and the capsule enhances as a ring. Cerebral oedema surrounding caseating lesions is usually less intense than in the case of pure granulomas.

If tuberculomas are discovered at the stage of caseation, they are often up to 5 cm in diameter. The associated CT changes of pressure effects and oedema are severe [51]. At the next stage, central necrosis of the tuberculoma develops. The fluid or semi-fluid centre of the mass does not enhance on CECT. Characteristically, a dense ring of enhancement surrounds a hypodense core. This ring is comprised of a compressed collagen capsule and the outer layers of the caseating granuloma (Fig. 2.10). Jinkins suggests that, from the very start, new fragile blood vessels develop in the capsule, and the passage of contrast material through leaky walls allows the blood–brain barrier to be breached and the granuloma to enhance [21].

Involution of tuberculomas during treatment is often a slow process, although some of them exhibit a reduction of size as little as 4–6 weeks after the inception of an anti-tuberculous regime. Failure to make clinical or radiological progress raises the suspicion of either drug resistance or misdiagnosis. Any paradoxical response that occurs, with enlargement of the lesion, is dealt with in a later section. Sometimes, small lesions occur and resolve without therapy [47]. In areas where tuberculosis and cysticercosis are both endemic, true diagnosis is problematic [40] (see section on *Differential Diagnosis of Tuberculoma*). In the early stages of therapy, enhancement

Fig. 2.10 a, b. Pre- and post-contrast computed tomography (CT) scans reveal an isodense, right-occipital mass (*arrows*). After contrast injection, there is strong ring enhancement around a caseating or necrotic centre (*arrowhead*). **c** Post-contrast CT demonstrates ring enhancement and solid tuberculomas in the right posterior cerebrum (*arrows*)

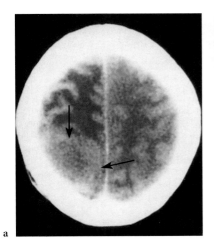 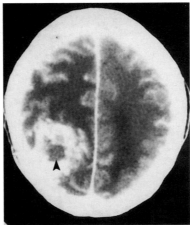 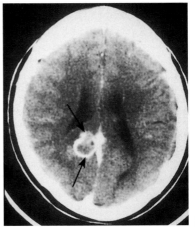

a b, c

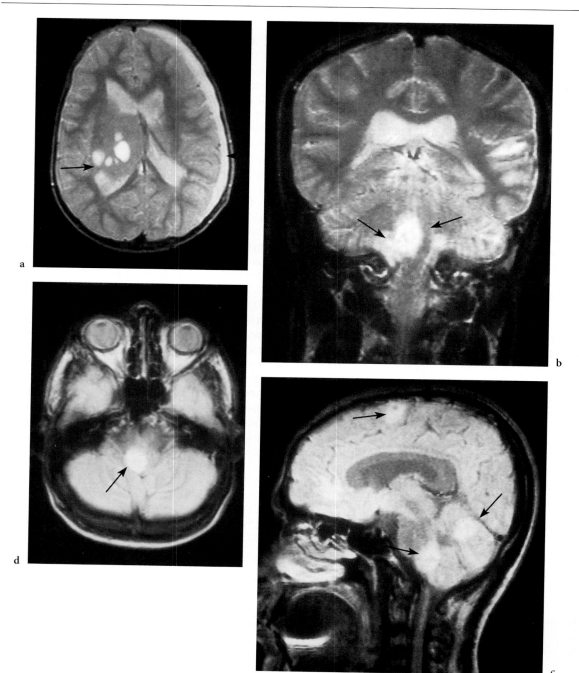

Fig. 2.11. a Axial, post-gadolinium magnetic resonance imaging (MRI). A group of right-sided thalamic tuberculomas. These are solid, and the lateral ventricle is effaced (*arrow*). Note also the extensive enhancement of meninges over the left convexity in this young patient with tuberculous meningitis (*arrowhead*). **b** Coronal, post-gadolinium MRI. There is an irregular, ovoid tuberculoma in the right side of the brain stem. There is some involvement of the right cerebellar hemisphere (*arrows*). **c** A sagittal, post-gadolinium study of a patient with three tuberculomas. All enhance but show some central relative hypodensity. The lesions are seen in the parasagittal, cerebellar and brain-stem locations (*arrows*). **d** An axial, post-gadolinium MRI scan reveals a single enhancing tuberculoma high in the brain stem (*arrow*)

on CECT sometimes continues to increase. Enhancement is a rough index of activity and, with treatment, it eventually wanes. Calcification develops, in some cases, during the healing process and is more obvious on CT than on MR images. An adequate course of chemotherapy is essential, and inadequate treatment or patient non-compliance leads to recrudescence of the tuberculoma. Tuberculomas are usually round, oval or lobulated, the latter shape being the result of aggregation of a number of smaller lesions.

In children, Cremin and Jamieson describe the formation of grape-like clusters of tuberculomas that may be associated with solid lesions elsewhere [9, 11]. Around the circumference, the ring enhancement often varies in thickness [20]. It is usually continuous but, when broken, is difficult to differentiate from metastasis [47]. The usual size is 2 cm or less but, in endemic areas, the lesion may be up to 8 cm in diameter. The larger lesions often have special characteristics and may show lamination due to alternating phases of granuloma formation and caseating necrosis.

Multiple lesions often show different stages of development. If single, and before ring enhancement develops, deep thalamic, midbrain and brain-stem lesions are difficult to differentiate from primary and secondary neoplasms and lymphoma. Lack of neovascularity on DSA is helpful in making the diagnosis in such cases.

The appearances of parenchymal tuberculomas on MR imaging examinations are described in the radiological literature. There are wide variations in the descriptions, almost certainly due to the varying maturity of the lesions described. Many of the studies were carried out before the availability of MR-T1 imaging with Gd contrast. Later descriptions are more consistent with each other. The state-of-the-art description is from Jinkins, Chang, Rodrigues and Gupta, who suggest the following classification of MR imaging findings [21]:

1. The non-caseating granuloma is T1 hypointense to brain tissue and T2 hyperintense, enhancing homogeneously with T1-Gd studies.
2. A solid, caseating granuloma is hypointense to isointense on T1 images and isointense to hypointense on T2 images, with a hypointense rim, depending on the degree of capsule development (Fig. 2.11). With T1-Gd studies, strong rim enhancement is seen. The two types of lesion just described are invariably surrounded by a zone of oedema of varying extent (Fig. 2.12). This oedema is hypodense on T1 and hyperintense on T2 images. The oedema does not enhance on injection of gadolinium.

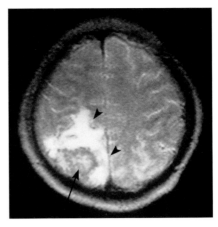

Fig. 2.12. An axial, non-enhanced, T2-weighted magnetic resonance image of an occipital tuberculoma of mixed signals (*arrow*). There is extensive surrounding oedema (*arrowheads*)

3. When central necrosis or liquefaction occurs, the central signal on T1 is hypointense. On T2, the necrotic material gives a fairly homogeneous, hyperintense signal, and the surrounding capsule appears hypointense. T1-Gd demonstrates intense rim enhancement of the lesion. In those cases of long-standing, laminated tuberculoma, no post-Gd studies have yet been published, so the enhancing characteristics are not yet available. These laminated lesions show alternating bands of iso- and hypointensity on T1, and alternating bands of hypo and hyperintensity on T2 images [40]. The reason for the shortening of the T2 signal in some tuberculomas is not clear but may be the result of the presence of paramagnetic free radicals in the enclosed macrophages, distributed inhomogeneously throughout the lesion [13, 21, 52].

Tuberculous Abscess

Although uncommon, true tuberculous abscesses develop from parenchymal tuberculous granulomas or the spread of tuberculous foci in the meninges to the brain substance in patients with TBM. Cremin and Jamieson have pointed out that two distinct types of necrosis occur in tuberculomas. Microscopically, those possessing a structure of fibrovascular elements, as demonstrated with reticulin stains, undergo gummatous necrosis, where the inflammatory granulomatous tissue undergoes necrosis. Cremin points out that this type of central necrosis gives a MR imaging signal on T2 studies that is isodense to brain tissue and is surrounded by a dense zone of oedema. Tuberculomas of this type do not develop into abscesses [9, 11]. Those tuberculomas that do

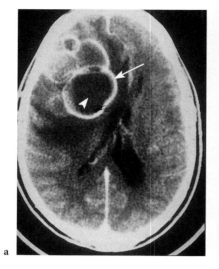
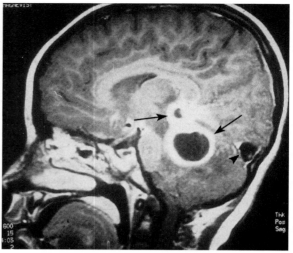

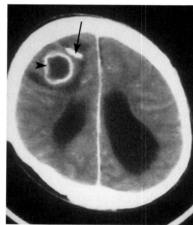

Fig. 2.13. a A group of right-frontal tuberculous abscesses in the sub-cortical white matter, causing midline shift. Post-gadolinium imaging demonstrates an intense enhancement of the thin ABCs wall (*arrow*), while the liquid contents remain of low signal (*arrowhead*). **b** Two deep, midline tuberculous abscesses in the region of the tentorium (*arrows*). There is a smaller collection posteriorly (*arrowhead*). **c** Two right-frontal tuberculous abscesses, one of which has been successfully drained (*arrow*). The second shows the characteristic enhancement of a thin wall surrounding hypodense fluid (*arrowhead*). This was in a late-stage case of tuberculous meningitis

convert into abscesses show a different structure on microscopy as they have no reticulin elements, being comprised entirely of cellular elements. The necrosis of these epithelioid cells, macrophages and polymorphonucleocytes passes through a phase of inspissation or caseation to liquefaction and the development of a true abscess. These are usually isolated lesions, occasionally occurring simultaneously with other solid tuberculomas. Tuberculous abscesses show the same MR imaging characteristics as pyogenic abscesses, being oval or round in shape with a thin, strongly enhancing wall that, on T1-Gd MR imaging examination, is in marked contrast to the hypodense liquid centre (Fig. 2.13).

A point of clinical importance is that, while solid or caseating tuberculomas contain few bacteria, the tuberculous abscess contains the mycobacterium in large numbers. If such an abscess ruptures into the ventricular system or the subarachnoid space, a devastating ventriculitis or meningitis ensues. Drainage of these lesions is, therefore, a dangerous procedure.

Seeding of daughter abscesses along the needle track has been described by De Castro [20] who points out that, in the West, abscesses are more likely to develop in older age groups and among the immunosuppressed.

Atypical Tuberculous Mass Lesions

Tuberculoma en plaque lesions occur more commonly as a complication of TBM than as isolated parenchymal tuberculomas. En plaque lesions also occur when a tuberculoma abuts onto the meningeal surface of the brain and a proliferation of granulomatous tissue extends into the adjacent meninges. When presenting as isolated tuberculomas, the clinical pattern is similar to that of other intracranial-space-occupying lesions [55].

A common site of such lesions is the tentorial edge, where the resemblance to meningioma causes difficulties in diagnosis. In these cases, angiography

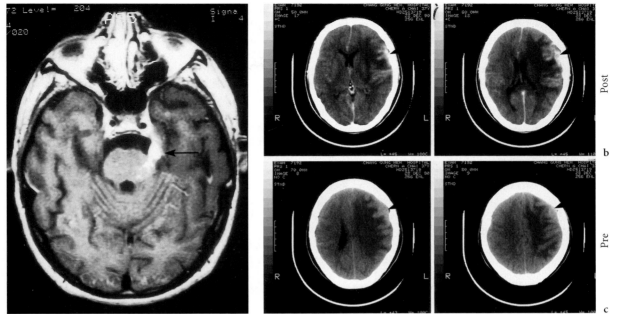

Fig. 2.14. a An enhancing en plaque tuberculoma in the posterior fossa (*arrow*). Difficult to differentiate from a meningioma. **b, c** Pre- and post-contrast computed tomography scans demonstrate a hyperdense lesion in the fronto-parietal area. After intravenous contrast injection, there is extensive enhancement of the adjacent meninges. This is associated with ring enhancement of a 1-cm tuberculoma with a central, hypodense nidus (*arrows*). Images by courtesy of Dr. Ng, Chang Gung Memorial Hospital, Kwei Shan, Tao Yuan, Taiwan

is necessary to demonstrate the lack of tumour circulation in the tuberculoma (Fig. 2.14). Other primary and secondary tumours need to be differentiated in the same way. When tuberculous meningeal mass lesions are confluent with the cerebral cortex, there is extensive gyral enhancement on CECT and T1-Gd images, and the adjacent cortex and white matter show oedema beneath the lesion. This oedema will be hypodense on CT and T1 MR imaging and hyperintense on T2, showing no enhancement on T1-Gd MR imaging. Graveli et al. describe a lesion, in the cavernous sinus, with all the imaging characteristics of a meningioma; this lesion proved, after removal, to be a tuberculoma [56].

Miliary Tuberculomas

In patients presenting with miliary pulmonary tuberculosis, haematogenous spreading may occur to any organ in the body and, in these organs, 2-mm to 3-mm granulomas are demonstrated histologically. In miliary tuberculosis of the central nervous system, similar granulomas are present, widely disseminated throughout the cerebrum, cerebellum, brain stem and meninges. In the meninges, they result in the development of TBM.

As on non-enhanced CT, the granulomas are isodense or slightly hypodense to brain tissue, and the lesions are difficult to recognise but are seen as tiny hyperdense foci on CECT. T1-Gd presents the granulomas as multiple enhancing foci, and T2 images show foci of hyperintensity throughout the axial central nervous system [21, 45]. Cases of miliary tuberculoma are uncommon but, in the future, Gd-enhanced MR imaging sequences will help to define the true incidence of these cases. Jinkins, in a study of 80 patients with intracranial tuberculosis examined by CT, reported only one case of miliary tuberculoma; the case recovered completely after therapy. However, the prognosis is usually grave and depends, to some extent, on the degree of involvement of the other organs of the body.

The Target Sign

There is general agreement that the radiographic appearances of intracranial tuberculomas are nonspecific and that the ability of tuberculous lesions to mimic other diseases of pyogenic, fungal neoplastic and parasitic origin leads to a wide range both of appearances and differential diagnoses [9, 11, 15, 19–21, 24, 40, 46, 47, 49, 50]. Wechman suggested that one particular CT pattern is specific to parenchymal tuberculoma [57]. He called this pattern the target sign. Van Dyk, in a further study, noted this same pattern in 10 of 30 patients with tuberculoma [48]. Of these 30 patients, TBM was complicated by cerebral tuberculoma in 14, and 16 had sporadic parenchymal tuberculoma. Of those with the target sign, three suffered from TBM. The target sign is comprised of a round or oval lesion, isodense or slightly hyperdense on non-contrast CT, with a central nidus of calcification. Alternatively, on CECT, the peripheral enhancing ring is seen, as well as a central small area of contrast enhancement. The resulting image, with alternating peripheral enhancement followed by a zone of isodense tissue containing an enhancing or calcified nidus in its centre, is likened, by Van Dyk and Wechman, to a target. Neither of the two authors had access to MR imaging techniques with which to study these lesions.

Van Dyk reviewed 5539 CT examinations of intracranial lesions concurrently with his tuberculoma patients and did not find the target sign in any other condition. All his tuberculoma patients were South Africans of Negroid stock. The target sign has only rarely been described in other parts of the world [46, 47].

The failure of this sign to appear in larger numbers outside Africa is almost certainly due to a number of factors, such as the response of the local population to tuberculous infection. The time of presentation of the patients to the local hospitals must also be considered, as the presence of central calcification suggests that these are long-term lesions, although the presence of enhancement indicates considerable peripheral activity.

The mean age of Van Dyk's patients presenting with the target sign was 12.4 years and, for those not showing this phenomenon, 21 years. Cremin and Jamieson, working in a different area of the Republic of South Africa, do not mention the target sign, but Drouat, working in Algeria, describes one patient, as does Vengaskar in India [46, 47].

Calcification is a late-stage development in parenchymal tuberculomas. The CT image of ring enhancement surrounding a non-enhancing zone indicates that caseation or caseation necrosis is present in cases exhibiting the target sign. The central nidus of calcification associated with inactivity is rarely seen in other areas of the world; this may be due to local or indigenous factors. MR imaging studies of the target sign in Spain have recently suggested that the sign is non-specific and is seen in patients with acquired immunodeficiency syndrome (AIDS), complicated by intracranial toxoplasmosis and primary lymphoma; the target sign was also seen in a non-AIDS pyogenic brain abscess in an elderly female [54]. In their patients, the CT studies demonstrated a target sign. In the case of the pyogenic abscess, both CT and

MR imaging were carried out. MR imaging examination after Gd contrast injection revealed ring enhancement of the lesion but no central dot. T2-weighted studies showed a high-signal lesion surrounded by a low-signal ring with a low-signal central dot, giving a target appearance. It is postulated that the central dot is due to the presence of haemosiderin. The authors propose that a target sign with central calcification may well be pathognomonic of tuberculoma, but those with a central enhancing dot on CT examination are not necessarily due to tuberculoma, and cases due to AIDS following intravenous drug abuse will become an increasingly common finding in the future [54].

Paradoxical Growth of Tuberculomas During Anti-Tuberculous Therapy

Since first described by Lees, McLeod and Marshall in 1980 [58], a number of cases have been cited where tuberculomas have developed or increased in size during apparently adequate anti-tuberculous therapy of non-resistant tuberculous organisms. None of these cases were Caucasian in origin but included patients of the Indian, Chinese, Vietnamese and, in one case, North American Negroid races.

The reasons for this phenomenon have, so far, not been explained. Some of the cases had concurrent lymph-node infection, and these lymph nodes also increased in size during therapy. The increase in the size of lymph nodes during treatment is well recognised. A possible explanation is a local hypersensitivity and inflammatory reaction resulting from the release of tuberculoprotein from dead or dying mycobacteria [59, 60]. Other examples of this response to the release of tuberculoprotein are the sudden unexpected deaths of patients with widespread pulmonary or miliary tuberculosis and the development of adult respiratory distress syndrome during treatment in patients with miliary tuberculosis [60].

In tuberculous regional lymphadenitis, the lymph nodes contain large numbers of *M. tuberculosis*. This is not so in the case of parenchymal cerebral tuberculomas, where tubercle bacilli are sparse. Alternative mechanisms need to be considered in these cases of paroxysmal growth of tuberculomas. The treatment requires a higher dose of anti-tuberculous drugs, combined with corticosteroids, and, in most cases, there is an improvement. However, a number of deaths have been recorded [58, 60–62].

The relapse time between the initial, apparently successful, treatment of the tuberculoma and the onset of new focal signs, convulsions or raised in-

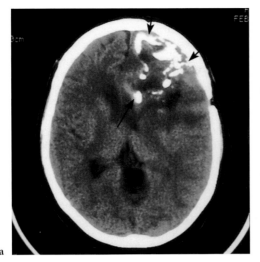 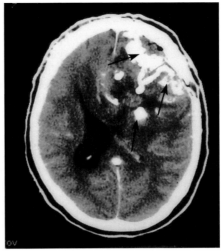

a   b

Fig. 2.15 a, b. Pre- and post-contrast computed tomography scans after craniotomy. There is extensive cortical and white-matter calcification and some cortical atrophy (*arrows*). Post-contrast scanning shows a number of centres of enhancement (*arrows*). These areas represent continued activity in this tuberculoma some months after commencement of anti-tuberculous chemotherapy

tracranial pressure due to the paradoxical expansion, varies between 1 month and 18 months. Patients have come from a wide range of age groups, from infants to the elderly.

It is important to realise that this pattern of disease occurs during the routine and apparently effective treatment of tuberculoma in both TBM and sporadic parenchymal cases. Often, as a result, the initial diagnosis is then questioned and alternatives such as malignancy considered. This is especially so if the tuberculoma is a single lesion deep in the cerebrum, midbrain or posterior fossa.

Teo has described a number of studies of cases reported in the literature [62]. In a study of 30 African patients, Van Dyk does not mention the paradox, as is also the case with Cremin and Jamieson, working in South Africa [9, 11, 48]. In Saudi Arabia, Abdul Jabber describes a Saudi male and a female whose nationality is not stated with the phenomenon. Jinkins, in a study of 80 patients from Saudi Arabia with TBM or parenchymal or complex tuberculous lesions, does not include any cases responding paradoxically [19, 49, 63].

Late-Stage Appearances of Parenchymal Tuberculomas

The behaviour of parenchymal tuberculomas during anti-tuberculosis therapy is related to the size of the lesion at the time of the initial diagnosis. Small single or multiple tuberculomas of less than 1 cm in diameter usually disappear completely during therapy, often within the first few months and almost invariably within a year. This is especially true in children [9, 11]. This is the case if the initial lesion is a solid granuloma, without central caseation or calcification. Tuberculomas above 2 cm in diameter take longer to resolve, often between 1 year and 2 years, when the lesion shows central necrosis or caseation or if the tuberculoma is a larger lobulated structure, as in those described by Bhargava [15]. Jinkins, in his study of 80 patients with parenchymal tuberculomas, described 57 patients with isolated granulomatous lesions and followed them up with serial CECT examination until therapy could be safely stopped, using failure to enhance on CECT to indicate healing. Many of these cases required between 18 months and 2 years of therapy before resolution. In his series, 14 of 57 eventually showed a normal CECT, 8 showed a residual, non-enhancing, calcified lesion and 12 displayed calcification with associated, overlying cerebral atrophy (Fig. 2.15). Seventeen displayed focal cerebral atrophy alone. One patient continued to enhance after 2 years of chemotherapy, and five patients were lost before follow-up [19]. This is a higher percentage of calcified lesions than in some other studies. Wilkinson [64] and Reed [65], in two separate studies, stated that 38% of late-stage TBM cases showed late-stage calcification, but only 1% and 6% of cases of parenchymal tuberculoma developed this phenomenon in their two studies, respectively. This is in agreement with Van Dyk, only one of whose 30 cases developed significant late calcification [48].

■ Differential Diagnosis of Intracranial Tuberculosis

It is clear from the radiological literature that there are no specific CT or MR imaging findings in cases of either TBM or parenchymal cerebral tuberculosis, and that the diagnosis rests on a combination of clinical assessment, imaging appearance and response to therapy. A wide range of pathological processes, including malignancy, pyogenic and fungal infections, parasitic infestations and a range of other disconnected conditions, from trauma to aneurysm, can mimic either TBM or parenchymal tuberculoma. In *Haemophilus influenzae* meningitis, basal meningeal enhancement is present and commonly leads to cerebral infarctions. Infarctions are also seen in aspergillosis and mucormycotic infections, where the source of the infection is the nasal cavity or the paranasal sinuses. In these two infections, the cause of the cerebral infarctions is due to the spread of the fungus along the vessel walls, and the infarctions are common in the cortical and subcortical regions; this is in contrast to the distribution in the basal ganglia in TBM. However, large vessels are occluded in patients with fungal or tuberculous infection, in which case extensive infarction of the anterior or middle cerebral artery territories will occur.

In the disseminated form of cerebral coccidioidomycosis (DCC), intense basal meningeal enhancement involving the sylvian systems is common and is often more intense than in TBM. However, cases where basal enhancement is absent even in the presence of hydrocephalus, occur in both conditions [9, 66]. In DCC, the basal ganglia and white-matter lesions are more diffuse than in TBM, and focal granulomas and basal-ganglia infarctions are rare [66]. Ventriculitis is also common in DCC whereas, in TBM, it is usually only present in terminal cases. The geographical distribution of the common fungal diseases, DCC, histoplasmosis and blastomycosis overlap the distribution of tuberculosis, giving rise to problems of differentiating them from one another. The patterns of the intracranial lesions vary and must be carefully studied in making a diagnosis. For instance, in histoplasmosis, the subependymal distribution of the disease along the ventricular margins is in contrast to the typical subcortical parenchymal lesions of TBM [43]. *Cryptococcus neoformans* may manifest both intense basal meningeal enhancement as well as arteritis, leading to basal-ganglia infarction, so that the radiological appearances are often indistinguishable from TBM. In *Cryptococcus*, however, the organism can be isolated from the CSF and recognised using simple laboratory techniques. Spirochaetal disease gives rise to both basal meningitis and to parenchymal granulomatous gumma formation. The presence of established cerebral atrophy and other clinical signs of syphilis differentiates these cases, as does the peripheral distribution of the granulomas. The granulomas are often attached to the meninges in syphilis, an uncommon finding in compound cerebral tuberculosis.

Tick-borne Lyme disease is the second spirochaetal disease that may affect the cerebrum. In these cases, granulomas in the basal ganglia are seen but, unlike those of tuberculosis, are diffuse and lack ring enhancement on CETC and T1-Gd MR imaging, so the two conditions are unlikely to be confused. True abscesses developing in bacterial, fungal and tuberculous disease cannot be separated from each other on the basis of their radiological appearances alone. Either histological evidence or the response to therapy has to be considered to make the differentiation. It is unusual for these abscesses to be sterile, so the infecting organism can usually be determined by aspiration and culture.

Intracranial Malignancies

Single or multiple malignant tumours may mimic tuberculosis. Of the primary intercranial tumours, low-grade astrocytoma and cystic astrocytoma give rise to the most difficulty. Both of these types of tumour tend to be isodense on CT and MR imaging and enhance homogeneously or incompletely. The ring enhancement of a tuberculoma, on CECT and T1Gd MR images, helps to differentiate it from a tumour, as the ring enhancement of a tumour is often incomplete and varies in thickness at points around its circumference. Both tumours and tuberculomas are surrounded by oedema but, in the case of a tumour, there is usually a more emphatic mass effect than in a tuberculoma of equivalent size. In many cases, either DSA or a trial of therapy will be necessary to make the diagnosis.

The same principles are true of secondary malignancy. Single intracranial metastases are often inhomogeneous on contrast-enhanced studies and show central necrosis similar to that of a tuberculoma. However, on enhanced CT and MR imaging examination, tuberculomas seldom present with haemorrhages within the lesion, which is often the case in secondary malignancies. Multiple metastases and glioblastoma multiforme, as well as multicentric, primary, intracranial neoplasms require angiography to make the diagnosis, as does meningioma en plaque. Compound meningeal tuberculosis is difficult to differentiate from leptomeningeal carcinomatosis but, in the case of the latter, the basal-meningeal enhancement tends to be patchy, with differing thicknesses and intensities, in contrast to the more usual homogeneous and continuous appearance of tuberculous compound leptomeningitis [67].

Primary lymphomas tend to be periventricular in position. They often cross the midline, passing through the corpus callosum, which a supratentorial tuberculoma never does. Lymphomas have limited mass effects, are structurally diffuse and show little or no oedema and no ring enhancement. In AIDS patients, lymphoma and toxoplasmosis can co-exist with intracranial tuberculosis, giving rise to diagnostic difficulties. Secondary lymphoma commonly affects the meninges, in contrast to the preference for a subcortical site of tuberculous lesions.

Cysticercosis

Cysticercosis and tuberculosis have similar geographical distributions; they often share the same pattern of symptoms at onset. Headache due to raised intracranial pressure or convulsions, either focal or generalised, are triggered by local space-occupying lesions. The cysticercosis infestation is widespread throughout the body and, in some cases, the diagnosis can be made from the histology of subcutaneous nodules in which the parasite is present. The diagnosis of cerebral cysticercosis is difficult and, as in cerebral tuberculosis, the lesions undergo a series of changes in appearance as they develop and eventually die. The embedded cysts have a characteristic mural node and, if this can be demonstrated, the diagnosis is apparent. MRI studies are helpful in this respect but, on CT, cysticercal cysts are often difficult to differentiate from tuberculomas.

The living cysticercal larva produces no reaction in the host tissues, and it is only while dying that the larva releases metabolites inducing a local reaction in the host. In the case of cerebral cysticercosis, a circumferential inflammatory reaction occurs, giving rise to intense ring enhancement on both CT and MR imaging and to a zone of oedema surrounding the lesion. At this stage, the cyst usually measures between 1 cm and 2 cm in diameter, and an enhancing or high-signal node is seen in its centre.

The death of the larva leads to lessening of the surrounding tissue reaction and of the oedema. This is followed by either dissolution of the cyst, with complete resolution of the lesion, or dissolution of the components accompanied by the development of punctate calcification. The calcification is best demonstrated radiologically on CT, but MR imaging studies differentiate the various stages of the development and death of the cyst more clearly. At all stages, differentiation from tuberculomas is difficult, and a trial of anti-tuberculous drugs may be necessary to make the diagnosis.

The distribution of the lesions in the cerebrum, brain stem and cerebellum is the same in the two diseases, although cysticerci may be more numerous than tuberculomas. Single cysticercal cysts, as with single tuberculomas, do occur. Cysticerci also develop as intraventricular lesions, unusual in the case of tuberculoma. In these cases, the cysticercal cysts are very difficult to visualise, as they are isodense to CSF on both CT and MR imaging and are usually diagnosed due to the accompanying hydrocephalus associated with interference of the circulation of CSF. Hydrocephalus may also be a feature when the CSF pathways are involved in the inflammatory response to a mature or dying cyst, causing obstruction to a foramen or to the aqueduct of Sylvius. There is no basal meningeal enhancement in cysticercosis, but very extensive cyst formation can occur in the basal CSF cisterns and Sylvian systems. These racemose cysts are thin walled and do not enhance. They are common in the cerebellopontine angle and sometimes cause an expansion of the CSF spaces. If present, they may help in differentiating coexistent intracerebral cysticercal cysts from tuberculomas. Lotz et al., in a combined study of the pathomorphology and MR imaging of intracranial cysticercosis, make the point that, intracranially, the condition is predominantly a disease of the subarachnoid space, which is the only environment where the larger cysts can survive. The smaller parenchymal lesions arising from dead or dying cysts are the lesions likely to be confused with tuberculomas [68 – 70, 75].

Toxoplasmosis

The parasite toxoplasmosis produces intracerebral pathology that may be confused with tuberculoma. Cystic or solid ring-enhancing lesions, often with a central enhancing nodule, are present. Toxoplasmosis is the most common infestation in AIDS patients, where tuberculosis may coexist, giving rise to problems of diagnosis. The distribution of lesions in the subcortex and the deep white matter is similar in both conditions. However, in toxoplasmosis, subependymal lesions are common, the ring enhancement is usually thicker and more irregular than in tuberculoma and haemorrhage into the lesion often occurs – a point of differentiation. A course of anti-toxoplasmic therapy will usually cause some reduction of size of the lesions within 2 – 3 weeks, and this may be the only way of differentiating them from tuberculomas [43].

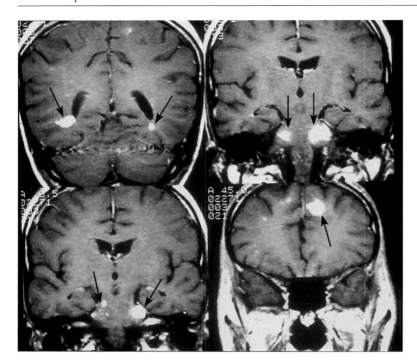

Fig. 2.16.
Coronal T1–gadolinium images. Multiple, enhancing, granulomatous lesions are seen in the cerebrum and brain stem (*arrows*). The appearance is indistinguishable from that of multiple tuberculomas. The patient was proved to have sarcoidosis

Neurosarcoidosis

Neurosarcoidosis occurs in 5% of cases of sarcoidosis and is usually a sub-acute condition clinically unlikely to be confused with TBM. However, the meningeal enhancement in neurosarcoidosis produces radiological images similar to those of TBM. Sub-frontal meningeal enhancement in a patient who is not acutely ill is a common manifestation, and the suprasellar cisterns, parasellar spaces and hypothalamic parenchyma are often involved, which can result in the development of diabetes insipidus. Neurosarcoid changes are usually diffuse and are more likely to be confused with tuberculous border-zone disease than with tuberculoma. In a few cases, sarcoid parenchymal granulomas do occur. There is little oedema surrounding these granulomas, and solid (rather than ring) enhancement is present (Fig. 2.16). Hydrocephalus occurs only when periventricular, infiltrating lesions have caused obstruction. MR imaging with Gd-labelled diethylene triamine penta-acetic acid demonstrates the presence of sarcoid material along the cortical vessels in the Virchow-Robin spaces. These deposits enhance markedly, as do scattered granulomas in the brain substance [71]. Destructive lesions of the calvarium are also a differentiating symptom; due to the integrity of the dural barrier, simultaneous intracranial tuberculosis and tuberculous osteitis is very uncommon. Moreover, histological study of the calvarial lesion will point to the correct diagnosis.

Other granulomatous disorders are unlikely to be confused with tuberculosis. Neurobrucellosis is a very rare disorder even in areas where the infection is endemic. Both the central and peripheral nervous systems can be affected. The CT scan is usually normal, but epidural granulomas have been reported (Fig. 2.17). However, the pathological mechanism is usually due to demyelination [72, 73].

Other Intracranial Lesions that Must be Differentiated from Tuberculosis

Tumefactive multiple sclerosis (TMS) presents as large, contrast-enhancing white-matter lesions surrounded by vasogenic oedema. These are usually low signal on T1 and high signal on T2 MR images, with only minimal ring enhancement on T1-Gd studies (Fig. 2.18). The surrounding oedema may be extensive. The clinical presentation will usually differentiate between TMS and tuberculoma; a history of an earlier acute spinal myelitis, with subsequent recovery, is often an important pointer, as is the simultaneous presence of lesions in different stages of development in the central nervous system [74].

Granulomatous masses are common in *Candida* meningitis, which sometimes complicates the AIDS, leukaemia and the lymphomas. These masses tend to be extra-axial and fail to enhance on T1-Gd images, differentiating them from tuberculomas.

Fig. 2.17.
a Post-contrast computed tomography scan revealing periventricular enhancement (*arrow*) and oedema (*arrowheads*). This was a case of cerebral brucellosis. **b** Diffuse, high-signal, thalamic lesions in a case of cerebral brucellosis (*arrow*)

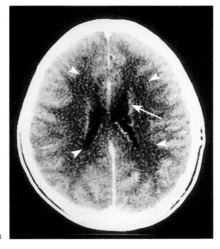

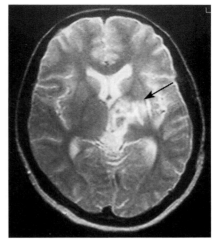

a

b

Cryptic, angiomatous malformations presenting as mass lesions develop a layered appearance as a result of episodes of local bleeding into the angioma. The presence of methhaemoglobin accounts for a layered void effect on T2 images. This contrasts with the layered, hypointense signal in some tuberculomas. If MR spectroscopy is available, the presence of methhaemoglobin in these lesions may be de-monstrated. Gupta, using spectrographic studies, has pointed out that tuberculomas have low levels of iron and other metallic elements [52].

Intracranial aneurysm may be differentiated from tuberculoma by DSA or MR imaging. Small tuberculomas in the subacute phase of TBM have proved difficult to differentiate from aneurysms of the Circle of Willis [68]. Aneurysm is an uncommon complication of tuberculous arteritis but can occur, leading to intracranial haemorrhage, epistaxis or bleeding from the aural canal [25,33]. The relationship of solid, enhancing tuberculomas to blood vessels may be a cause of confusion in the absence of a MR-imaging facility. MR images will confirm the solidity of a tuberculoma and demonstrate the flow void in an aneurysm.

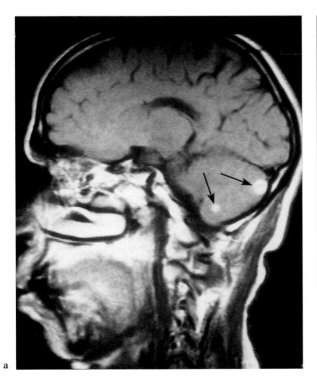

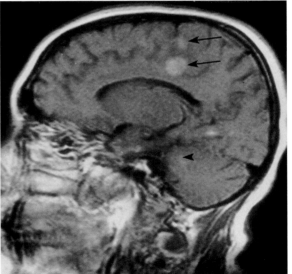

b

Fig. 2.18 a, b. Sagittal, post-gadolinium magnetic resonance imaging demonstrates two cerebellar tuberculomas (*arrows*). Scan b is of a case of multiple sclerosis (MS). There are similar lesions in the cerebrum but, in MS, they are slightly less well defined (*arrows*); there is a poorly defined lesion in the cerebellum (*arrowhead*)

a

■ References

1. Dastur DK, Manghani D, Udani PM (1995) Pathology and pathological mechanisms in neurotuberculosis. Radiol Clin North Am 33:733–752
2. Dastur DK (1972) Neurotuberculosis. In: Minckler J (ed) Pathology of the nervous system, Vol. 3. McGraw-Hill, New York, pp 2412–2422
3. Kirkpatrick JB (1991) Neurologic infections due bacteria, fungi and parasites. In: Davis RL, Robertson DM (eds) Textbook of neuropathology. Williams and Wilkins, London, pp 719–803
4. Reid H, Fallon RJ (1992) Bacterial infections. In: Adams JH, Duchen WL (eds) Greenfields neuropathology. Edward Arnold, London, pp 302–334
5. Rich AR (1944) The pathogenisis of tuberculosis. Charles C. Thomas, Springfield
6. Lincoln EM (1935) Haematogenous tuberculosis in children. Am J Dis Child 50:84–103
7. Rich AR, McCordock HA (1933) Pathogenisis of tuberculous meningitis. Bull Johns Hopkins Hosp 52:5–37
8. Proctor B, Lindsay JR (1942) Tuberculosis of the ear. Arch Otolaryngol Head Neck Surg 35:221–249
9. Jamieson DH (1995) Imaging of intracranial tuberculous in childhood. Pediatr Radiol 25:165–170
10. Schoeman J, Hewlett R, Donald P (1988) MR of childhood tuberculous meningitis. Neuroradiology 30:473–477
11. Cremin BJ, Jamieson DH (1996) Childhood tuberculosis: modern imaging and clinical concepts. Springer, Berlin Heidelberg New York
12. Rutherford GS, Hewlett RH (1994) Atlas of correlative surgical neuropathology and imaging. Kluwer, London
13. Kioumehr F, Dadsetan MR, Rooholamini, Au A (1994) Central nervous system tuberculosis: MRI. Neuroradiology 36:93–96
14. Arimitsu T, Jabbari B, Buckler RE, et al. (1979) CT in a verified case of tuberculous meningitis. Neurology 29:384
15. Bhargava S, Tandon PS (1980) Intracranial tuberculomas: a CT study. Br J Radiol 55:935
16. Chu NS (1980) Tuberculous meningitis: CT manifestations. Arch Neurol 37:458
17. Schroth G, Kretzschmar K, Gawehn J, Voigt K (1987) Advantage of magnetic resonance imaging in the diagnosis of cerebral infections. Neuroradiology 29:120–126
18. Witrak BJ, Ellis GT (1985) Intracranial tuberculosis manifestations on CT. South Med J 78:386
19. Jinkins JR (1991) Computed tomography of intracranial tuberculosis. Neuroradiology 33:126–135
20. De Castro C, De Barros N, Campos Z, et al. (1995) CT scans of cranial tuberculosis. Radiol Clin North Am 33:753–769
21. Jinkins JR, Gupta R, Chang KH, Rodriguez-Carbajal J (1995) MRI of central nervous system tuberculosis. Radiol Clin North Am 33:771–786
22. Cremin BJ (1995) Tuberculosis: the resurgence of our most lethal infectious disease – a review. Pediatr Radiol 25:620–626
23. Bonafe' A, Manelfe C, Gomez MC, et al. (1985) TBM: contribution of CT to its diagnosis and prognosis. J Neuroradiol 12:302
24. Gupta RK, Jena A, Sharma A, et al. (1988) MR imaging of intracranial tuberculomas. J Comput Assist Tomogr 12:280–285
25. Leiguarda R, Berthier M, Starkstein S, et al. (1988) Ischemic infarction in 25 children with tuberculous meningitis. Stroke 19:200–204
26. Gupta RK, Gupta S, Singh D, Sharma B, et al. (1994) MR imaging and angiography in TBM. Neuroradiology 36:87–92
27. Wallace RC, Burton EM, Barrett FF, et al. (1991) Intracranial tuberculosis in children: CT appearance and clinical outcome. Pediatr Radiol 21:241–246
28. Dastur DK, Lalitha VS, Udani PM (1970) The brain and meninges in tuberculous meningitis. Neurology (India) 18:86–100
29. Artopoulos J, Chamelis Z, Christopoulos S, et al. (1984) Sequential CT in tuberculous meningitis in infants and children. Comput Radiol 8:271–277
30. Chang K-H, Han M-H, Roh J-K, et al. (1990) Gd-DTPA enhanced MR imaging in intracranial tuberculosis. Neuroradiology 32:19–25
31. Medical Research Council (1948) Streptomycin treatment of tuberculosis. Lancet 1:582–596
32. Lehrer H (1966) Angiographic triad of tuberculous meningitis: a radiographic and clinico-pathological correlation. Radiology 87:829–835
33. Cross DT, Moran CJ, Brown AP, et al. (1995) Endovascular treatment of epistaxis in a patient with tuberculosis and a giant petrous-carotid aneurysm. Am J Neuroradiol 16:1084–1086
34. Rochas-Echeverri LA, Soto-Hernandez JL, Garza S, et al. (1996) Predictive value of digital subtraction angiography in patients with tuberculous meningitis. Neuroradiology 38:20–24
35. Takahashi S, Goto K, Fukasawa K, et al. (1985) Computed tomography of cerebral infarction along the distribution of the basal perforating arteries. Radiology 155:119–130
36. Foix C, Hillemand P (1925) Les arteres de l'axe encephalique, jusqu'au diecephale inclusivement. Rev Neurol 2:705–739
37. Plets C, De Reuk J, Vander Eeken H, et al. (1970) The vascularisation of the human thalamus. Acta Neurol Belg 70:687–768
38. Hsieh AY, Chia LG, Shen W-C. (1992) Locations of cerebral infarctions in TBM. Neuroradiology 34:197–199
39. Damasio H (1983) A computed tomographic guide to the identification of cerebral vascular territories. Arch Neurol 40:138–142
40. Gupta RK, Jena A, Singh AK (1990) Role of MR in the diagnosis and management of intracranial tuberculomas. Clin Radiol 41:120–127
41. Vallejo JG, Ong LT, Starke JR (1994) Clinical features, diagnosis and treatment of tuberculosis in infants. Pediatrics 94:1–7
42. Kingsley DPE, Hendrickse WA, Kendall BE, Swash M, Singh V (1987) Tuberculous meningitis: role of CT management and prognosis. J Neurol Neurosurg Psychiatry 50:30–36
43. Atlas SW (1991) MRI of the brain and spine. Intracranial Infection. Raven Press, New York, pp 511–534
44. Salgado P, Del Brutto OH, Talamas O, et al. (1989) Intracranial tuberculoma: MR imaging. Neuroradiology 31:299–302
45. Shen WC, Cheng TY, Lee SK (1993) Disseminated tuberculomas of spinal cord and brain demonstrated by MRI with gadolineum-DTPA. Neuroradiology 35:213–215
46. Draouat S, Abdenabi B, Ghanem M, Bourjat P (1987) Computed tomography of cerebral tuberculoma. J Comput Assist Tomogr 11:594–597
47. Vengsarkar US, Pisipaty RP, Parekh B, Panchal VG, Shetty MN (1986) Intracranial tuberculoma and the CT scan. J Neurosurg 64:568–574
48. Van Dyke A (1988) CT of intracranial tuberculosis, with specific reference to the "Target sign." Neuroradiology 30:329–336
49. Jinkins JR, Al Kawi MZ, Bashir R (1987) Dynamic computed tomography of cerebral parenchymal tuberculomata. Neuroradiology 29:523–529

50. Al Deeb S, Yaqub BA, Sharif HS (1992) Neurotuberculosis: a reveiw. Clin Neurol Neurosurg 94:S30

51. Baudrillard JC, Auquier F, Bernard MH, Lerais JM, Toubas O, Beranger C (1984) Tuberculome intracerebrale. Apropos un cas, aspect tomodensitometriques. Radiology 65: 385–387

52. Gupta RK, Pandey R, Khan EM, Mittal P, Gujral RB, Chhabra DK (1991) Intracranial tuberculomas: MRI signal intensity. Correlation with histopathology and localised proton spectroscopy. Magn Reson Imaging 11: 443–449

53. Abugali N, van de Kuyp PF, Annable W, Kumar M (1994) Congenital tuberculosis. Pediatr Infect Dis J 13:738–741

54. Bargallo J, Berenguer J, Garcia-Barrionuevo J, et al. (1996) The "Target sign": is it a specific sign of CNS tuberculoma? Neuroradiology 38:547–550

55. Ng SH, Tang LM, Lui TN, et al. (1996) Tuberculoma en Plaque. Neuroradiology 38:453–455

56. Graveli AB, Redondo A, Salama J, et al. (1998) Tuberculoma of the cavernous sinus. Neurosurgery 42:179–182

57. Welchman JM (1979) CT of intracranial tuberculomata. Clin Radiol 30:567–573

58. Lees AJ, MacLeod AF, Marshall J (1980) Cerebral tuberculomas developing during treatment of tuberculous meningitis. Lancet 1:1208–1211

59. Leading article (1984) Immune reactions in tuberculosis. Lancet 2:204

60. Campbell IA, Dyson AJ (1971) Lymphnode tuberculosis: a comparison of various methods of treatment. Tubercle 58:171–179

61. Chambers ST, Hendrickse WA, Record C, Rudge P (1984) Paradoxical expansion of intracranial tuberculomas during chemotherapy. Lancet 2:181–184

62. Teoh R, Humphries MJ, O'Mahony G (1987) Symptomatic intracranial tuberculoma developing during the treatment of tuberculoma: a report of 10 patients with a review of the literature. QJM New series 63 241:449–460

63. Abduljabbar M (1991) Paradoxical response to chemotherapy for intracranial tuberculoma: two case reports from Saudi Arabia. J Trop Med Hyg 94:374–376

64. Wilkinson HA, Ferris AJ, Muggid AL (1971) Central nervous system tuberculosis: a persistent disease. J Neurosurg 34:15–22

65. Reed MH, Ferguson CA (1978) The radiology of intracranial tuberculosis in children. Can Assoc Radiol J 29: 113

66. Dublin AB, Phillips HE (1980) CT of disseminated cerebral coccidioidomycosis. Radiology 135:361–368

67. Kumar A, Montanera W, Willinsky R (1993) MR features of tuberculous arachnoiditis. J Comput Assist Tomogr 17: 127–130

68. Gucuyener K, Baykaner MK, Keskil IS, et al. (1993) Tuberculoma in the suprasellar cistern: possible CT misinterpretation as aneurysm. Pediatr Radiol 23:153–154

69. Rajshekhar V, Haran RP, Prakash GS, Chandy MJ (1993) Differentiating solitary small cysticercus granulomas and tuberculomas in patients with epilepsy. J Neurosurg 78: 402–407

70. Jena A, Sanchetee PC, Gupta RK, et al. (1988) Cysticercosis of the brain shown by magnetic resonance. Clin Radiol 39:542–546

71. Williams DW, Elster AD, Kramer SI (1990) Neurosarcoidosis: Gadolinium-enhanced MR imaging. J Comput Assist Tomogr 14:704–707

72. Shakir RA (1986) Neurobrucellosis. Postgrad Med J 62:1077–1079

73. Larbrisseau A, Maravi A, Aguilera E, Martinez-Lage JM (1978) Can J Neurol Sci 5:369

74. Miller DH, Ormerod IEC, Rudge P, et al. (1989) The early risk of multiple sclerosis following isolated acute syndromes of the brain-stem and spinal cord. Ann Neurol 26:635–639

75. Lotz J, Hewlett R, Alheit B, Bowen R (1988) Neurocysticercosis: correlative pathomorphology and MR imaging. Neuroradiology 30:35–41

CHAPTER 3

Tuberculous Radiculomyelopathy and Myelitic Tuberculomas

■ Introduction

Until the advent of computed tomography (CT) and magnetic resonance imaging (MRI), the radiological study of spinal neurotuberculosis was held back by the limitations of conventional myelography, the only method of examination of the spinal cord available at that time [1]. By its nature, myelography could only demonstrate surface lesions of the spinal cord and variations in the dimensions of the myelum, as well as thickening and deformity of the nerve roots and cauda equina and, if present, spinal canal block. Except in its early stages, the pathological process of tuberculous radiculomyelopathy hindered myelography. The excessive glutinous exudates associated with spinal meningitis cut off the normal circulation of cerebrospinal fluid (CSF), making lumbar puncture and the introduction of intra-thecal contrast agents difficult and, in the later stages, impossible.

Post-mortem studies demonstrate that these exudates are extensive, often filling the spinal canal almost completely and compressing the cord and other spinal contents. The associated swelling of the cord and spinal nerves rapidly produces spinal block [2]. In late-stage cases, gliotic, collagen and fibrotic pathological tissues form, causing irreversible changes in the theca and the myelum. Clinical examination reveals many different patterns of neural dysfunction of the trunk and limbs, depending on the underlying distribution of the pathological lesions. In patients with combined tuberculous meningitis (TBM) and spinal meningitis (TBSM), peripheral nervous system deficits may be obscured by the low level of the patient's consciousness. The clinical expression of the disease varies considerably from patient to patient. Acute onset with back pain, paraesthesia, muscular weakness and sphincter dysfunction are common features. However, an insidious onset can occur, with a progressive pattern of symptoms mimicking intraspinal tumour, polyradiculopathy or spinal demyelination. Such chronic onset has been described and may occur many years after apparently resolved intracranial TBM [1]. In treated cases, inactive fibrotic and glial tissues remain in the spinal canal, often combined with cavitation in the spinal cord, representing areas of previous spinal infarction or healed tuberculous myelitis.

In all cases, it is essential to investigate both the brain and the spinal lesion, as concomitant intracranial and intraspinal lesions are common [3]. In a small number of cases, CT or MRI at the level of a spinal block will reveal tuberculous osteomyelitis of a vertebral body or, rarely, an isolated, tuberculous, epidural lesion.

Wadia and Dastur classified tuberculous radiculomyelopathy into two groups:

1. Primary, arising from a focus of tuberculosis (TB) outside the central nervous system (CNS)
2. Secondary, arising from intracranial TBM or from spinal tuberculous osteomyelitis

In a series of 70 cases, they found the primary type to be more common [4, 5]. The secondary type of spinal TB radiculopathy (TBSM) is caused either by spreading down from intracranial TBM or by spreading out and up from a focus of spinal TB osteomyelitis, commonly in the thoracic or lumbar region.

More recently, Dastur reaffirms that 50 % of cases are of the primary type and over 30 % are of the spread-down type from intracranial TBM [2]. This hypothesis is supported by the findings of Gupta [6]. Of 20 consecutive patients with intraspinal tuberculosis, 75 % were of the primary type and 25 % secondary to intracranial TBM. None of the cases had vertebral tuberculous osteomyelitis. Geographical and racial differences may affect the mechanism of spread, as Chang et al., in a study of 13 cases, describe 85 % (11/13) associated with TBM, one case secondary to spinal tuberculous osteomyelitis and only one primary case of an extramedullary tuberculoma arising low in the thoracic spine [1].

Downward spreading gives rise to the production of exudates that surround and compress the spinal cord. As in the case of intracranial meningitis, arteritis develops in the small vessels supplying the spinal cord. This, in turn, causes localised areas of ischaemia in the cord with ischaemic myelitis. Local haematological spread gives rise to the development

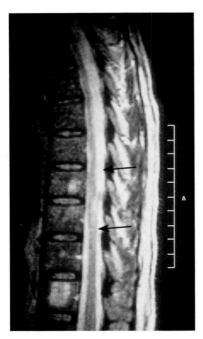

Fig. 3.1. Sagittal, T1, post-gadolinium scan of the thoracic spine. Markedly thickened spinal meninges and thick, enhancing exudates compress the thoracic spinal cord and displace it anteriorly (*arrows*). A case of spinal tuberculous meningitis

of intra-axial tuberculomas in areas supplied by these vessels. Swelling of the cord is also an important factor in the production of ischaemia, and this swelling, combined with the resistance of the surrounding exudates, compounds the overall effect (Figs. 3.1, 3.2). The deposition of surface exudates on the spinal radicles leads to thickening and deformity of nerve roots in the acute stages and, as in the case of late-stage intracranial TBM, fibrosis of these deposits results in permanent damage, with the development of chronic, adhesive arachnoiditis and radiculo-myelopathy.

All the layers of the theca and the axial nervous system can be affected by tuberculous infection. Both leptomeningeal TB and tuberculous radiculomyelitis are descriptive terms in current use but, as not all the intraspinal elements are necessarily simultaneously involved, the term spinal neurotuberculosis, as used by Dastur, seems a better description.

Extension beneath the posterior longitudinal ligament of the spine of a spinal tuberculous osteomyelitic abscess of a vertebral body commonly results in a tuberculous spinal epidural abscess. These abscesses are usually anterior to the cord, as TB confined to the posterior elements of the spine are uncommon.

The dura mater may prove a barrier against the initial lesion but, in some cases, penetration of the dura follows with the development of spinal tuber-

culous meningitis. As in the case of intracranial meningitis, there are few defences, and spread of the infection through the arachnoid–pial complex is rapid. Granulomas develop along the surfaces of both the arachnoid mater and the surface of the cord, leading to thickening of the membranes and, in areas of cord involvement, to fusiform expansion of the cord. Pitting and excavation of the surface of the spinal cord occurs beneath these granulomas, involving the neural tracts in the areas involved. Granulomatous investment of the spinal nerve roots causes sensory changes in the dermatome supplied by the affected root and to peripheral motor weakness, but the clinical signs may be difficult to elicit if intracranial TBM is present.

Myelitis is the result of either granuloma formation in the cord or of ischaemia following arteritis or thrombosis of small arteries and veins. It is often of a patchy nature, although a true transverse myelitis sometimes occurs.

These variable patterns of neurological deficit are often repeated at multiple levels, as the infection spreads both cranially and caudally along the subarachnoid space. The myelitic lesions are usually confined to short lengths of the cord with intervening normal segments, but cord oedema or tuberculous myelitis can involve considerable lengths of the myelum. In these cases, either associated fusiform swelling is present or, where local ischaemia or venous thrombosis is complicated by cavitation, there is loss of volume of the cord [1, 6, 7].

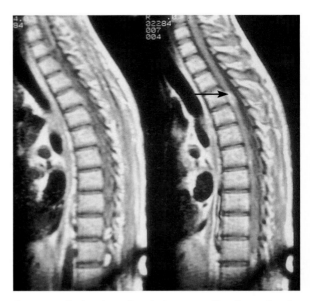

Fig. 3.2. A single tuberculous lesion expanding the cord at the Th4 level. Ring enhancement with a central, lower signal due to a tuberculoma (*arrow*)

Spinal block is common at the level of any tuberculous, spinal osteomyelitic abscess, or epidural or subarachnoid granuloma. In the case of abscess, particles of extruded, fragmented, vertebral bone, the associated epidural caseation and the commonly occurring gibbus formation all play a part in narrowing the spinal canal and in compressing the cord at the site of infection.

Spinal block also develops in the absence of osteomyelitis, as granulomatous tissue and thick exudate evolve at any level in the spinal canal and may do so at multiple sites. It most commonly occurs at the level of the conus medullaris or low in the thoracic canal [1, 6]. As impedances develop, spinal puncture becomes increasingly difficult, and a dry tap may be the result. The CSF becomes thick, at low pressure and xanthochromic due to its high protein content. Injecting intrathecal contrast fluid is difficult, and flow of the contrast is impeded by thickened and adhesive nerve roots and glutinous exudates. If MRI is not available, upper cervical spinal puncture is an alternative, but the same difficulties can be encountered in the cervical region.

The clinical presentation of TBSM is similar to a large number of other conditions, ranging from tumour to demyelinating disorders and polyneuropathies. Tuberculous myeloradiculopathy should always be included in the differential diagnosis of spinal lesions and, although rare, cases of primary TBSM do occur, as well as those arising as an extension of intracranial TBM or from tuberculous spondylitis with epidural spinal abscess. Tuberculous disease in other systems occurs in only 10 % of cases of TBSM [1], so the absence of pulmonary, lymphnode or gastrointestinal TB in no way excludes the possibility of tuberculous radiculomyelopathy.

■ Imaging Methods in Spinal Neurotuberculosis

Plain Film Examination

Plain film examination is often of little help, except in those cases where associated tuberculous spondylitis is present. If symptoms are due to primary tumour of the axial system, then occasionally expansion of the spinal canal or intervertebral foramina, such as that due to neurofibroma, will be recognised. Narrowing of the spinal canal due to old trauma or secondary vertebral neoplasm can be demonstrated, and the presence of remnants of oily contrast medium are characteristic in cases of chemical arachnoiditis. However, in cases of radiculomyelopathy, whatever the cause, it is unusual for changes in the structure of the axial skeleton to be visible.

Water-Soluble-Contrast Myelography

CT and MRI are not available in the majority of hospitals worldwide but, using a basic radiography unit, myelography of the spinal axial nervous system can be achieved even without a tilting table. In the majority of cases, it is possible to define the lesion and the extent of the extramedullary disease. The disadvantage of the method is that, although the structures of the dura–arachnoid–pial system are outlined, only the surface of the myelum is defined. Variations in the volume of the myelum are noted, but the presence of pial inflammation and intramedullary granulomatous or ischaemic lesions is not demonstrated. Also, it is not known whether lesions of the subarachnoid space and nerve roots are actively inflamed or represent scar tissue.

As in the case of intracranial tuberculous meningitis, the changes occurring in TB are non-specific. Bacterial and fungal inflammatory diseases are mimicked, as are parasitic disease, tumour, arteriovenous malformation, sarcoidosis and polyradiculopathies. An attempt should be made to examine the full length of the neural canal as, in STBM, multiple lesions are common, with skip areas of normal cord and theca intervening.

In cases of tuberculous radiculomyelopathy, a normal myelogram is uncommon [6]. The common patterns of the disease are as follows:

1. Irregular filling of the subarachnoid space due to the presence of granulomatous exudates, granulomas and thickening of the dentate ligaments.
2. Thickening of the nerve roots of the cauda equina and the paired nerve roots, particularly in the lower thoracic and lumbar regions.
3. Partial or total extramedullary blockage at the level of the conus medullaris or in the lower thoracic region. Blockage at the higher levels of Th5, Th1–C7 and C5 occur but are less common.
4. Long, vertical, band-like filling defects, perhaps the result of thickening of the anterior midline septum.
5. Variations in the dimensions of the myelum, due to myelitis and oedema. Most intramedullary tuberculomas are too small to cause expansion of the cord.
6. Large mass lesions due to arachnoid or pial tuberculomas, simulating spinal extramedullary tumours. These, in practice, are usually found posterior to the cord and in the lower thoracic region.
7. Epidural spinal abscess due to the extension of tuberculous vertebral osteomyelitis or, rarely, isolated epidural abscess without vertebral involvement [6].

8. Multiple filling defects in the contrast column, either fine and widespread or larger and coarser due to granulomatous lesions. Thecal granulomatous tissue also gives rise to surface irregularities and variations in the dimensions of the thecal sac [1, 6, 7].

Lumbar puncture allows the examination of the CSF at the time of introduction of the contrast medium. In acute cases, where the clinical picture of TBM or TBSM has not fully developed, the cell content of the CSF may be polymorpho-leucocytic. This will suggest a bacterial meningitis. However, once the immune system has been triggered, the characteristic pattern of CSF pleomorphism, raised protein and low sugar levels rapidly develops. As exudates are formed, lumbar puncture becomes more difficult and, if a spinal blockage develops, then a dry tap will occur. In the presence of extensive lumbar disease, the introduction of contrast medium will be painful for the patient, with extreme lumbar root pain developing after the introduction of the fluid, and sedation will usually be necessary during the procedure. If there is a spinal block, and no CT or MRI facilities are available, then spinal puncture at the C1/C2 level should be carried out and the upper part of the spinal canal examined with contrast medium. In contrast to the appearances of a spinal tumour, the margins of a tubercular spinal blockage are usually irregular, as opposed to the sharp outline of most tumours. Thickening of the elements of the cauda equina is unlikely to be confused with the more serpentine appearances of an arteriovenous malformation. Other granulomatous lesions and masses due to syphilitic gummata or neurosarcoid will need to be ruled out, as well as those due to parasitic diseases, such as schistosomiasis. Similar appearances of coarse filling defects caused by leptomeningeal carcinomatosis and the leukaemias in the area of the cauda equina and lumbar thecal sac raise diagnostic difficulties, but the general clinical picture and findings outside the nervous system will usually provide pointers to the correct diagnosis in these cases.

CT and Combined Water-Soluble-Contrast Myelography with CT

CT examination has some disadvantages as, in order to pinpoint multiple lesions at different levels, a very large number of axial images are necessary. Sagittal reconstructions are not of sufficient quality to demonstrate small lesions within the myelum, the relatively poor tissue differentiation between CSF, exudates and myelum being another negative factor. However, gross volume changes of the myelum can be

recognised, and Chang et al. describe cross-sectional changes in the cord, a pear-shaped cross section in the lower thoracic region being a common finding [1].

Improved images, when the site of the major lesion or lesions is clinically recognised, can be obtained by combining CT with intrathecal and intravenous contrast injection, but the problem remains that multiple lesions will not be recognised if they lie outside the area included in the scanning field. MRI, offering both multi-planar examination and the possibility of including multiple segments of the spinal canal by repositioning the patient during the examination session, has many advantages over CT scanning, while the application of gadolinium (Gd) MRI improves tissue differentiation.

In those centres without access to MRI facilities, myelography remains the best first examination despite its limitations in focusing on disease within the myelum. Recent MRI studies [6, 8] suggest that multiple tuberculomas of the cord are more common than previously realised and are not discovered by myelography. Once the diagnosis of TB has been made, these lesions respond to anti-TB therapy with a similar time scale to that of intracranial tuberculomas. CT examination a few hours after the introduction of the intrathecal contrast agent is a useful adjunct to myelography. The myelographic examination points to the areas of interest, and multiple axial slices in these areas produce valuable information as to the position, size and shape of the axial system and the presence of any extra-axial mass lesions, or spinal tuberculous osteomyelitis. The limitations of the technique arise from the poor definition of small, intramedullary lesions. These are characteristically isodense or slightly hypodense on CT imaging, and administration of intravenous contrast agents adds little information. It may be of value in enhancing epidural tuberculous granulation tissue or any paravertebral abscess, so its use should be considered in all cases.

In those patients in which myelography has demonstrated a spinal blockage some hours before, CT may outline intrathecal contrast that has passed above the block, defining its upper margin and giving useful information about the extent of the intraspinal granulation tissue. This is especially important if surgical decompression of the lesion is being considered.

Magnetic Resonance Imaging

In differentiating between the tissues of the various structures within the spinal canal, and in its multi-planar image acquisition, MRI is excellent in defining the changes of tuberculous radicular pathology. This is especially true in the area of the cauda equina and lumbar nerve roots [6, 7, 9, 10], although some authors still consider myelography and water-soluble-contrast CT (WSCCT) to have advantages [1]. However, in the delineation of inflammatory changes in the thecal tissues, the cord and the pia mater, as well as of intradural extramedullary granuloma, T1–Gd MRI study is superior to both water-soluble-contrast myelography (WSCM) and CT myelography.

The characteristic findings in active tuberculous lesions are isodense or slightly hypodense foci on T1-weighted images, and entirely hyperdense or annular hyperdense lesions with a hypodense centre on T2-weighted images. Gd-contrast, T1-weighted study is characterised by intense enhancement of tuberculomas, thecal inflammatory areas and granulomatous masses. The enhancement of the thickened theca is also well seen. On T1-weighted MRI, the change that is almost universally present in spinal tuberculous meningoradiculopathy is the loss of differentiation between the spinal cord, the CSF and the spinal meninges. These types of lesions may be present either segmentally or throughout the whole length of the spinal theca. However, these findings are not specific and are often present in a number of other conditions, as well as in TB [1, 6, 7, 10–16]. Variations in the calibre of the cord are seen. There may be an increase in volume, probably secondary to oedema of the myelum, and this may be accompanied by high-signal areas on T2-weighted images, which do not enhance after addition of Gd contrast agents. Narrowing of the cord is due to compression by excessive subarachnoid or subdural exudates.

Tuberculomas of the cord express a wide spectrum of appearances on T2-weighted imaging but are commonly high signal or isointense. They enhance on post-Gd, T1-weighted studies as discrete lesions or show rim enhancement, which differentiates them from areas of cord oedema.

The distribution of lesions seen on post-Gd studies varies from patient to patient and follows no particular distribution pattern. In some, long segments of the dura–arachnoid system are involved. In others, there are skip lesions with intervening areas of normal meninges. Marked plaque-like thickening of the meninges often occurs at the site of a spinal block, as do large, enhancing, granulomatous masses. These extramedullary masses usually lie posterior to the myelum. Isolated epidural granulomatous masses are described by Gupta [6] in the absence of both TBSM and tuberculous spondylitis.

In the MRI examination of the cervical spine, areas of the brain stem and medulla oblongata are invariably included in the field of examination. Tuberculomas may be present in these areas and, if isodense, are difficult to visualise without T1-Gd MRI

studies. Tuberculous radiculopathy of the cauda equina is not well demonstrated by non-contrast MRI examination. This is in contrast to non-specific lumbar arachnoiditis, where MRI has been shown to be a useful tool [9]. In suspected lumbar radiculopathy, T1-weighted, Gd-contrast MRI is often only carried out in the sagittal plane. There is a case for including a coronal, post-Gd study in the protocol to improve the definition of both the cauda equina, the emerging nerve roots and the associated pathological changes.

WSCM is still a valuable method in the imaging of the changes of both active tuberculous radiculopathy and chronic adhesive tuberculous radiculopathy. Despite its limitation of failing to image changes in the myelum, the superior definition of long stretches of nerve roots makes it an important method of investigation, one that is available to all radiologists.

T1-Gd MRI remains an important factor in the differentiation of active tuberculous granulomatous disease from chronic fibrotic adhesions and in separating the appearances of oedema from tuberculoma, as areas of both fibrotic tissue and oedema fail to enhance on T1-Gd MRI examination [1, 6]. Although unusual in the acute stage, syrinx formation and cavitation of cord lesions has been described [6]. This phenomenon is more common in the thoracic cord than in other areas. Loculation of the CSF, resulting from local obliteration of the subarachnoid space, is a common finding in both acute and subacute presentations.

Tuberculomas appear isodense or slightly hypodense on unenhanced T1 images and, therefore, may not be visualised. T2 images often show homogeneous low-signal appearances, but mixed signal patterns with central high signals are also described [6, 17]. This may be the result of accumulation of fibrotic lipid and macrophage material, which may explain similar appearances in intracranial tuberculomas. In two cases examined by Jena and colleagues, non-contrast T2 images revealed low-signal lesions [17].

Contrast-enhancement patterns in T1 studies vary in the intramedullary lesions. Either nodular or rim enhancement is described [1, 6, 17]. Although Chang asserts that conventional myelography remains the primary method of radiological investigation in spinal tuberculous radiculomyelitis [1], in a series of 16 cases of TBSM, Gupta describes five patients for whom the conventional myelogram was normal but subsequent T1-Gd MRI confirmed the presence of the disease.

The MRI findings may be summarised as follows:

- Intramedullary

  1. Cord oedema
  2. Cord tuberculomas (Fig. 3.3 a, b)
  3. Cord cavitation

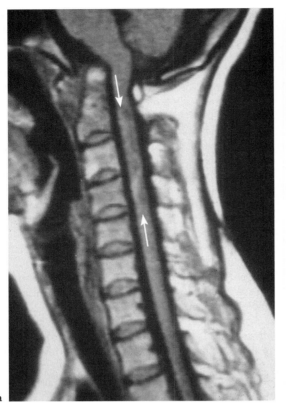

a

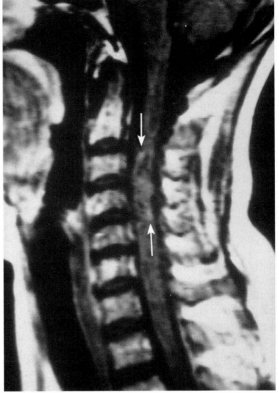

b

▲
Fig. 3.3 a, b. An intramedullary, tuberculous lesion extending over three cervical segments, with a mixed signal on T1 and a high signal on T2. Biopsy should be avoided, if possible, in these cases (*arrows*)

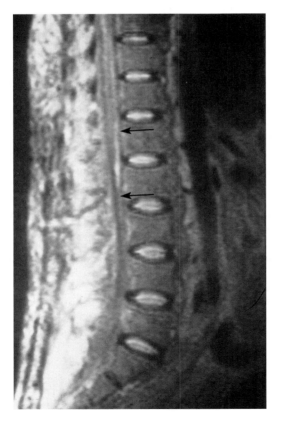

◀ **Fig. 3.4.** Sagittal, T1, post-gadolinium scanning reveals local enhancement of the meninges and the cauda equina in a case of spinal tuberculous meningitis (*arrows*)

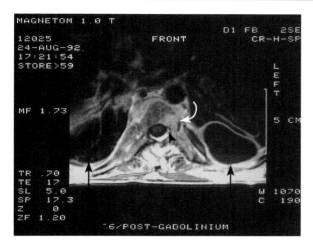

Fig. 3.5. Axial, mid-thoracic, post-gadolinium scan. There are two large para-vertebral abscesses with ring enhancement (*arrows*). The cord is displaced anteriorly by an epidural collection (*arrowhead*). There is tuberculous spondylitis in the vertebral body and transverse process (*curved arrow*)

- Meningeal

  1. Fluid loculation
  2. Obliteration of the subarachnoid space
  3. Meningeal enhancement (Fig. 3.4)
  4. Adherent and thickened nerve roots
  5. Meningeal tuberculomas
  6. Intradural, extramedullary mass lesions (Fig. 3.5)

■ Differential Diagnosis

Intraspinal TB is a rare cause of spinal meningitis and radiculomyelopathy but, with the advance of MRI techniques, more and more cases are being discovered. As opposed to some other spinal infections, TB tends to involve all the intraspinal elements simultaneously, although cases of isolated TB myelitis and isolated extradural abscess have been described [6,8].

The imaging findings are not specific to TB and may be seen in a wide range of diseases, notably in other infections as well as fungal, neoplastic, granulomatous, parasitic, demyelinating and iatrogenic conditions.

Spinal Arachnoiditis

Chemical arachnoiditis was, in the past, the most common cause of lumbar nerve-root adhesion. With the replacement of oily intrathecal contrast media by isotonic substances, it is seen less frequently.

It may be suspected in the presence of oil-contrast residues in the thecal sac or nerve-root sleeves. The arachnoiditis is confined to the lumbar region. Confirmation of the condition is made by demonstrating nerve-root deformity, thickening and adhesion on WSCM or CT myelography. The appearances on MRI study have been documented by Ross et al. [9].

It is also seen after spinal surgery or spinal anaesthesia. Infection is sometimes a cause of arachnoiditis after these interventions, but TB has been described as the infecting agent in 15% of cases of this subset. Tuberculous arachnoiditis tends to be seen in a younger age group, the common age distribution for other causes of spinal arachnoiditis being 30–50 years.

Other causes are subarachnoid haemorrhage, trauma and secondary tumour infiltration [7]. In spinal arachnoiditis, the change on water-soluble-contrast computed-tomographic myelography (WSCCTM) is of central clumping of the nerve roots of the cauda equina without thickening of the dura. Alternatively, there may be an empty thecal sac, the nerve roots being displaced posteriorly and adherent to the peripheral dura. In a third group, thickening and adhesion of the nerve roots to one another produces a spinal blockage on WSCM and, on WSCCTM, an attenuating mass partially filling the dural sac. In this group of patients, myelography by the cervical route demonstrates partial flow of contrast around the block at the lumbar level, with accumulation of long streams of contrast between the nerve roots. This effect has been described as "the dripping candle appearance" by Ross et al. [9]. In tuberculous arachnoiditis, factors other than adhesion of the nerve roots due to chemical arachnoiditis or low-grade infection are at play.

The response to tuberculous infection involves all the elements of the spinal canal contents. The resulting marked thickening of nerve roots, dura and surface of the cord give rise to appearances that in most cases are readily distinguishable from non-specific spinal arachnoiditis. Thickening and irregularity of the dural sac are almost invariably present in TBSM, although, in the acute phase, normal myelography coupled with abnormal MRI has been described [6]. The organisation of the subarachnoid exudates in TBSM changes the pattern of flow of contrast medium through the theca, and the development of nodular tubercles on the surfaces of the dura, nerve-roots and cord is clearly seen on myelography.

Non-specific spinal arachnoiditis (NSA) is usually confined to the lumbar region, an uncommon occurrence in TBSM. The surface of the cord and conus medullaris are not involved in the process whilst, in TBSM, changes in these structures, as well as lesions at higher levels, are further indications of the nature of the condition. The failure of the collagenous and fibrotic lesions of the nerve roots in NSA to enhance on T1-Gd MRI is a further distinguishing feature, but conventional and CT myelography remain valuable methods of investigation in those centres without MRI.

In the chronic form of TBSM, similar fibrotic and collagenous lesions occur, which also fail to enhance. A history of TBM or TBSM in the past may be the only method of differentiation, but the presence of a spinal blockage or extramedullary lesions at higher levels in the spinal canal remains an important differentiating factor [1, 6]. It has recently been shown that spinal nerve roots will enhance when the blood–nerve barrier breaks down, and this may occur due to any non-specific pathological insult. Such insults may include trauma, ischaemia, inflammation, demyelination and axonal degeneration. In the majority of these cases, there will be no evidence of nerve-root thickening, deformity or adhesion [18].

In young patients, the rare condition of hypertrophic interstitial polyneuritis must be considered when the imaging characteristics of thickening and surface irregularity of the spinal roots are present [7, 19]. The clinical lack of evidence of an infectious disease and the relatively slow progress of the condition should differentiate it from TBSM [1, 9].

Infective Leptomeningitis

Isolated spinal meningitis is unusual, as the majority of spinal cases are secondary to the spread of intracranial meningeal infection. The most common agents are viral or pyogenic organisms, which have a natural capacity to spread to the spinal subarachnoid space (Fig. 3.6). This is also the case with fungal infections, notably disseminated coccidioidomycosis. Spirochaetal infections are the result of haematogenous spread. The clinical presentation of the meningitides, with fever, neck, back and radicular pain, often linked with sensory loss and muscular weakness, leads to the examination of the CSF. In the acute stage of TBSM, the early CSF findings are of a polymorphonuclear cell pattern with a slightly raised protein content, suggesting a pyogenic origin of infection. The typical lymphocytic pleomorphosis and high protein levels of TBSM develop later, underlining the need for repeated CSF examinations [7].

CSF study gives us the opportunity to search for other infecting agents, such as fungi and syphilis, and for other causes of spinal meningitis, such as secondary malignancy. Immediate search for acid-fast bacilli should be carried out, but the return of positive smears is, unfortunately, low. Rapid culture methods are helpful, but even these lose valuable

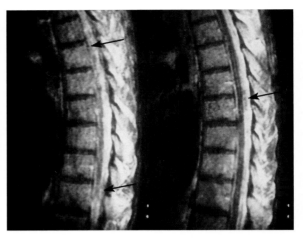

Fig. 3.6. Sagittal scans of the thoracic spine demonstrate irregular, low-signal thickening of the meninges at a number of levels (*arrows*). Bacteriological study of the cerebrospinal fluid confirmed enterococcal meningitis

time and, in areas where TB is endemic, anti-tuberculosis chemotherapy is started early. In cases where there is co-existent or recent TBM, the onset of spinal symptoms is virtually diagnostic of TBSM, and conventional and CT myelography will show a supportive (but non-specific) picture.

In recently published studies, a predilection for young age groups in TBSM is emphasised, the majority of cases being 30 years old or younger [1, 6, 10]. In non-granulomatous infections, the mean age is higher [13]. It must, however, be emphasised that the present upsurge of reactivated TB in older age groups in the West may well alter these age patterns in the near future.

MRI changes of dural thickening, linear enhancement of the cord surface and nodular enhancement of the nerve roots in the cervical, thoracic and lumbar regions are common to pyogenic meningitis, disseminated coccidioidomycosis and syphilis [10, 12, 20]; these diagnoses are rapidly confirmed by bacteriological, immunological and biochemical examination of the CSF and serum. Linear enhancement confined to the nerve roots is also described in aseptic meningitis and in immune-mediated meningitis [10, 20]. In patients with acquired immunodeficiency syndrome (AIDS), infection of the CNS by the cytomegalovirus (CVM) is a fairly common occurrence. The resulting polyradiculomyelitis is accompanied by a pattern of strong enhancement of the conus and cauda equina nerve roots, which are thickened, but without irregularity or nerve-root clumping. The CSF protein level is raised, and there is a polymorphonuclear reaction. Serum CVM antibody titres are often raised [21].

In some cases of bacterial meningitis, there is no demonstrable abnormality on T1-Gd MRI examination [13]. In TBSM, the imaging appearances are invariably advanced at the time of presentation [10]. In differentiating between these varying infections, much weighs on the clinical interpretation of the illness and its presenting features, the radiological imaging providing documentation of the extent of the disease.

Meningeal Carcinomatosis

Both TBSM and meningeal carcinomatosis share many symptoms seen on clinical imaging by WSCM, CT myelography and MRI examination [1, 11, 20]. The neoplasms commonly metastasising to the leptomeninges are primary carcinomas of the breast and lung, as well as lymphomas and melanomas. In most cases, they will have already manifested themselves elsewhere in the body, before meningeal involvement occurs (Fig. 3.7).

There will, however, be a small group of individuals in whom the primary tumour has not yet revealed itself. In all types of meningeal carcinomatosis, the clinical manifestations of back and root pain coupled with sphincteric disturbances overlap with those of TBSM. Multiple cytological examination of the CSF for malignant cells is required, as the sensitivity is low. On a single test, only 45 % are positive and, on a second test, up to 64 % of samples show malignant cells [20]. Once TBSM is established, the characteristic cytological changes of TB are present in a much higher percentage of cases. The initial polymorphonuclear response may lead to confusion with septic meningitis, but not with carcinomatosis. Lymphomas may also produce high levels of leucocytes in the CSF, but in unusually high numbers (Fig. 3.8) [22]. The mass lesions associated with lymphomas are often epidural and may have a paravertebral element, with extension of the mass through an intervertebral foramen.

The blood count will usually show the changes associated with the type of lymphoma concerned,

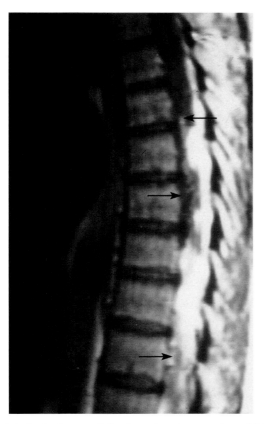

Fig. 3.7. Sagittal scan of the thoracic spine reveals multiple, low-signal filling defects. (*arrows*). These resulted from meningeal carcinomatosis

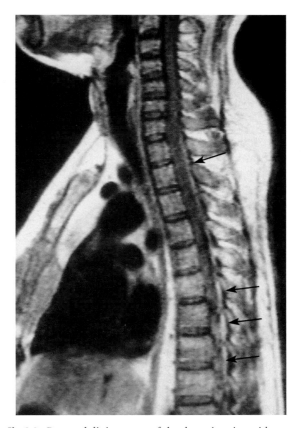

Fig. 3.8. Post-gadolinium scan of the thoracic spine with posterior meningeal enhancement in the upper area and patchy enhancement in the lower areas (*arrows*). A case of spinal meningeal lymphoma with meningeal infiltration

while bone-marrow puncture and MRI of the spinal segments concerned will demonstrate marrow infiltration. This is often also the case in meningeal carcinomatosis, where marrow signals of an inhomogeneous, nodular type will be discovered during MRI studies of the affected segment and in other areas of the spine [23, 24]. Both Chang and Krol describe the WSCM findings in meningeal carcinomatosis [1, 11]. Similar findings of meningeal thickening, nodular lesions, nerve-root thickening, surface changes in the conus medullaris and bunching of the elements of the cauda equina, as well as vertical, band-like filling defects are common to both meningeal carcinomatosis and TBSM. Chang suggests that the nodular lesions of meningeal carcinomatosis are more discrete, that those of TBSM do not demonstrate so sharp an outline and that the band-like defects are less prominent in malignant involvement of the leptomeninges. Involvement of the lumbar roots by thickening and surface nodules is also over shorter distances in TBSM than in malignant disease. A posterior mass in the subarachnoid space at the level of the conus medullaris is highly suggestive of TB, as is a change in the cross-sectional appearance of the myelum in the low thoracic region to "pear shaped" [1]. Enhanced MRI examination in both conditions are often similar. If TB is active, linear and nodular enhancement will occur while, in leptomeningeal metastasis, both linear arachnoid and pial enhancement are common and nodular enhancement is characteristic of carcinomatosis. In these cases, only accompanying changes of bone-marrow secondary deposits will point to the true diagnosis [20].

In cases of metastatic spread of intracranial tumours by tumour cells „dropping down" to the spinal subarachnoid space, similar imaging patterns will arise. The intracranial tumour will usually have manifested itself, and this underlines the necessity of imaging the brain in all cases of spinal disease [8, 20, 24].

Intramedullary Tumours

Clinically, tumour and tuberculoma share the same pattern of presentation. It is important to use every method of diagnosis available to avoid spinal biopsy. In a few cases of spinal tuberculoma, CSF study may be abnormal and point to the diagnosis. Other screening tests, Mantoux reaction, chest X-ray and sputum tests may be productive.

In the majority of cases, the radiologist will be confronted by one or more intramedullary masses. Spinal tuberculomas are usually less than 5 mm in size and not large enough to expand the cord (Figs. 3.9–3.11). CT imaging is usually ineffectual, due to poor tissue differentiation.

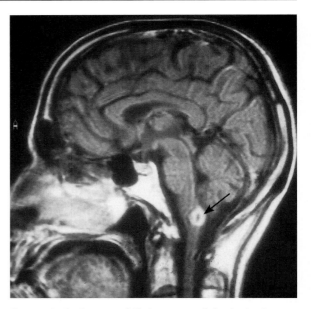

Fig. 3.9. Sagittal post-gadolinium scan of the brain demonstrating a cord tuberculoma at the cervico-medullary junction. Ring enhancement with a hypodense centre and expansion of the cord (*arrow*)

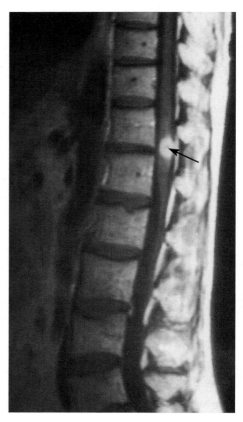

Fig. 3.10. A high-signal tuberculoma low in the thoracic cord. Note the central necrotic nidus (*arrow*)

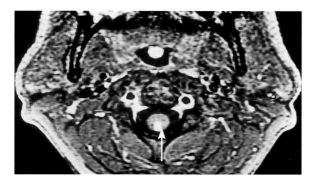

Fig. 3.11. An axial, T1, post-gadolinium scan of the neck, with fat suppression, demonstrates a small, intensely enhancing, solid tuberculoma of the cervical cord (*arrow*)

The introduction of MRI study with T1-Gd imaging has lead to many published instances of intramedullary tuberculoma. These are usually multiple lesions and are commonly associated with intracranial TBM or with TBSM [6, 8] (Fig. 3.12). Cases of isolated intramedullary spinal tuberculoma have been described [6, 17, 25], as have disseminated tuberculomas in the brain and spine in the absence of meningitis [8]. The MRI characteristics are similar to those of intracranial tuberculomas and, although usually small in size, lesions of up to 2 cm in diameter have been found [6]. These would show expansion of the cord on WSCM.

Low or normal signal is seen on T1-weighted imaging, and high, low or normal signal on T2-weighted imaging. Rim or homogeneous enhancement is usual on T1-Gd MRI acquirements. In cases with associated leptospinal TBM, some areas of T2-weighted high signal in the cord seem to be due to oedema or ischaemia, and these areas show no enhancement after Gd injection.

Jena describes a case with cord expansion and low intensity on T1- and hypointensity on T2-weighted imaging but showing a central area of high intensity on T2 images. In a second case, a cluster of small lesions expanded the cord, the lesions being hypointense on both T1 and T2 acquisitions [17]. T1-Gd MRI studies are, as yet, few in number but, as in the case of intracranial tuberculoma, intense rim enhancement surrounding a low-density area has been described [10].

Cord cavitation close to a tuberculoma in the presence of TBSM is also reported,, a change probably related to local ischaemic myelitis [6]. Pernaute describes a case of tuberculoma associated with a syrinx without spinal meningitis (Fig. 3.13) [26].

The most common primary tumours of the myelum, astrocytomas, ependymomas and haemangioblastomas, must be differentiated from tuberculomas. Astrocytomas are often not so sharply demarcated as tuberculomas, tend to be larger than 5 mm when first discovered and will expand the cord. Cystic elements in the tumour or syringomyelia are more

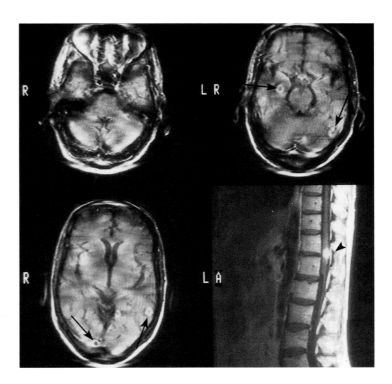

Fig. 3.12.
Multiple supra- and infratentorial tuberculomas demonstrate ring enhancement (*arrows*). There is a single tuberculoma in the thoracic cord (*arrowhead*)

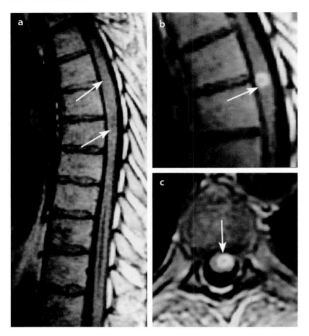

Fig. 3.13 a–c. A non-contrast study demonstrates expansion of the cord by an isodense lesion, with an associated area of syringomyelia beneath it (a, *arrows*). Sagittal and axial post contrast scans show the ring enhancement of a tuberculoma (*arrows*). Images by courtesy of Dr. Pernaud, University Hospital, Marques de Valldecilla, Santander, Spain

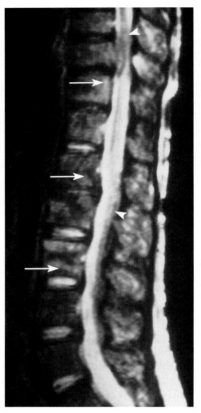

Fig. 3.14. Sagittal thoraco-lumbar scan demonstrating multiple, high-signal bone-marrow metastases (*arrows*). There is also irregular thickening in the meninges, due to further deposits in a case of nasopharyngeal carcinoma (*arrowheads*)

common than in tuberculoma. T1-Gd MRI enhancement is often inhomogeneous and may give rise to problems if it is confined to the periphery of the tumour.

Haemangioblastomas are usually small, enhance intensely and are difficult to differentiate from small, isolated tuberculomas unless the tuberculoma demonstrates ring enhancement. Ependymomas occur anywhere in the cord and enhance, but often incompletely, due to the presence of cystic elements in the tumour [27].

Secondary Malignancy

In cases of seeding from an intracranial primary tumour or secondary deposits from a distant primary focus, the primary lesion will often have already declared itself [24]. Multiple small, secondary deposits in the myelum are a problem. However, they are often associated with skeletal secondaries, which will be demonstrable by either MRI or isotope examination. In those cases where differentiation by imaging proves impossible, a trial of anti-tuberculosis chemotherapy should be considered (Fig. 3.14). CNS myeloma produces both mass lesions and leptomeningeal infiltration. Diffuse, myelomatous leptomeningitis is rare, but the appearances are similar to those of infective, carcinomatous and granulomatous leptomeningitis with diffuse enhancement of the theca and lumbar nerve roots. The presence of characteristic vertebral-body changes of multiple myeloma and the laboratory findings will differentiate this condition from TBSM [28].

Fungal Diseases

Fungal diseases introduced locally by inoculation though a skin wound show a pattern of infection more likely to be confused with tuberculous spondylitis than with TBSM. Fungal spread into the spinal canal through the intervertebral foramina or through the interspinous spaces is characteristic, as is localised bone destruction (Fig. 3.15). The accompanying leptomeningeal, inflammatory changes are usually over a short segment of the adjacent theca and are often posterior to the cord.

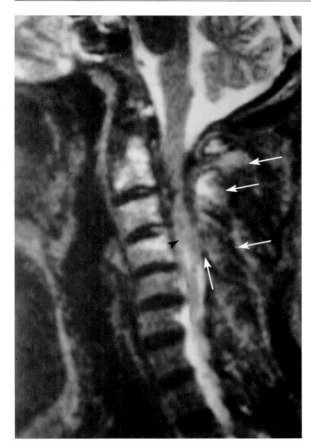

Fig. 3.15. Mixed signals in extensive mycetoma of the posterior cervical soft tissues (*arrows*). The fungus has extended into the spinal canal, both anteriorly and posteriorly, resulting in cord compression (*arrowheads*)

Disseminated fungal infection produces an imaging appearance similar to that of TB. As in TBSM, the progress of the disease may be either acute or chronic. Extensive thickening of the meninges in the basal cisterns and over considerable contiguous areas of the cervical theca are seen. In disseminated coccidioidomycosis, cervical meningeal thickening, of such a degree as to cause flattening of the spinal cord, is sometimes present.

The cervical spine lesions are the result of spread down from intracranial fungal meningitis, which shows features similar to TBM, including parenchymal lesions. The two conditions can be differentiated by culture of the organisms from the CSF and by complement fixation antibody titre studies of CSF. Meningeal biopsy at the time of any necessary shunt placement for accompanying hydrocephalus also gives an opportunity to confirm the diagnosis.

As is the case in all fungal diseases, blood vessels are invaded and infarctions occur. Wrobel describes two cases of anterior spinal-artery occlusion in patients

with DCC showing extensive, cervical meningeal enhancement on T1-Gd MRI studies but with no obvious increase in the signal in the cord on T2-weighted images [10, 29]. Histoplasmosis is another fungal disease that can develop in a disseminated form. In 25% of those with this type of the disease, the CNS is involved. Spinal histoplasmosis is unusual and appears to be the result of haematogenous dissemination rather than spread down from an intracranial focus.

Lesions in the cervical and lower thoracic regions occur. Local cord and meningeal inflammatory changes are see as a high signal on T2-weighted images and as areas of surface and intrinsic nodular enhancement with T1-Gd MRI. Without histological examination, it is impossible to differentiate these appearances from those of tuberculomas and TBSM [30]. In reported cases of meningeal fungal infection in patients infected with the AIDS virus, the usual sites involved are intracranial. Toxoplasmosis, cryptococcosis and candidiasis are the common fungal agents. Isolated spinal fungal infection has so far not been described. The lowered inflammatory response in these patients may be the underlying reason for the lack of spinal leptomeningeal reaction [31].

Tick-Borne Disease

Lyme disease due to *Borrelia burgdorferi* is a systemic inflammatory disease, endemic in both the USA and Europe, and is spread by the bite of a tick, *Ixodes ricinus*. It is prevalent in Eastern Europe and the Mediterranean regions. Exposure to the tick is likely to happen during camping and hiking vacations. When the CNS is involved, the CSF changes of lymphocytic pleomorphism and raised protein are similar to those seen in TBM. Usually, the clinical onset is milder than in TB, but radiculopathy and myelopathy can occur. The MRI appearances differ from TBSM in that enhancement is not so dramatic and is usually confined to the pial surface of the cord [32].

Other Granulomatous Diseases

Neurosarcoidosis

Sarcoidosis is a non-caseating, granulomatous disease with systemic manifestations. Neurosarcoidosis usually presents in the intracranial structures, and spinal neurosarcoidosis is a rare complication of the disease [33–35].

Changes in the myelum and the meninges are similar, on imaging, to both tumour and tuberculosis. As it is potentially curable with steroid therapy, it is important to differentiate it from other conditions.

Neurosarcoidosis occurs in 5–15% of patients with systemic sarcoidosis and may be the first indication of the disease [28, 29].

In the spine, sarcoid granulomas expand the cord and infiltrate the meninges. The resulting abnormalities are visible on myelography, WSCCT and MRI, and the resulting images are not specific to the disease. While the intracranial manifestations of sarcoidosis are well documented [36, 37], few cases of spinal neurosarcoidosis have been described, and the more recent advances in imaging techniques were not available in many of the studies. Frozen sections taken at the time of biopsy have proven unreliable and have been misinterpreted as glioma, as astrocytes are often present and granulomatous tissue has been overlooked [33]. Excision of the lesion has led to deterioration in the neurological condition of the patient. In all cases of biopsy of the cord or meninges, samples for TB culture and granulomatous histology should be taken.

Expansion of the myelum and surface nodules have been described on conventional myelography [33–35]. MRI examination has confirmed granulomas in the myelum, the pia mater and the dura, and these can extend over a number of spinal segments. As is the case with intracranial neurosarcoidosis, these lesions enhance on T1-Gd MRI studies [38, 39].

CSF examination reveals a raised protein level and a lymphocytic pleomorphism but, in the case of sarcoidosis, the CSF sugar level is usually normal, a finding that distinguishes it from TB. If spinal sarcoidosis is suspected, the brain should also be imaged. Other sarcoid foci are sometimes present, with a characteristic pattern of lesions in the hypophyseal and periventricular regions, although more widespread distribution is sometimes seen [36, 38, 39].

Isotope imaging with Ga-67 reveals sarcoid deposits in other organs, and the hilar lymph nodes may be enlarged on chest radiographs. Biopsy of the conjunctiva, lymph nodes or liver, or trans-bronchial biopsy, leads to a positive diagnosis in a high proportion of cases.

Neurosyphilis

Syphilitic Gummata

Spinal gummata are exceedingly rare but have similar imaging characteristics to tuberculomas. The more common expression of syphilis is hypertrophic leptomeningitis, a chronic condition often affecting the cervical segments (Fig. 3.16). In addition to the meningeal lesion, tertiary changes of neurosyphilis will be present, in most cases. Enhancing lesions in the myelum corresponding to posterior column

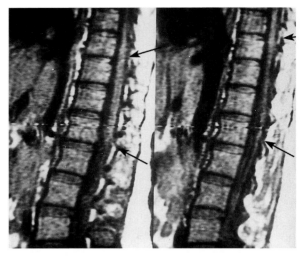

Fig. 3.16. Extensive meningeal thickening and enhancement posteriorly (*arrows*). The result of syphilitic pachymeningitis

pathology have described [10, 40]. Testing serum and CSF Venereal Disease Research Laboratory (VDRL)-antigen levels is part of the protocol in all cases of CNS disease.

Parasitic Diseases

Schistosoma

Schistosoma mansoni (SM), *S. haemotobium* (SH) and the Eastern form, *S. japonicum*, all cause granulomatous lesions in the CNS [41]. Sporadic cases are being reported more frequently in non-endemic areas as immigration and accessibility by air travel increases. SM or SH ova are deposited in the brain, cord or meninges. SH ova are presumed to pass through the vertebral plexus of veins and, in cases of hepato-splenic schistomatosis, SM passes through pulmonary arterio-venous shunts to reach the CNS. *S. japonicum* is more likely to infest the brain than the spinal cord [42, 43]. Although rare, the condition should be considered in any case of myelitis where the patient has recently travelled in an endemic area. Young males are the most commonly affected. The clinical presentation is similar to localised spinal TB, and the lesion is usually confined to the lower thoracic spine and conus medullaris [42–44]. Lower back pain, lower extremity paresthesia and loss of sphincter function are the usual symptoms. Myelography and MRI studies show local enlargement of the cord and, with T1-Gd MRI, both pial and intramedullary enhancement are seen.

Although lymphocytic pleomorphism and raised protein levels are found in the CSF, there is also an eosinophilia. Serum and CSF antibodies against SM or SH are found [41, 44].

Neurocysticercosis

Cysticercosis of the spine is an extremely rare cause of intramedullary lesions. Lotz et al., in a combined study of the pathology and imaging of intracranial cysticercosis, emphasise that, in the cranium, the disease is more often in the subarachnoid spaces than in the parenchyma. In the basal-cistern complex, racemose cysts are a common form of the infestation, and these can extend to involve the upper cervical subarachnoid space [45]. Intramedullary lesions in the spinal cord are a rare form of space-occupying lesion but must be differentiated from tuberculomas. Myelographic and CT examination will show expansion of the cord over a number of segments if the lesion is intramedullary, and subarachnoid filling defects if the cysts are leptomeningeal. Intramedullary cysts are usually found in the lower thoracic region, and the MRI characteristics are of a multiseptate lesion similar in appearance to a cystic neoplasm with enhancing margins. The description by Gupta of tuberculomas associated with cord cavitation necessitates the inclusion of tuberculoma in the differential diagnosis. Laboratory testing for a cysticercosis-specific antibody is positive in a high proportion of cases [6, 45, 46].

Demyelinating Disease

Multiple Sclerosis

In all cases of suspected spinal myelitis or space occupation, CT or MRI of the brain should be carried out, as silent intracranial lesions are sometimes present (Fig. 3.17). Spinal lesions in multiple sclerosis (MS) are often preceded by an episode of acute myelitis, followed by recovery. Later, signs of intracranial or spinal MS recur. Dissemination in time is an important feature of MS lesions [21, 47, 48]. The clinical presentation is of great importance in MS, as the enhancing spinal lesions are impossible to differentiate, using imaging methods, from granulomas or tumours of the cord.

■ References

1. Chang KH, Han MH, Choi YW, et al. (1989) Tuberculous arachnoiditis of the spine: findings on myelography CT and MR imaging. AJNR 10:1255–1262
2. Dastur D, Manghani DK, Udani PM (1995) Imaging of tuberculosis and craniospinal tuberculosis: pathology and pathogenic mechanisms of neurotuberculosis. Radiol Clin North Am 33:733–752
3. Tandon PN (1978) Tuberculous meningitis (cranial and spinal). In: Vinken PJ, Bruyn GW (eds) Infections of the nervous system. (Handbook of clinical neurology, vol 33) Elsevier, Amsterdam pp 195–262
4. Wadia NH (1973) Radiculomyelopathy associated with spinal meningitides (arachnoiditis) with special reference to the tuberculous variety. In: Spillane JD (ed) Tropical neurology. Oxford University Press, London, pp 63–72
5. Wadia NH, Dastur DK (1969) Spinal meningitides with radiculo-myelopathy. Part 1: clinical and radiological features. J Neurol Sci 8:239–260
6. Gupta RK, Gupta S, Kumar S, Koli A, et al. (1994) MRI in intraspinal tuberculosis. Neuroradiology 36:39–43
7. Kumar A, Montanera W, Willinsky R, et al. (1993) MR features of tuberculous arachnoiditis. J Comput Assist Tomogr 17:127–130
8. Shen W-C, Cheng T-Y, Lee S-K, et al. (1993) Disseminated tuberculomas in the spinal cord and brain demonstrated by MRI with gadolinium-DTPA. Neuroradiology 35:213–215
9. Ross JS, Masaryk TJ, Modic MT, Delamater R, et al. (1987) MR imaging of Lumbar arachnoiditis. AJR 149:1025–1032
10. Gero B, Sze G, Sharif H (1991) MR imaging of intradural inflammatory diseases of the spine. AJNR 12:1009–1019
11. Krol G, Sze G, Malkin M, Walker R (1988) MR of cranial and spinal meningeal carcinomatosis: comparison with CT and myelography. AJR 151:583–588
12. Sharif H (1992) Role of MR imaging in the management of spinal infections. AJR 158:1333–1345
13. Donovan Post MJ, Sze G, Quencer RM, et al. (1990) Gadolineun-enhanced MR in spinal infection. J Comput Assist Tomogr 14:721–729
14. Sze G (1988) Gadolineum-DTPA in spinal disease. Radiol Clin North Am 26:1009–1024
15. Dillon WP, Norman D, Newton TH, et al. (1989) Intradural spinal cord lesions: Gd-DTPA enhanced MR imaging. Radiology 170:229–237

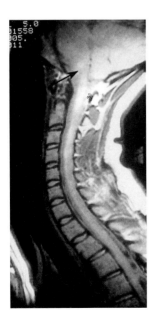
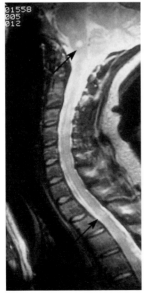

Fig. 3.17. Enhancing lesions in the cord and the brain stem (*arrows*). A case of multiple sclerosis

16. Sze G, Abramson A, Krol G, et al. (1988) Gadolineum-DTPA in the evaluation of intradural extramedullary spinal disease. AJNR 9:153–163

17. Jena A, Banerji AK, Tripati RP, et al. (1991) Demonstration of intramedullary tuberculomas by magnetic resonance imaging: a report of two cases. Br J Radiol 64: 555–557

18. Jinkins JR (1993) MR of enhancing nerve roots in the unoperated lumbosacral spine. AJNR 14:193–202

19. Rao CVGK, Fitz CR, Harwood-Nash DC (1974) Dejerine-Sotas syndrome in children (hypertrophic interstitial polyneuritis). AJR 122:70–74

20. Phillips ME, Ryals TJ, Kambhu SA, Yuh WTC (1990) Neoplastic vs inflammatory meningeal enhancement with Gd-DTPA. J Comput Assist Tomogr 14:536–541

21. Hansman Whiteman ML, Dandapani BK, Shebert RT, Donovan Post MJ (1994) MRI of AIDS-related polyradiculomyelitis. J Comput Assist Tomogr 18:7–11

22. McAllister MD, O'Leary DH (1987) CT myelography of subarachnoid leukemic infiltration of the lumbar thecal sac and lumbar nerve roots. AJNR 8:568–569

23. Williams MP, Olliff JFC, Rowley MR (1990) CT and MR findings in parameningeal leukaemic masses. J Comput Assist Tomogr 14:736–742

24. Blews DE, Wang H, Kumar AJ, Robb PA, et al. (1990) Intradural spinal metastases in pediatric patients with primary intracranial neoplasms: Gd-DTPA enhanced MR vs CT myelography. J Comput Assist Tomogr 14:730–735

25. Rhoton EL, Ballinger WE, Quisling R, Sypert GW (1988) Intramedullary spinal tuberculoma. Neurosurgery 22: 733–736

26. Sanchez Pernaute R, Berciano J, Rebollo M, Pascual J (1996) Intramedullary tuberculoma of the spinal cord with syringomyelia. Neuroradiology 38:S105–S106

27. Slasky BS, Bydder GM, Niendorf HP, Young IR (1987) MR imaging with gadolineum-DTPA in the differentiation of tumour, syrinx and cyst of the spinal cord. J Comput Assist Tomogr 11:845–850

28. Quint DJ, Levy R, Krauss JC (1995) MR of myelomatous meningitis. AJNR 16:1316–1317

29. Wrobel CJ, Meyer S, Johnson RH, Hesselink JR (1992) MR findings in acute and chronic coccidioidomycosis meningitis. AJNR 13:1241–1245

30. Desai SP, Bazan C, Hummell W, Jinkins JR (1991) Disseminated CNS histoplasmosis. AJNR 12:290–292

31. Mathews VP, Alo PL, Glass JD, Kumar AJ, McArthur JC (1992) Aids-related cryptococcosis: radiologic-pathologic correlation. AJNR 13:1477–1486

32. Demaerel P, Wilms G, Van Lierde S, et al. (1994) Lyme disease in childhood presenting as primary lepto-meningeal enhancement without parenchymal findings on MR. AJNR 15:302–304

33. Hitchon PW, Ul Haque A, Olson JJ, et al. (1984) Sarcoidosis presenting as an intramedullary spinal cord mass. Neurosurgery 15:86–90

34. Huang H, Haq N (1987) Spinal leptomeningeal sarcoidosis. Neuroradiology 29:100

35. Kelly RB, Mahoney PD, Cawley KM (1988) MR demonstration of spinal cord sarcoidosis: report of a case. AJNR 9:197–199

36. Hayes WS, Sherman JL, Stern BJ, Citrin CM, Pulaski PD (1987) MR and CT evaluation of intracranial sarcoidosis. AJR 149:1043–1049

37. Greco A, Steiner RE (1987) Magnetic resonance imaging in neurosarcoidosis. Magn Reson Imaging 5:15–21

38. Nesbit GM, Miller GM, Baker HL, et al. (1989) Spinal cord sarcoidosis: a new finding at MR imaging with Gd-DTPA enhancement. Radiology 173:839–843

39. Williams DW, Elster AD, Kramer SI (1990) Neurosarcoidosis: Gadolinium-enhanced MR imaging. J Comput Assist Tomogr 14:704–707

40. Tashiro K, Moriwaka F, Sudo K, et al. (1987) Syphilitic myelitis with it's MRI verification and successful treatment. Jpn J Psych Neurol 41:269–271

41. Scrimgeour EM, Gajdusek DC (1985) Involvement of the CNS in schistosoma mansoni and S. Haemotobium infection. Brain 108:1023–1038

42. Murphy KJ, Brunberg JA, Quint DJ, Kazanjian PH (1998) Spinal cord infection: myelitis and abscess formation. AJNR 19:341–348

43. Silbergleit R, Silbergleit R (1992) Schistosomal granuloma of the spinal cord: evaluation with MR imaging and intraoperative sonography. AJR 158:1351–1353

44. Dupuis MJ, Atrouni S, Dooms GC, Gonsette RE (1990) MR imaging of schistosomal myelitis. AJNR 11:782–783

45. Lotz J, Hewlett R, Alheit R, Bowen R (1988) Neurocysticercosis: correlative pathomorphology and MR imaging. Neuroradiology 30:35–41

46. Castillo M, Quencer RM, Donovan Post MJ (1988) MR of intramedullary spinal cysticercosis. AJNR 9:393–395

47. Miller DH, Ormerod IEC, Rudge P, et al. (1989) The early risk of M.S. following isolated acute syndromes of the brain and spinal cord. Ann Neurol 26:635–639

48. Posner CM, Paty DW, Scheinberg L, et al. (1983) New diagnostic criteria for MS: guidelines for research protocols. Ann Neurol 13:227–231

CHAPTER 4

Tuberculous Spondylitis

■ Introduction

Tuberculous spondylitis (TS) is an osteitis of vertebrae; it results from infection by *Mycobacterium tuberculosis*. Any part of the vertebral column can be infected, as can the paraspinal tissues, both anterior, posterior and extradural. Usually, the vertebral body is the primary site of infection but, rarely, the posterior elements of the spinal column are the first structures to be affected [1–7].

When untreated, the infection spreads from the vertebral body to the disc space and the paravertebral soft tissues, notably to the areas beneath the anterior and posterior, longitudinal spinal ligaments (Fig. 4.1). Extension outwards of the infection leads to abscess formation in the anterior and posterior spinal muscles. These collections may become large and often communicate with the subligamentous abscesses. In the case of posterior collections, continuity with the extradural compartment is often direct, by way of the intravertebral foramen.

Posterior abscess formation is often discernible clinically as a fluctuant swelling on the back, close to the spine. Occasionally, such a collection may rupture through the skin. Anteriorly, involvement of the psoas sheath occurs, and unimpeded spread, caudally through the psoas and iliopsoas muscles to the pelvis, is commonly seen. Some of these psoas-sheath abscesses surface as a swelling in the inguinal region. Accompanying spasm in the psoas muscle causes the hip to be held in a flexed position to relieve the associated pain. As these large collections do not cause the severe symptomatic changes present in pyogenic abscesses, they are generically known as cold abscesses.

The dura mater generally forms an effective defensive barrier against spread of the infection from the extradural to the subarachnoid space. However, in a small number of cases, spinal tuberculous meningitis, myelitis or radiculomyelopathy occurs [8].

In the cervical region, the anterior spread of soft-tissue infection develops into a retropharyngeal abscess (Fig. 4.2). In the thoracic spinal region, the pathway of the soft-tissue infection is guided by muscle planes, the pleural boundaries and mediastinal structures. The abscess may extend over a number of spinal segments. The cranial extension is limited, usually to not more than one segment but, caudally, the paravertebral soft-tissue swelling can be extensive (Fig. 4.3). Rupture into the pleural cavity occurs, leading to tuberculous empyema; extrapleural extension of infection around the chest wall also occurs. The posterior extremities of the ribs and the costovertebral joints are often destroyed, in these cases. Rarely, tuberculous mediastinal abscesses rupture into the oesophagus or even the aorta. Extradural abscess and granulation tissue cause compression of the cord and, in many cases, of cervical, thoracic and upper lumbar lesions; symptoms of neurological compromise follow [1–3, 5, 6, 9–15]. In children, occupation of 60% of the spinal canal may occur before neurological signs develop [9]. In the area of the cauda equina, there may be no signs of nerve-root compression with this extent of disease. As in the case of tuberculous infections elsewhere in the body, the imaging patterns are in no way specific for the disease.

Primary and secondary malignancy, lymphoma, pyogenic and *Brucella* infection may produce similar appearances. Fungal infections, parasitic disease and other granulomatous disorders must also be considered in the differential diagnosis. Clinical, laboratory and histological findings must be weighed in the effort to distinguish between a broad spectrum of disease entities. Although the association of thoracic kyphotic deformity with paresis was noted by Delachamps in 1570 [9], this complication of TS is known as Pott's disease (Fig. 4.4). The disease is named after the Englishman Sir Percival Pott who, in 1779, wrote "Remarks on that kind of palsy of the lower limbs, which is frequently found to accompany a curvature of the spine, together with its method of cure" [9]. One hundred years later, in 1882, Robert Koch isolated *M. tuberculosis* from cases of tuberculosis and showed it to be the infecting organism. TS is a curable disease and, if untreated, the resulting morbidity is catastrophic for the patient. The spinal deformity and paresis are avoidable complications

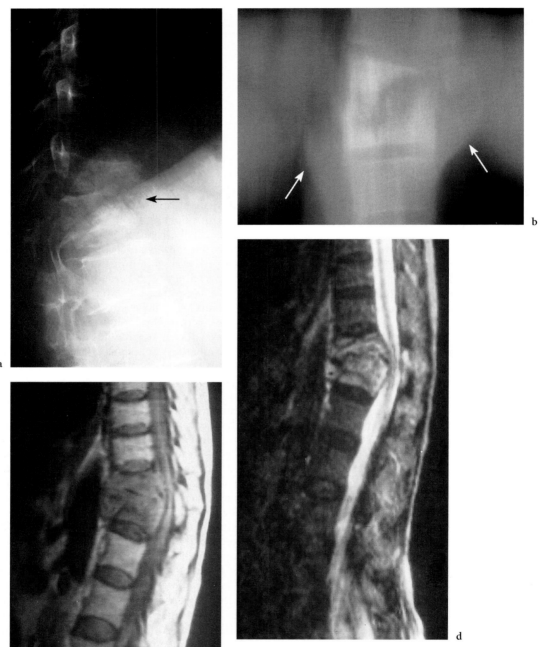

Fig. 4.1. **a** Plain lateral radiograph of classical tuberculous spondylitis. A thoracic vertebral lesion is destroying the lower half of the body of T10 (*arrow*). The disc has herniated into the vertebral-body abscess. There is kyphosis. **b** Plain anterior–posterior tomography demonstrates partial destruction of the bodies of two thoracic vertebrae. The disc space has disappeared. There is some bone sclerosis in this long-standing lesion. There is an extensive, paravertebral abscess on both sides (*arrows*). **c**, **d** Sagittal T1 and T2 scans. Two thoracic vertebral bodies are almost totally destroyed. The disc space is replaced by an intra-osseous abscess. An epidural spinal abscess compresses the spinal cord, which is also stretched, due to kyphosis. In T1 images, the infected vertebrae show a low signal. In T2 images, there is an increased signal in the bodies, the intra-osseous abscess and the epidural collection. The disc can no longer be recognised

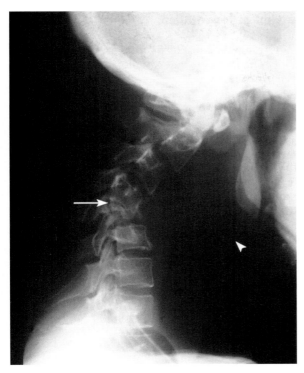

Fig. 4.2. Plain radiograph demonstrating marked kyphosis due to partial destruction of the bodies of C4–C5. Note the posterior displacement of the C5 body, indicating posterior element involvement (*arrow*). An anterior, retropharyngeal tuberculous abscess displaces the airway forward (*arrowhead*)

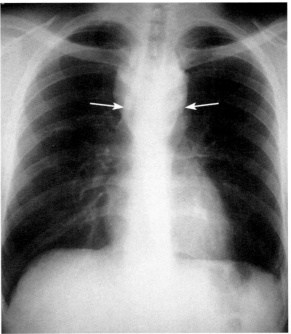

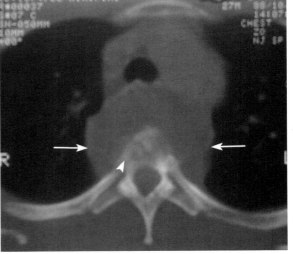

Fig. 4.3 a, b. Plain chest radiography. Widening of the upper mediastinal shadow resulting from a well-defined paravertebral abscess, extending over five spinal segments (*arrows*). **b** Computed tomography of the upper thorax demonstrates the posterior mediastinal abscess (*arrows*) and partial destruction of the body of T4 (*arrowhead*)

if the diagnosis is made early enough in the disease process. Unfortunately, this is not often the case. In the developing world, where patient and family tolerance of disease is high and medical facilities are scarce, the disease is often diagnosed in an advanced state with evidence of vertebral-body destruction, paraspinal infection and paresis already established. In the Northern Hemisphere, because of the decline in the number of patients with the disease, chances are high that, in the initial stages it may be overlooked and not considered in the differential diagnosis. In a patient presenting with persistent back pain and limitation of spinal mobility, TS will be low on the list of differential diagnoses and may not even be considered [3].

TS is a condition that develops slowly over months or years and, in the early stages, the radiographic changes are subtle but, if overlooked, lead to serious disability. Morbidity is high, while deaths are confined to 1% of patients, usually those with cervical TS or those in whom the infection spreads to become miliary disease.

The ongoing epidemic of tuberculous infections worldwide is raising clinicians' awareness of the disease. After about 40 years of decline, lasting until 1986, the number of reported cases in the USA began to increase annually at a rate of 3% per year for adult patients [16]. In children, the increase has been much more dramatic, increasing in the under-5-years age group by 39% between 1987 and 1990 [17]. In the USA in 1986, 17.5% of all cases of tuberculosis were extrapulmonary and, of these, 10% were musculoskeletal

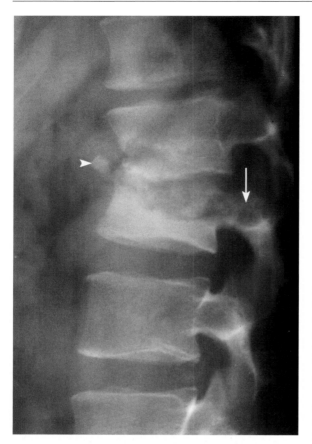

Fig. 4.4. Radiography demonstrates a lesion involving two vertebrae. The lower vertebral body shows extensive destruction that extends into the pedicle (*arrow*). The disc space is narrowed, and the lower half of the upper vertebral body is involved in the tuberculous process. Fragments of bone have been extruded into an anterior abscess (*arrowhead*)

[18]. Of this last group, 50% of cases had spinal tuberculosis [5, 6]. In Africa, India and Asia, spinal tuberculosis is a disease of the young. A high proportion of cases occur in patients under the age of 10 years [5]. Among immigrant and non-Caucasian groups in the Northern Hemisphere, young adults are the group most commonly affected, the average age being 39 years. However, amongst Caucasians in Europe and North America, an older age group is affected [3].

The increasing number of acquired immunodeficiency syndrome (AIDS) patients with a co-infection of tuberculosis has also increased the number of cases of extrapulmonary tuberculosis. Statistics show a higher occurrence of extrapulmonary infections in AIDS patients than in the general population [5, 16, 18].

■ Clinical Presentation

TS is an insidious form of osteomyelitis, and it is, sadly, often the case that pathological changes are advanced by the time the diagnosis is made. Persistent, localised pain in the back is the common early sign, and evidence of systemic disease is usually absent. The back pain is often present for months or even years. Increasing pain, lack of spinal mobility, abdominal pain resulting from paraspinal abscess or the development of fluctuant, subcutaneous swellings are other prodromal signs. Weight loss and night sweats may be the only constitutional signs of the disease [19]. In a small number of cases, there may be little in the way of presenting symptoms until sudden onset of paresis.

Paresis may also be preceded by slowly developing symptoms of neurological compromise. Weakness in the limbs, decreased sensation and sphincteric disturbances develop slowly, so that a tumour of the spinal cord is often suspected. In the case of cervical spine lesions, an anterior, paraspinal abscess or retropharyngeal abscess may cause hoarseness of the voice or difficulty in swallowing as the presenting complaints (Fig. 4.5).

Initial laboratory investigations are of little help, as the blood picture is usually normal. The erythrocyte sedimentation rate, if abnormal, will suggest an infective lesion, but it will also be raised in pyogenic infections [20 – 22]. The chest radiograph shows signs of active tuberculosis in less than 50% of cases. Mantoux skin testing is usually positive, but an anergic response may be misleading, as a small number of children and the immunosuppressed show a negative Mantoux reaction in the presence of active tuberculosis [9, 17].

Sites of Infection

In the majority of cases, the lesion is in the thoracic spine or in the thoraco-lumbar region. The lumbar spine is less commonly affected, and the cervical spine and the sacrum are rarely affected [1, 2, 5, 6, 23]. The atlanto-axial region is involved in less than 1% of cases (Fig. 4.6).

In the cervical spine, between 10% and 12% of cases occur between C2 and C7 (Fig. 4.7). Around 60% of cases are thoracic and 30% lumbar. Exact percentages vary from one study area to another. Weaver's 123 cases included a higher percentage of cervical spine lesions than the average 15%, some of these being skip lesions. Liu, in a series of 29 cases, describes no cervical spine cases [12].

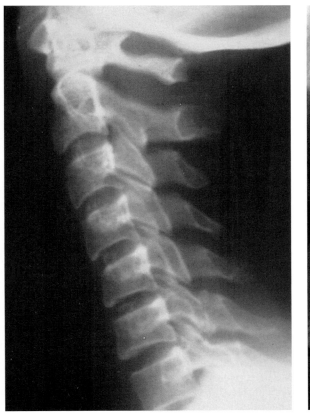

a

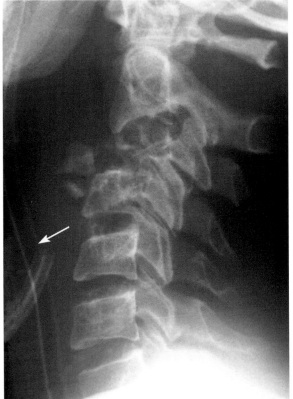

b

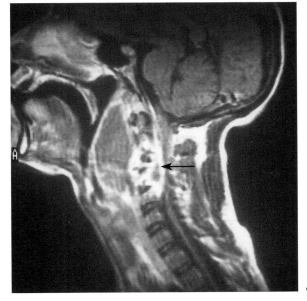

c

Fig. 4.5 a – c. A young man presented with neck pain. Plain radiography of the cervical spine shows no bone change, and the disc spaces are preserved. The neck was held rather straight. **b** Four months later, the body of C3 is almost totally destroyed, as are the lower margins of C2 and the posterior part of the body of C4. There is subluxation. Note the position of the nasogastric tube, due to a retropharyngeal collection (*arrow*). **c** The post-gadolinium scan outlines the retropharyngeal, tuberculous abscess. The spinal lesion is more extensive than is apparent from the plain films, involving the upper four cervical vertebrae and an extensive epidural component (*arrow*)

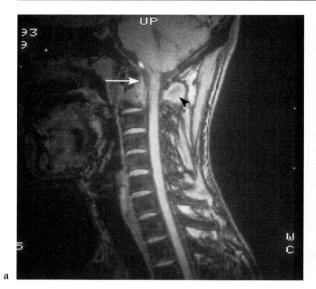

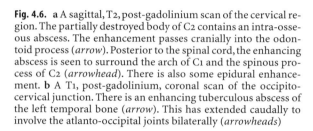

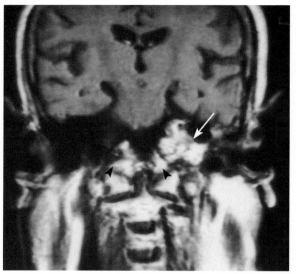

a

b

Fig. 4.6. **a** A sagittal, T2, post-gadolinium scan of the cervical region. The partially destroyed body of C2 contains an intra-osseous abscess. The enhancement passes cranially into the odontoid process (*arrow*). Posterior to the spinal cord, the enhancing abscess is seen to surround the arch of C1 and the spinous process of C2 (*arrowhead*). There is also some epidural enhancement. **b** A T1, post-gadolinium, coronal scan of the occipitocervical junction. There is an enhancing tuberculous abscess of the left temporal bone (*arrow*). This has extended caudally to involve the atlanto-occipital joints bilaterally (*arrowheads*)

Pathological Basis of the Images

The initial Rich focus multiplies in the cancellous bone or yellow marrow to form a group of tubercles [24]. As in other sites in the body, the core of the lesion contains multinucleated giant cells and epithelioid cells surrounded by lymphocytes. The bone of the vertebral body becomes decalcified and oedematous, both processes influencing the appearance of the bone in plain film, computed tomography (CT) and magnetic resonance imaging (MRI) studies [2, 4, 6, 25]. As the bone destruction continues, caseating material replaces the bone. This, in turn, becomes necrotic and inter-osseous abscesses develop. These, again, influence the imaging patterns and are recognisable on axial scanning [1, 2, 4, 6]. Abscesses contain caseating material, calcified bone fragments and pus and are encapsulated by fibrotic walls containing neovascularity, which enhance with contrast agents [4, 6].

In the healing phases and, rarely, in active disease, osteoblastic change accompanies the usual osteolysis and leads to recognisable bone sclerosis [3, 11]. New bone formations eventually develop and, in those cases where severe vertebral collapse has not occurred, the vertebral body may regain its original height (Fig. 4.8).

Anatomical Basis of Pathways of Infection

Although the haematological pathway has been accepted as the main pathway of infection in TS, there has been considerable controversy over whether the mycobacterium or any other organism reaches a vertebral body via the arteries or veins [7, 22, 25–28]. The nutrient vessels of the vertebral body were demonstrated in detail by Wiley and Trueta, who concluded that it was highly unlikely that the mode of spread of infection to the spine was by venous pathways; instead, spread occurs via arteries [29]. Their work gained support from Ratcliffe in his more recent paper [26]. The major support for a theory of venous spread came from Bateson [27], who described a venous plexus, arising from the spinal venous plexus, with branches throughout the laminae, pedicles and transverse processes of the vertebrae. The spinal venous plexus also receives blood from the centre of the vertebral body and from the vertebral end plates via the basivertebral vein and the anterior external plexus, which is a circumferential venous path running along the margins of the vertebral end plates.

The arguments against spread of infection through these venous pathways is based on the fact that the hydrostatic pressure in the system is such that passage of material to the vertebra from the plexus is highly unlikely and would be against the flow in what is primarily a drainage system. Trueta also pointed out that, in cases of vertebral osteomyelitis, no cases of intracranial, extradural infection occurred; such infection might be expected if infected material had gained access to the spinal venous plexus. In cases of spinal osteomyelitis, the usual focus is beneath the end plate, a fact which also supports access of the infecting material through the spinal arteries [29].

Ratcliffe describes the branches of the spinal arteries in detail. Anatomically, the area of the end plate and just beneath it is known as the vertebral metaphysis, while the main part of the body is called the equatorial zone. These two areas have distinct blood supplies. The arterial supply of the metaphysis is via branches from the spinal arteries, which in turn arise from the paired segmental arteries and the lumbar and intercostal vessels. The arteries entering the

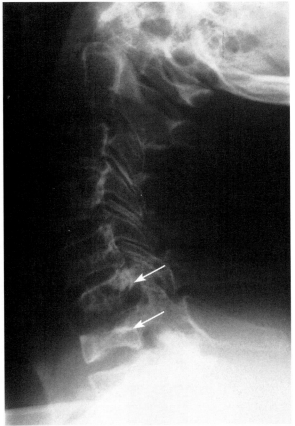

a

substance of the metaphysis are small end vessels called the metaphyseal arteries (MA). These are branches of the metaphyseal anastomosing arteries (MAA), which circumnavigate the vertebrae just beneath the vertebral end plate. Any infected material passing through this system will embolise in the cancellous bone anteriorly and beneath the end plate. Branches of the MAAs also pass superiorly and inferiorly, joining the upper and lower MAAs together and crossing the intervertebral disc spaces to link up with the metaphyseal systems above and below. In this way, infection can spread between adjacent vertebrae [26].

The equatorial area of the vertebral body receives its blood supply via nutrient arteries and branches of the spinal arteries, which enter the body through a posterior foramen. These arteries branch widely through the substance of the central part of the vertebral body. It is likely, in those cases where there is rapid osteolytic destruction of the core of the body, that the mycobacterium enters by way of these nutrient arteries. This may be the case where a single vertebral body is affected in the initial stages of TS, with later spread to other vertebrae via subligamentous spread [20] (Fig. 4.9).

Two recent cases illustrate the problem of the spread of pelvic infection to the spine. For some time, bacillus Calmette-Guerin (BCG) has been used in the treatment of superficial carcinoma of the bladder. Intravesical BCG is infused, and side effects are rare. In two cases, TS developed after therapy in the T11 – T12 region and, in another case, in the lumbosacral region [30, 31]. The isolated organism in one of these cases was *M. bovis*, the same as that employed in the manufacture of the BCG used in the treatment. In these cases, it was not clear which haematological pathway was involved. TS has been reported in the past after BCG inoculation, so an arterial passage may have occurred. However, the pelvic origin again raises the possibility that, in certain circumstances,

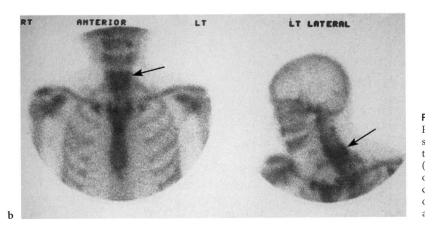

b

Fig. 4.7 a, b.
Radiography demonstrates tuberculous spondylitis destroying the lower part of the body of C6 and the upper part of C7 (*arrows*). **b** The technetium bone scan outlines the lesion, but the anatomical detail is poor. However, the full extent of the bone and soft-tissue infection is apparent (*arrows*)

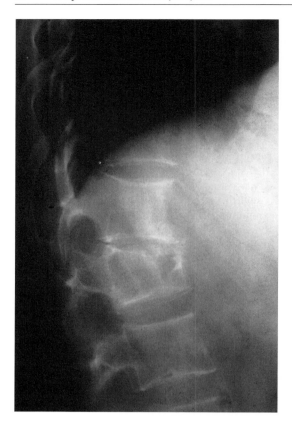

◀ **Fig. 4.8.** A tuberculous lesion of the thoraco-lumbar junction. The first lumbar vertebral body is partly destroyed, with some kyphosis. The disc space is narrowed. Both bone destruction and bone sclerosis are present in this long-standing lesion

▼ **Fig. 4.9 a, b.** Plain radiograph of the lumbar spine demonstrates tuberculosis confined to a single vertebral body (*arrow*). **b** The corresponding sagittal, magnetic resonance imaging scan demonstrates the vertebral-body infection, with relatively little anatomical change. The disc spaces are also only slightly abnormal, with a diminished signal and loss of the intra-nuclear cleft (*arrow*)

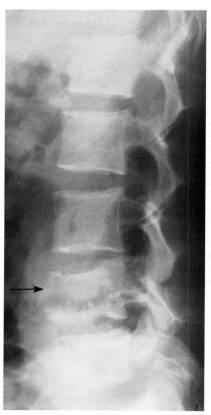

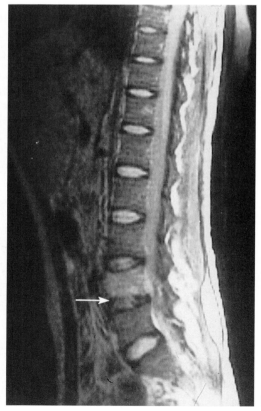

a

b

infected material can pass to the spine through Batson's plexus.

Other pathways of vertebral infection have been postulated. Direct spread along lymphatic channels from infected pre-vertebral lymph nodes may be the source, in some cases [32]. Weaver suggests that, in some of his cases, the primary site of infection may have been paraspinal, with later spread to the spine [3]. Direct, as opposed to haematological, spread from the lung has also been proposed as a source of spinal infection in a small number of cases [33]. Whelan reports one case of spinal tuberculous meningitis with extension of the infection to the vertebral body [4].

■ Methods of Imaging TS

Plain Radiography

There are a number of differing patterns in the development of TS, which are reflected in plain-radiographic appearances. Four of these depend on the site of the initial focus of infection.

Metaphyseal Infection

Infection of the bone adjacent to the vertebral end plates enters through the spinal arteries and their subdivisions, the MAAs and MAs [26, 29]. This gives rise to a Rich focus [24] in the area close to the upper or lower anterior margins of the vertebral body [1, 2, 4–6].

Initial plain-radiographic changes are difficult to discern but are the result of decalcification in this area. This equates with diminution of the intensity of the "white-stripe" boundary of the vertebral body [3, 23]. This early change is best seen on the lateral view as, on anterior/posterior images, the area is often obscured by the overlying neural arches (Fig. 4.10).

As the metaphyseal infection progresses, the overlying cortex is destroyed and the intervertebral disc space is invaded. Bulging of disc space upwards or downwards into the softened vertebral body occurs, leading to a degree of loss of vertebral-body height. This may be accompanied by slight narrowing of the disc space, although this is a later event than in pyogenic vertebral osteomyelitis, where infection of the disc space is accompanied by destruction of the disc tissue by proteolytic enzymes [4].

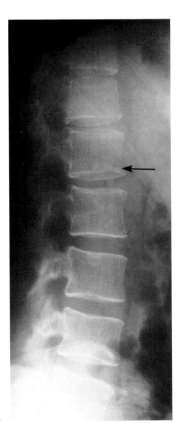 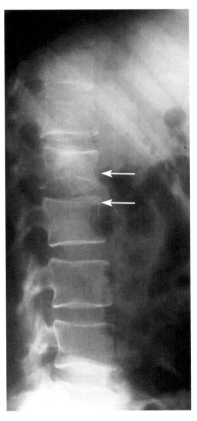

Fig. 4.10 a, b.
Early tuberculous spondylitis. The lower end plate of L1 shows some loss of the "white stripe" and a Schmorl's-node appearance anteriorly (*arrow*). There is minimal narrowing of the disc space. **b** Two months later, there is a metaphyseal lesion of the whole lower end plate and early changes in the upper plate of L2 (*arrows*)   a

b

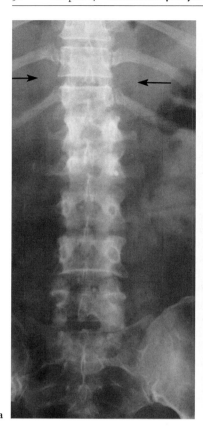

a

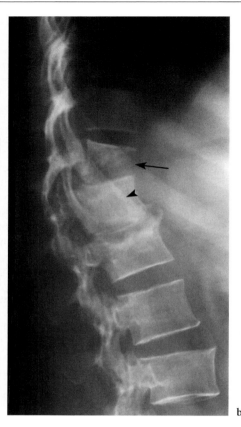

b

Fig. 4.11 a, b.
Anterior–posterior and lateral radiographs in a case of established tuberculous spondylosis affecting three vertebral bodies. The lower half of the T12 vertebral body has been destroyed, leading to kyphosis (*arrow*). There is an equatorial lesion of the L1 body, with cavitation (*arrowhead*). Extensive metaphyseal disease on either side of the narrowed L1–L2 disc space. **b** There is loss of the psoas shadow on the right side and widening of the thoracic paravertebral shadows indicating the extent of the soft-tissue infection (*arrows*)

Narrowing of the disc space is sometimes less apparent in non-whites and the disc space is often preserved until a later stage of the disease [3, 7, 20, 25]. As the destruction of the metaphyseal bone continues, spread of infection though the intermetaphyseal communicating vessels leads to involvement of the metaphyseal region of the vertebral body above or below, and similar appearances develop. (Fig. 4.11). Sequestration of the intervertebral disc into the two consecutive vertebral bodies is the next stage and, because the infected area is mainly in the anterior part of the vertebral bodies, kyphosis and wedging of the vertebrae follow. Unfortunately, by the time of presentation of the majority of patients, these changes have already occurred.

Equatorial Infection

Entry of the infection into the central portion of the vertebral body is via the nutrient artery branches of the spinal arteries or through the basivertebral veins [26, 29]. In these cases, there is decalcification of the central part of the vertebral body; this decalcification is discernible on the lateral view. The vertebral end plates are initially intact. The spread of the infec-

tion destroys cancellous bone and the surrounding anterior and lateral cortex of the vertebral body. There is often early angular collapse of the vertebrae, and anterior, subligamentous spread leads to extension of the infection to the adjacent disc spaces and vertebral bodies. In the initial stages, the lesion may be difficult to see because of the overlying neural arch while, on the lateral view in the lumbar region, overlying gas in loops of bowel may cause confusion (Fig. 4.12).

Paravertebral Infection

Paravertebral, infective masses are usually present at the time of presentation of the patient although, with the early application of MRI in back pain, one may expect more instances where TS is diagnosed before the development of a paraspinal mass [20]. In the thorax, these masses are readily seen, as they lie between the spine and the pleural reflections of the lung so that their density is in contrast to the lucent lung tissue. Apart from the early stage, when they are not of sufficient size to be apparent, these abscesses are seen as fusiform densities abutting on the spinal shadow, often extending over a number of vertebral

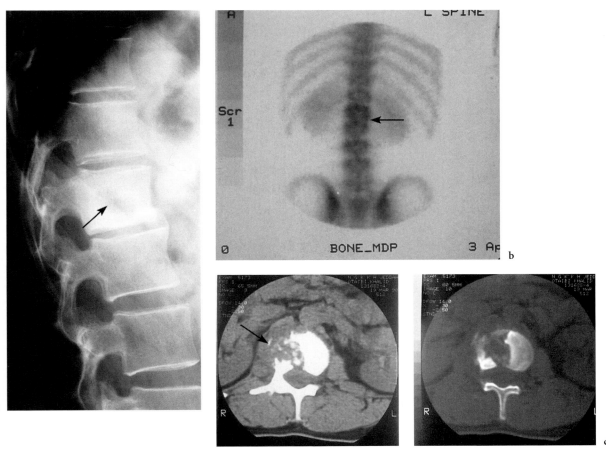

Fig. 4.12. a Plain lateral radiography indicates a central bone defect in the body of L1 (*arrow*). **b** The lesion exhibits only moderate increase in uptake in the vertebral body on a technetium-contrast scan (*arrow*). **c** Computed tomography reveals a surprising degree of bone destruction, with extrusion of bone fragments into an isodense paravertebral abscess (*arrow*). Biopsy retrieved tissue that cultured positive for alcohol acid-fast bacilli

levels above and below the affected spinal segment. On radiographs of the lung, they will only be seen if the exposure is sufficient to penetrate the mediastinum, the dorso-lumbar junction being a particularly difficult area in which to visualise them (Fig. 4.13).

In the lumbar region, paraspinal masses are detected when they obliterate the retroperitoneal tissue planes or if they contain calcification. They may be difficult to detect [34]. In Weaver's 123 cases, 58 % had detectable paravertebral abscesses. Calcification is unusual in the present day, when patients are more likely to come forward for help at an earlier stage of their illness. However, if not apparent on plain films, it is often visible on CT images and is important supporting evidence of the diagnosis of TS. It is not, however, pathognomonic and has been recorded in childhood discitis with osteomyelitis [35]. Psoas abscesses may reach considerable size, displacing the intra-abdominal contents and, rarely, rupturing into the pelvic organs.

A second type of paravertebral tuberculosis is sometimes seen, where the paravertebral infection is the main presenting sign. This is known as subligamentous TS. Extensive, subligamentous, paraspinal masses characterise this type of infection, with minimal or late involvement of the vertebral bodies or disc spaces. The subligamentous collections exert pressure on the anterior aspects of the vertebral bodies, and concavity of the anterior margins results. The radiographic appearance is similar to that seen in aortic aneurysms [23].

Posterior-Element Infection

This is usually a manifestation of extension of the bone destruction of established vertebral-body disease into one or both of the vertebral pedicles [4, 6, 11, 12, 14]. This is an important development, as the treatment protocol must then be changed. Pedicle

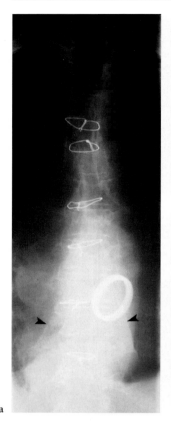

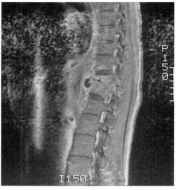

Fig. 4.13 a, b.
On plain radiography, the spine is partially obscured by wire sutures and a synthetic heart valve, but the T8–T9 disc space cannot be seen, and the paravertebral shadow is widened on both sides (*arrowheads*). **b** On post-gadolinium, T1 MRI the heart valve gives rise to significant interference. The body of T9 is almost completely destroyed, and there is an intra-osseous abscess (*arrow*) and an extensive anterior spinal abscess (*arrowhead*). The cord is compressed by an epidural element of the infection

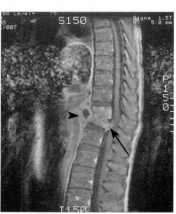

a

b

c

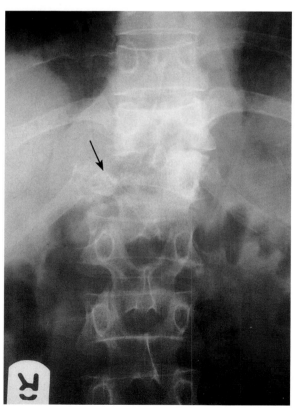

destruction indicates spinal instability, and the patient is in danger of dislocation of the vertebral body posteriorly, with resulting spinal paresis. Any surgical intervention must initially be by a posterior approach, with fixation of the posterior elements [36] (Fig. 4.14).

A second type of posterior-element infection occurs when the first focus of infection is confined to this area. Commonly, this is seen in a pedicle or is sometimes isolated to a spinous process; however, it may involve the whole of the neural arch [7, 15, 20, 22, 28, 37, 38]. This type of presentation is much less likely than neural-arch disease due to direct spread from the infected vertebral body and seems to be more common in non-Caucasian patients [4, 37], although it has been reported to occur in European and North American drug users [22, 39] (Fig. 4.15).

In India, original figures for the rate of occurrence of posterior element tuberculosis suggested a level of 2% in cases of TS [40]. More recently, a series of 228 cases of Pott's disease included 22 cases with the

Fig. 4.14. Plain radiographic examination demonstrates severe, destructive change in T11 and T12. The posterior elements of T12 are infected, as is the body. The right pedicle and costo-vertebral joint cannot be seen (*arrow*). The spine is, therefore, unstable

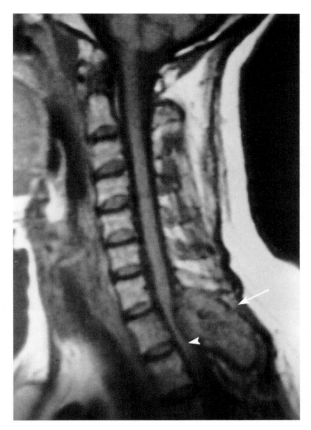 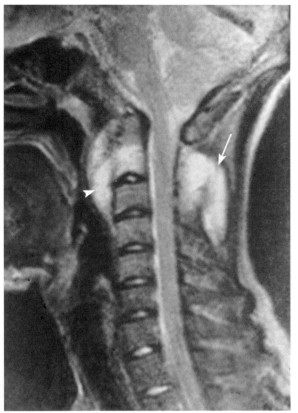

Fig. 4.15. T1 MRI before contrast indicates diminished signal in the spinous process of the seventh cervical vertebra (*arrow*). A posterior, epidural tuberculous abscess is compressing the cord (*arrowhead*). Alcohol acid-fast bacilli were seen on fine-needle aspiration

Fig. 4.16. Post-gadolinium MRI of tuberculous spondylitis affecting the body and spinous process of C2 (*arrow*). There is an anterior, retropharyngeal abscess (*arrowhead*)

infection confined to the lamina and pedicles, an unusually high incidence of 10 % [28]. In another group of cases, Naim Ur Rahman describes five patients with disease confined to the neural arch and observes that it is an infrequent entity. In recent publications from North America, three cases of isolated neural-arch TS have been described [22, 37, 38], as have two cases of isolated spinous-process TS [20]. This unusual presentation is likely to be initially confused with neoplastic disease. There is a second, diverse group of presentations, which seem to be related to the duration of the disease.

Infection of a Single Vertebral Body

This unusual presentation raises diagnostic problems, as single-vertebra disease is more usually associated with numerous conditions other than TS. This is especially so when the adjacent disc spaces are preserved (Fig. 4.16).

This type of infection may represent an early stage of TS disease and is, perhaps, related to initial introduction of the mycobacterium into the equatorial region via the nutrient arteries or the basivertebral veins. Weaver speaks of a central, lytic destruction of the vertebral body, with eventual sequestration of the disc into the hollowed-out vertebral body [3]. A radiological picture of vertebra plana can also evolve, with preservation of the related intravertebral discs [7] (Fig. 4.17).

Two recent cases demonstrated pathological changes in the vertebral body, with normal intravertebral discs and posterior elements [20]. Initially, lymphoma or neoplasm was considered in these cases. In one case, tuberculosis was confirmed by biopsy but, in a second, the diagnosis was not confirmed until adjacent vertebrae, the disc space and paravertebral tissues were involved in the infectious process, giving rise to a characteristic picture [20] (Fig. 4.18).

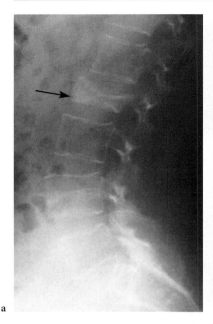
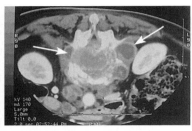
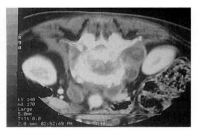
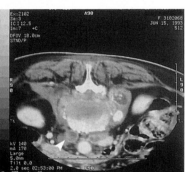
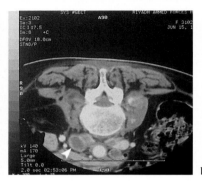
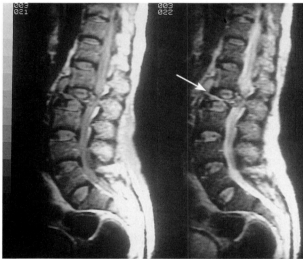

Fig. 4.17. a Plain view of the lumbar spine in an elderly, osteoporotic woman. There is vertebra-plana-type collapse of the body of L2 (*arrow*). The adjacent disc spaces are preserved. **b** Contrast-enhanced computed tomography of the region, acquired prior to aspiration biopsy, with the patient lying prone. Partial destruction of the body of L2 is associated with bilateral psoas abscesses (*arrows*) and para-aortic collections (*arrowheads*). The spinal canal is effaced by extruded bone and epidural infection. **c** A near-midline, sagittal, T2-weighted scan confirms normal intravertebral discs with visible neural clefts. The body of L2 is collapsed, and a high signal is seen (*arrow*). The spinal-canal contents are compressed. Alcohol acid-fast bacilli were found on immediate bacteriological screening of the aspirate

Infection of Adjacent Vertebrae, with Disc-Space and Paravertebral Involvement

This is both the usual and the classical presentation of TS. The changes are often already present at the time of the initial radiographs. In active, untreated disease, the vertebral-body lesions are osteolytic, and partial destruction of the adjacent metaphyseal regions will lead to a degree of collapse of the upper vertebral body into the lower [3]. The intervening intervertebral disc will, in adults, be intact and will have dislocated into the caseating substance of the vertebral bodies.

In the few cases of low-grade infection, in inadequately treated cases and in those where some degree of healing is occurring, the density of the vertebral bone will vary from lytic to sclerotic [3]. In cases of TS of the thoracic spine, the paraspinal involvement is easily seen, usually as a fusiform swelling on both sides of the spine. There may be variations of this pattern, and the abscesses are sometimes rounded in form and may be asymmetrical. It is usually the case that the size of the paravertebral swelling is large in relationship to the extent of vertebral-body destruction. In pyogenic abscesses, if a paravertebral collection is present it is usually on a much smaller scale.

Fig. 4.18 a, b.
Anteroposterior (AP) and lateral radiographs of a case of classical Pott's disease of the lower half of T12 and the upper margin of L1. Note the paravertebral soft-tissue collection on the AP study (*arrows*) and the degree of kyphosis on the lateral view (*arrowhead*)

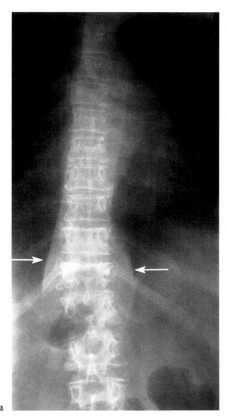
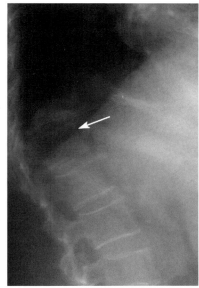

a

b

In the lumbar region, paraspinal abscesses are more difficult to detect, as the contrast between the abscess and the lung, which is so helpful in the case of the thorax, is absent. Indistinct or absent psoas-muscle soft-tissue shadows are a helpful indication but, in the early stages, small collections may not be visible. In long-standing cases, concavity of the anterior margins of the vertebral bodies is an indication of prevertebral granulomatous tissue or pus. Very large psoas abscesses can develop and, in certain cases, the pain that they cause may be one of the presenting symptoms (Fig. 4.19). These collections commonly occur in the groin and, rarely, they perforate into one of the pelvic organs.

A Primary Site of Infection with Multiple, Adjacent, Vertebral Involvement or with Skip Lesions

As vertebral-body infection continues, subligamentous spread involves disc spaces and vertebral bodies above or below the original focus of infection. A number of contiguous segments become involved. In a small number of cases, around 4%, distant skip lesions develop, often high in the thoracic spine or in the cervical spine [3, 6] (Fig. 4.20).

There appear to be some racial differences in this type of presentation. Descriptions from India observe that multiple vertebral bodies are sometimes involved, with preservation of the intervening disc spaces. This is unusual in North American or European pa-

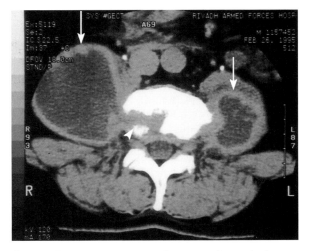

Fig. 4.19. Post-contrast computed tomography study demonstrating bilateral, large psoas abscesses. These show thick, irregular edge enhancement (*arrows*). There is destructive change in the right side of the vertebral plate (*arrowhead*)

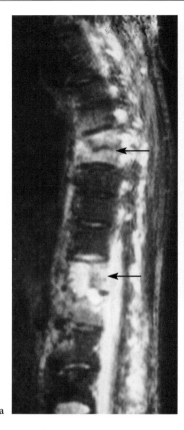

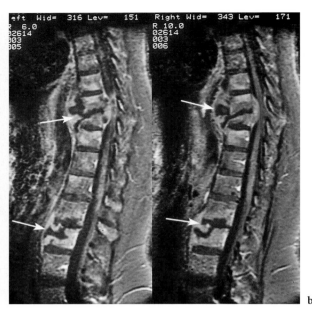

Fig. 4.20 a, b. T2-weighted magnetic resonance imaging of a patient with tuberculous spondylitis at two levels (*arrows*). **b** Post-gadolinium, T1 scan of a patient with lumbar and thoracic skip lesions (*arrows*)

tients [3, 7, 13, 23, 28]. In another type of distribution of the lesions, multiple single-vertebral-body infections may occur at different levels [23]. In the case of high cervical-spine infection, any accompanying abscess is seen as a retropharyngeal collection causing an indentation in the posterior pharyngeal wall and is detectable on lateral plain radiographs of the neck [21].

Conventional Tomography

Although conventional tomography has been superseded in recent times by CT and MRI scanning methods, there are many areas of the world where these newer techniques are not available and where the physician must rely on less advanced techniques. While the advantage of tomography is the absence of images of overlying structures, the loss of contrast between various tissues limits its value (Fig. 4.21). Spinal areas where it is of considerable use, in the absence of CT facilities, include the occipito-cervical junction, where lateral and anterior/posterior studies enable the extent of bone destruction and any subluxation between the first and second cervical vertebrae to be monitored. The cervico-thoracic junction and the dorsal spine in general are other areas where

the images of overlying structures make plain-radiographic interpretation difficult. In some centres where CT is available, tomography is still used as an adjunct in the management of TS [9, 10].

Myelography (Water-Soluble Contrast Myelography)

Again, in the industrialised nations, myelography has largely been superseded by CT, CT-myelography or MRI. Its value is limited in those patients who have no encroachment on the spinal canal. Although posterior bulging or displacement of the vertebral body is sometimes recognisable by plain-film examination, there is a large group of patients who exhibit either posterior, subligamentous abscesses or extradural granulomatous masses encroaching on the spinal-canal contents, and this development is not apparent on plain-film or tomographic examination.

In these conditions, water-soluble contrast myelography (WSCM) will demonstrate the characteristic changes of extradural space occupation, ranging from slight displacement of the contrast column to total spinal blockage. The examination is also of value in documenting the degree of improvement during treatment (Fig. 4.22).

Fig. 4.21.
Conventional tomography is still important where more sophisticated methods are unavailable. The osseous lesions are well demonstrated (*arrows*), as is the narrow disc space (*arrowhead*)

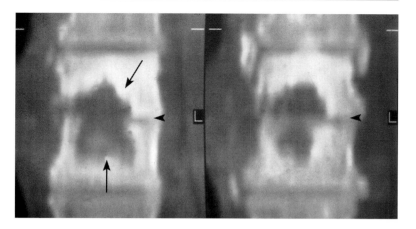

CT Examination

CT is an ideal axial-scanning medium for bone but is less efficient for soft tissues. Recent advances in both software and hardware development enable scans to be acquired in almost real time, while new methods of collimation and reductions in slice thickness have improved image quality.

Fig. 4.22. a A T1-weighted, sagittal scan demonstrates a low-signal tuberculous lesion affecting two thoracic vertebral bodies (*arrow*). **b** The conventional myelogram demonstrates vertebral-body lesions with kyphosis and compression of the spinal-canal contents (*arrow*). **c** Myelography in another patient with a total spinal blockage due to tuberculous epidural disease at the T8 level (*arrow*)

Helical CT produces scans rapidly, with minimal patient movement, but the capital-cost outlay has, until now, limited the introduction of the technique [6]. Reformatting of images in the sagittal plane produces images of a detail adequate enough to visualise moderate changes in the vertebral bodies and disc spaces (Fig. 4.23).

One of the limitations of CT is that the chosen field may not include the whole of the pathological zone. This is especially so in the case of TS, where even careful study of the plain radiographs may underestimate the number of vertebral bodies involved and where skip lesions may not have been recognised, either clinically or radiographically. The axial images demonstrate excellent bone detail and also define those areas of soft-tissue calcification not seen on

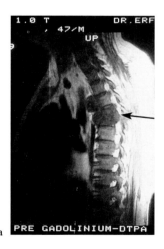

a

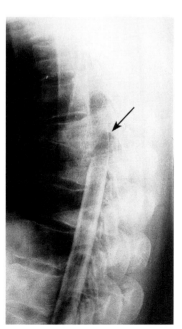

b

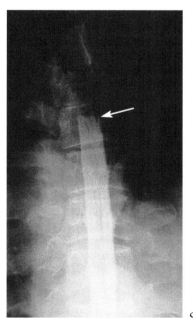

c

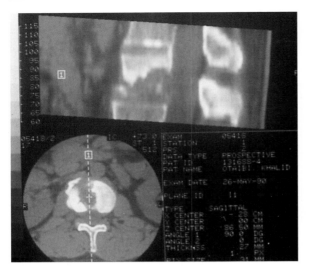

Fig. 4.23. Tuberculous spondylitis. Computed tomography examination through the centrally destroyed vertebral body. Sagittal reconstruction reveals the narrow disc space, fragmentation and no obvious epidural component

plain films or MRI. After injection of intravenous (IV) iodinated contrast medium, the soft-tissue areas require a second series; however, even after this, the contents of the spinal canal may be difficult to discern, an essential factor in assessing extradural, tuberculous lesions. An important use of CT is the production of precise images for use as guides to percutaneous biopsy and percutaneous abscess drainage, either of the vertebral body itself or of infected paraspinal soft tissues.

Early Changes of TS on CT Imaging

Focal low-density lesions in the vertebral bodies, showing homogeneity and usually with regular boundaries, are the characteristic early changes. As the disease progresses, fragmented bone will be seen within the cavities, which eventually develop into intra-osseous abscesses containing caseating material or necrotic pus. Elevation of the anterior bone cortex is often seen just below the disc space, with a thin band of less dense material between the cortex and the vertebral body. The elevated bone produces a crescent-like shape.

As the infection spreads cranially or caudally, destruction and fragmentation of the cortical bone of the end plate occurs. This change is seen on both axial and sagittally reconstructed images. The first sign of paravertebral extension of the infection is a loss of clarity in the fat planes surrounding the vertebra and those lying between the muscle bundles.

Established and Advanced Disease

Within the vertebral body, there is loss of the normal bone architecture, with extensive fragmentation of bone. These fragments are often sequestrated into surrounding tissues. There is loss of vertebral height, which can be measured on the pre-scan "scanogram" or on sagittal reconstruction. Loss of the supporting strength of the end plate leads to sequestration of the intervertebral disc into the substance of the vertebral body.

As destruction of the vertebral body proceeds, infection extending posteriorly will destroy the pedicles, producing instability of the spinal segment. This is less common in adults than in children and appears to be seen more often in patients from India. It is important to recognise this development, as posterior spinal fixation will be necessary if paraparesis is to be avoided.

Infection spreading laterally from a paravertebral site sometimes involves the costovertebral joints and destroys the posterior elements of the ribs at one or more levels. These infected foci may then spread extrapleurally around the chest wall or intra-pleurally to form an empyema. Destruction of the posterior part of the ribs is also commonly seen in foci of infection initially confined to the lamina, pedicle or transverse process [4].

In infection of the paravertebral soft tissues, the characteristic lesions are thick-walled, multi-locular paravertebral abscesses which may be either anteriorly or posteriorly placed. These exhibit enhancement on contrast studies, due to their vascularity and their inflammatory nature, and may contain fragments of calcification on the pre-contrast images. In the abdomen, these abscesses often involve the psoas muscle sheaths and may extend caudally a number of segments below the infected vertebral bodies [4, 6, 23].

Subligamentous spread of infected material is also characteristic, so infection of vertebral bodies and disc spaces above and below the original focus is common. If this tissue is granulomatous, it may not enhance with contrast and, if it is pus, it will remain of low attenuation but with an enhancing rim [1]. Skip lesions may also present, at this stage [3, 6].

As these inflammatory tissues encroach on the spinal canal, areas of extradural, granulomatous tissue or abscesses develop. Displacement or compression of the dural sac and its contents follows. In the lumbar region, this is not necessarily accompanied by neurological deficits, but these are common when the granulomas invade the narrower, thoracic spinal canal [12]. Passage of infected material from a paraspinal abscess through the intervertebral foramen to compress the dural sac is not an uncommon occurrence.

In patients who present late for investigation, in addition to the patterns previously described, kyphosis is often a feature. This may be severe enough to make axial scanning difficult. End-plate destruction and vertebral-body wedging are often advanced and, in some late-stage patients, total destruction of a vertebral body will have occurred. In these cases, it is only possible to elucidate the full extent of the destruction by counting the number of ribs and relating this number to the number of verte-bral bodies involved. A coronal CT reconstruction may be necessary in order to solve this problem.

In some late stage patients, there may be both osteolytic and osteoblastic changes, with both destructive and sclerotic areas present in the vertebral bodies. Although rare unless the patient has received some anti-tuberculous chemotherapy, this pattern is easily confused radiologically with metastatic neoplasm. In rare cases, anterior fusion across the disc space occurs spontaneously without treatment.

TS is a chronic disease and, even with medical treatment, areas of low-grade, granulomatous infection may persist, leading to worsening of kyphosis and late onset of spinal paresis. These cases are difficult to image axially, but enhancing abscesses or granulomatous tissue should be searched for, as further medical treatment may be required.

In non-compliant patients who have taken part of a course of anti-tuberculous medication, a situation of recurrent paraspinal abscesses and intermittent spondylitic infections lasting a number of years is

Fig. 4.24 a – d. Various computed tomography (CT) presentations of tuberculous spondylitis. **a** Non-contrast CT shows fragmentation of the whole body, with extension into the left pedicle. **b** Non-contrast CT showing numerous cloacae varying in size, and expansion of the collapsing anterior margins. **c** Post-contrast CT showing anterior subperiosteal disease (*arrow*) associated with destruction in the body and extrusion of fragments into the spinal canal (*arrowhead*). **d** Post-contrast CT demonstrating a marginal anterior osteolytic lesion with an associated anterior abscess (*arrow*). There is a psoas abscess on the right (*arrowhead*)

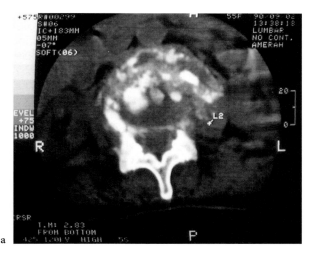

a

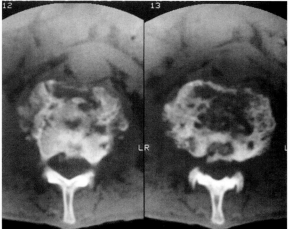

b

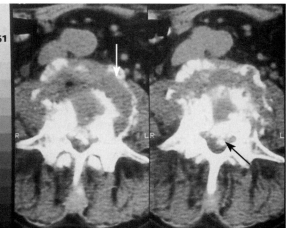

c

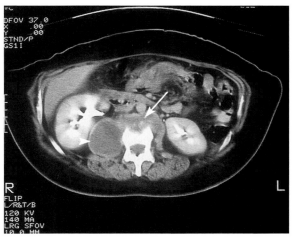

d

often seen. Secondary infection in these patients often leads to the development of systemic amyloid disease, with subsequent renal or cardiac failure. Although not specific to TS, a number of different patterns of bone destruction have been ascribed to tuberculous infection and, when present in a young patient in conjunction with paraspinal abscesses containing fragments of calcification, these patterns are extremely suggestive – but not pathognomonic – of TS.

Jain et al. have described four distinct patterns of destruction in their cases:

1. Fragmentary
2. Osteolytic
3. Subperiosteal
4. Localised and sclerotic (Fig. 4.24)

Type 1 is the common appearance described by most authors, in which the end plates are destroyed and the disc space is involved. This is, presumably, the result of initial infection via the metaphyseal arteries, with the infection spreading through the intermetaphyseal collateral vessels to the vertebra above or below. In the osteolytic type, the infection is initially confined to the equatorial core of the vertebral body, and this may be the basis of single-body infection with preservation of the disc space. Single-body infection was seen in 7 of Jain's 30 cases. This mechanism of infection also seems to be the case in type 4, where he describes a central, low-attenuation cloaca surrounded by a sclerotic margin. In type 3, there was subperiosteal disease with fragmentation of the anterior margin of the metaphysis and separation of a crescent of cortical bone. This latter may be an early stage of the type-1 pattern of involvement. All of Jain's patients showed paravertebral masses, low density in the case of abscess or caseation, and higher in granulation-tissue masses.

Type-4 disease is uncommon and, despite the presence of associated soft-tissue masses, tuberculosis may not be considered, initially, as the diagnosis. Recovery of histological material from these patients is also difficult, as the lesion is encased in normal cancellous bone, while biopsy of the soft-tissue mass often reveals necrotic material only (Fig. 4.25).

MRI Examination

With continuing improvement of software, coils and scan sequences, MRI imaging has become the imaging mode of choice for investigating the spine [41–44]. Inflammatory diseases of the spine are no exception to this rule, and the characteristic findings and methods of MRI examination are well documented [1, 2, 6, 9, 10, 12, 25, 41, 42, 45–47].

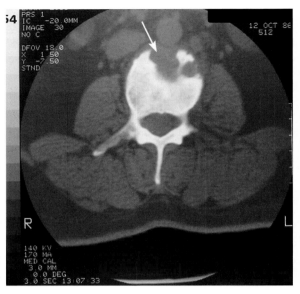

Fig. 4.25. Non-contrast computed tomography. Anterior-marginal cloacae. The lesion is difficult to differentiate from localised *Brucella* and is in a difficult situation to biopsy percutaneously (*arrow*)

The advantages of MRI include multiplanar images, good tissue differentiation, excellent visualisation of the bone marrow, the spinal canal and its contents and the paravertebral soft tissues. These advantages outweigh the poor definition of bone and the inadequate imaging of calcified tissue.

Spin-echo sequences with short recovery time/excitation time (TR/TE) ratios (T1 weighted) require short scanning times. T2-weighted sequences with longer TR/TE ratios lose some of their value, due to involuntary movement artefacts and to patient movement during the longer scanning times. T1-weighted images with fat suppression, acquired immediately after IV injection of paramagnetic contrast agents, highlight inflammatory tissues, and scans in all three planes are of particular value in demonstrating the full extents of the lesions of TS [2, 6].

In addition to these advantages over other methods of imaging, MRI does not expose the patient to ionising radiation – an important factor, especially when multiple follow-up examinations are taken into consideration. Unfortunately, access to centres with an MRI facility is very limited for patients in the developing world, and they must rely mainly on conventional radiography with all its limitations.

In the first paper describing the MRI findings in TS, Roos et al. examined patients with advanced disease [45]. These patients exhibited the classical triad of vertebral end-plate destruction, loss of disc-space height and paraspinal abscesses. Since that time, the application of MRI to the investigation of back pain in general radiological practice is beginning to reveal TS in an early stage in patients who do not demonstrate the features of established disease.

In the adult, unlike in pyogenic infection, intervertebral disc and disc-space infection is not an early feature of TS, and there is quite often no initial loss of disc-space height. In other cases, initially only a single vertebral body is involved. This increases the overlap in appearance of infectious and neoplastic disease and poses increased problems for the radiologist. With the advent, in the West, of early MRI scanning for patients with back pain and the increasing numbers of cases of tuberculosis in North America and Europe, these "atypical" presentations will, undoubtedly, become common.

Vertebral-Body Changes

The T1-weighted image changes reflect the pathological increase in water content of the bone marrow due to oedema of the inflamed tissue. Infected areas exhibit a lowered signal intensity. This is, normally, a homogeneous diminution of signal, although heterogeneous change and even patchy increase of T1 signal has recently been described [25, 46] (Fig. 4.26). The T2-weighted image changes reveal an increased signal in the affected areas, and these correspond to the lowered or increased signal seen in T1 sequences (Fig. 4.27).

The characteristic spread of infection though the MAAs and MAs underlies the early change of T1 and T2 images in the anterior part of the vertebral end plates. Less typically, the posterior areas show the initial pathological change, probably related to infection entering through the nutrient branches of the spinal arteries [26]. In equatorial infection, a more usual picture is T1 and T2 changes throughout in the whole of the vertebral body, a change giving rise to problems of diagnosis if only one vertebral body is affected [7, 25].

In later stages of TS, the central equatorial bone-marrow signal is replaced by a global low-intensity signal representing an inter-osseous abscess. On post-gadolinium (Gd) contrast images, there is intense rim enhancement of the surrounding tissues. Cortical bone destruction is best seen on second-echo T2 images, and this change is often related to a localised inflammatory focus (Fig. 4.28).

Disc and Disc-Space Images

In the early stages of TS, disc changes are subtle. In T1 images, the disc assumes the same signal as the

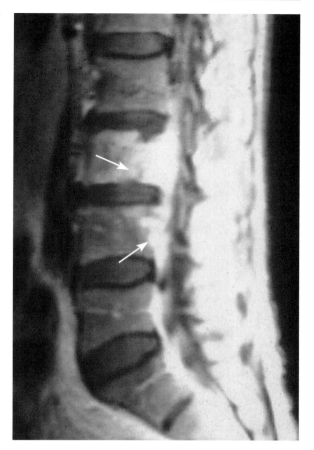

Fig. 4.26. Tuberculous spondylitis producing unusual, patchy, high-intensity signals in the bodies of L3 and L4 on T1-weighted magnetic resonance imaging (*arrows*)

adjacent vertebral-plate infection, but the disc itself does not, at this stage, demonstrate morphological change. Blurring of the disc-space margins indicates involvement of the disc space by way of subligamentous spread of infection. T2 acquisitions are characterised, in adults, by loss of the internuclear cleft. High-intensity signal in the disc is uncommon but does occur infrequently, as opposed to the early disc involvement in pyogenic infection (Fig. 4.29).

Subligamentous Spread

Bulging of the anterior or posterior subligamentous soft tissues is best seen on sagittal imaging. The collections are isointense with other structures on T1 scans but may be outlined by displaced anterior fat planes. Posteriorly, the extradural collections and ligaments merge with the image of the dura so, although the cord may be seen to be displaced, the true extent of the infection may not be apparent on T1

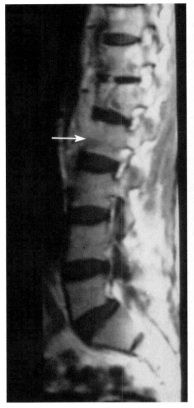
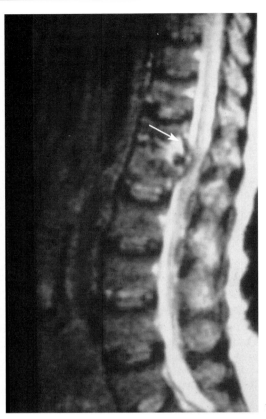

Fig. 4.27 a, b. T1- and T2-weighted studies of the lumbar region in a case of tuberculous spondylitis. Total loss of the L1–L2 disc on the T1 image, coupled with extensive destruction of the adjacent regions of the vertebral bodies (*arrow*). **b** In T2 images, no disc signal is present, and there is an intra-osseous abscess extending epidurally (*arrow*)

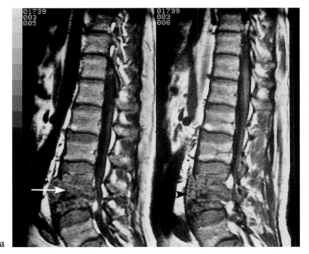
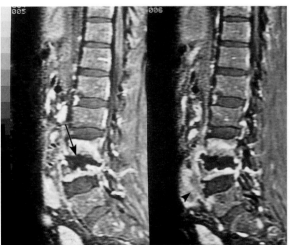

Fig. 4.28 a, b. Pre- and post-gadolinium T1 scans of L3–L4 tuberculous spondylitis. In T1 images, there is absence of the intervertebral-disc signal (*arrow*). The whole of L4 and the lower half of L3 show a reduction in the marrow signal. There is an anterior collection (*arrowhead*). **b** Post-gadolinium scans demonstrate almost total destruction of the body of L4. There is an extensive abscess with margin enhancement. The central, low-intensity signal represents caseating material (*arrow*). The collection beneath the longitudinal spinal ligament enhances (*arrowhead*)

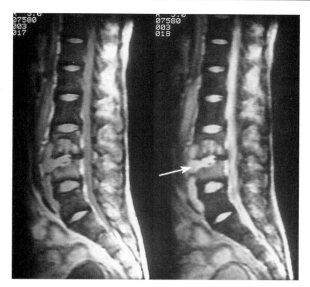

Fig. 4.29. Sagittal, T2-weighted magnetic resonance imaging. Tuberculous spondylitis with a high-intensity signal in the bodies of L3 and L4. The disc space shows a high-intensity signal in the anterior two thirds coupled with loss of the normal shape and of the nuclear cleft (*arrow*)

imaging. Smith et al. describe two cases where the epidural collection was posteriorly placed [25].

With T2 studies, the high signal of the cerebrospinal fluid may obscure the extent of the diseased extradural tissues, but any anterior granulation tissue will be seen as an intense signal beneath the anterior longitudinal ligament. T1-weighted, Gd-enhanced images with fat suppression demonstrate the true extent of inflammation. Sagittal images acquired im-

mediately after contrast injection are followed by axial and coronal scans. The margins of subligamentous disease enhance and, if they contain pus, the central core will demonstrate a low signal. The overlying dura mater will enhance if involved. The degree of cord compression and displacement is clearly seen.

Paravertebral Abscesses

Relatively large, multilocular collections with thick, irregular walls, showing isointensity or low-intensity signals on T1-weighted acquisitions, are characteristic of TS. The contents of the abscess show a high signal intensity on T2-weighted images, and the full extent of the abscess, often stretching over three or four spinal segments, is demonstrated. T1-Gd, fat-suppressed images confirm the enhancement of the abscess margins (Fig. 4.30).

Due to their characteristic of registering a signal void, small calcifications are difficult or impossible to recognise on these images. In TS, this is a distinct disadvantage, as tuberculosis is one of the few conditions where calcification is present, although it is not pathognomonic of the disease [35]. Small fragments of bone sequestrated into the spinal canal, which are important in planning surgical intervention, are best examined by CT scanning [11].

Fig. 4.30 a, b. Multi-level tuberculous spondylitis on a post-gadolinium, sagittal scan involving three thoracic and two lumbar vertebrae (*arrows*). The true extent of the paravertebral disease is best demonstrated on a coronal scan (*arrowheads*)

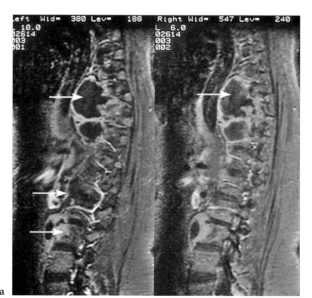

a

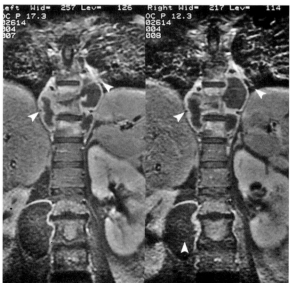

b

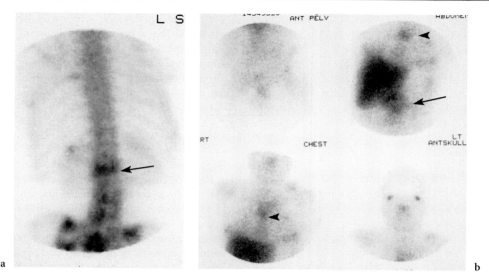

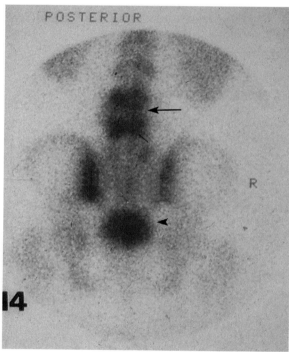

Fig. 4.31. **a** A technetium scan demonstrates an L3 spondylitis (*arrow*). **b** Gallium scans of the same young woman confirm the L3 lesion (*arrow*) and demonstrate a second lesion in the mid-thoracic spine on a 72-h scan (*arrowhead*). **c** Technetium scan of L3–L4 tuberculous spondylitis in a male (*arrow*). Note the accumulation of tracer in the bladder (*arrowhead*)

MRI imaging also demonstrates skip lesions, and sagittal T1 imaging of the whole spine, including the sacrum, should be part of the protocol in patients with TS. Lesions of the posterior elements of the spine are readily identified on all three MRI modalities: T1, T2 and T1-Gd. They seem to be more common than previously realised and do not only occur in non-Caucasians. It seems that IV-drug abusers are more susceptible to both TS and other infectious lesions presenting in this atypical manner [39, 46].

Isotope Imaging

Scintigraphic examination following IV injection of ^{99}mTc-methylene diphosphonate (MDP) is widely used as a diagnostic tool in suspected spinal infection and has many positive features as an investigative agent. Increased uptake of the isotope in an area of bone destruction is seen at a very early stage at a time when conventional radiographs appear normal. Whole-body scanning will reveal bone changes at more than one site.

The commonly used protocol of sequential injection of ^{67}Ga citrate immediately after the technetium bone scan and scintigraphic examination 48 h later has numerous advantages. First, in conjunction with the clinical picture, it suggests the infective nature of the lesions and, second, it will demonstrate any associated soft-tissue lesions and document multi-focus disease. The disadvantage of poor anatomic detail in the scintigraphic images can be countered by focusing other methods of examination on the abnormal areas revealed by the scan (Fig. 4.31).

Although some authors have used ^{99}Tc and ^{67}Ga scanning with enthusiasm [48], there have also been disappointing reports [3, 49]. In 56 patients with confirmed TS, Weaver and Lifeso reported 64% with positive and 35% with negative ^{99}Tc scans. Only ten of these patients underwent ^{67}Ga scanning, with seven normal and three abnormal results. Weaver argues that the early bone lesion of TS is purely lytic and that this accounts for the high rate of negative technetium studies.

Sharif et al. demonstrated 100% positive technetium scans in a group of 13 cases of proven TS, but no distinction between these and similar changes seen in brucellar spondylitis could be made in ten of the scans [1]. It should be emphasised that the ability of ^{99}Tc and ^{67}Ga scans to show the multiplicity of affected vertebra and, in the case of ^{67}Ga, to suggest their infective nature, is of particular value in the investigation of suspected TS.

■ Differential Diagnosis

Pyogenic Vertebral Osteomyelitis and Pyogenic Disc-Space Infections

In recent years, the target group for both pyogenic and tuberculous vertebral-body and disc-space infection has been expanding. As medical technology advances, there is a larger pool of immunosuppressed, elderly or debilitated patients, as well as the increased number of AIDS patients and IV-drug abusers. The likelihood increases of the radiologist being confronted by cases of spinal infection (Fig. 4.32).

Disc-space and vertebral-body infection are commonly caused by *Staphylococcus aureus*, although an increasing number of different organisms has been reported [48]. Often, in pyogenic spondylitis (PS), there is a source of infection elsewhere in the body, septicaemia, a recent operation or invasive procedure, decubitus ulcers or a chronic renal or prostatic infection. The development of back pain and fever in a debilitated patient, contrasting with the more usual history in TS, where the symptoms develop in a relatively fit patient, shows a more insidious onset.

TS favours the thoracic and thoraco-lumbar region while, in pyogenic infection, there is a predilection for the lumbar region. In five published groups totalling 58 patients, the focus of infection was in the lumbar spine in 39, the thoracic spine in 12 and the cervical spine in 4, with 4 patients with involvement at more than one level [24, 35, 43, 47, 50].

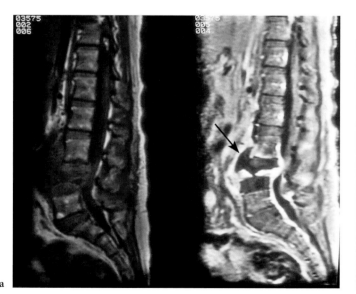
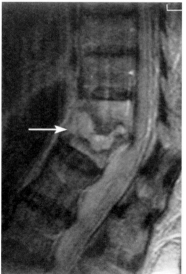

Fig. 4.32. a A classical tuberculosis spondylitis lesion in a diabetic, demonstrated by pre- and post-gadolinium, T1-weighted scans (*arrow*). **b** Thoracic magnetic resonance imaging of pyogenic spondylitis in a diabetic. There is early destruction of the vertebral bodies and disc space. There is no anterior spread and little epidural involvement (*arrow*)

Plain radiographs are not helpful in either condition in the early stages of the disease. There is a latent period of up to 8 weeks before plain-film changes can be recognised. The pattern in PS of early loss of disc-space height, associated with irregularity of the margins of the end plates, is unusual in TS, where the disc space is preserved in the early stages of the disease and the first sign of end-plate involvement is loss of the white cortical stripe.

The early changes on CT examination in TS and PS are likely to be confused, as fragmentation of the end-plate zone is frequently apparent in both conditions. Any accompanying soft-tissue mass is often well developed in TS at the time the patient presents for treatment. The accompanying soft-tissue masses of PS are usually small and close to the vertebral body, and are often confined to the subligamentous areas. Loss of fat planes and oedematous changes in surrounding muscles are common to both conditions. The presence of calcification in the soft tissues is highly suggestive of tuberculosis as the cause of the infection but can rarely occur in pyogenic infection [35]. MRI appearances of vertebral-body and disc-space infection are well defined [42]. In T1-weighted images, a confluent decrease in signal intensity from the vertebral bodies and disc spaces, with a loss of definition of the disc–vertebral-body margin is seen. T2-weighted images, in PS, show an increased signal intensity in the vertebral bodies adjacent to the involved disc and an increased signal in the disc, accompanied by morphological changes in the disc itself. These include loss of the nuclear cleft and changes in the shape of the disc accompanying the increased T2 signal. This signal increase may occur throughout the whole body of the disc or be confined as a streak of signal intensity in one area (Fig. 4.33).

This pattern of signal in T2 images is unusual in TS. Whereas the T1 decrease in signal is seen, the disc change in T2 images includes loss of the intranuclear cleft, but a discernible increase in the signal of the disc is unusual in adults. However, in established disease, total or partial enhancement of the disc occurs with T1-Gd imaging. Radionuclide examination is of value in demonstrating the presence of a spinal lesion and, in the case of scanning using ^{67}Ga, in suggesting that the lesion is infective and pinpointing any other sites of infection in the body. In the case of PS, [99]mTc-MDP bone scans have a sensitivity of 90%, a specificity of 78% and an accuracy of 86%, while combined ^{67}Ga and [99]mTc-MDP studies increase the specificity to 100% and the accuracy to 94% [42]. The isotope studies confirm bone changes before they are apparent on plain-film examination. However, because of the poor delineation of anatomical structure in these studies, even when using single-photon-emission computed tomography (SPECT), it

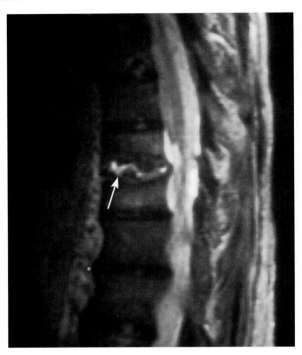

Fig. 4.33. T2-weighted, sagittal magnetic resonance imaging in a pyogenic discitis. The high-intensity signal of the infection is confined to the disc space and the epidural plane (*arrow*)

proves impossible to differentiate between TS and PS by scintigraphy alone.

Spinal Neoplastic Disease

Secondary metastatic neoplasm of the vertebrae may, in certain circumstances, simulate vertebral infection, giving rise to difficulty in diagnosis. This is particularly the case where a single vertebra or two adjacent vertebrae are involved and when no clinical evidence of the primary tumour is present. In those conditions that commonly metastasise to the spine (prostatic, lung and breast cancers, melanoma, lymphoma and myeloma), the clinical presentation will often provide the answer.

Plain-film characteristics will also be helpful in differentiating malignancy from TS in the majority of cases, while isotope bone scans and CT and MRI examinations reveal a pattern of bone-marrow involvement distinctive for metastasis or infection [43, 44].

Preservation of the disc space has always been held as a significant pointer towards a diagnosis of malignant vertebral disease as opposed to infection. However, it must be remembered that, in the earlier stages of TS, the disc space will be preserved (Fig. 4.34).

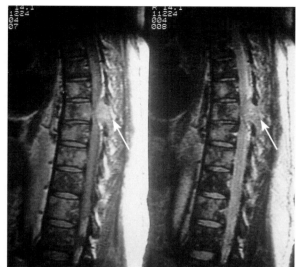

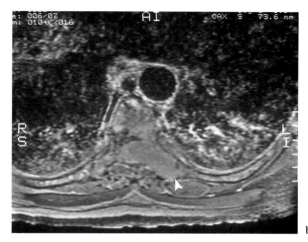

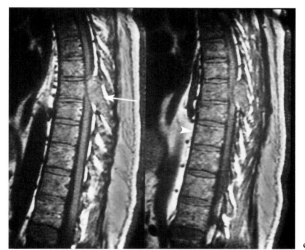

Fig. 4.34. a,b Pre-contrast sagittal and axial scans demonstrate a low-signal mass lesion in the posterior elements of a thoracic vertebra (*arrows*). The axial image shows the extent of the lesion in the spinal canal (*arrowhead*). **c** Post-gadolinium, T1 scanning reveals that the lesion does not enhance (*arrow*). On all of the images, the bone-marrow signal was noted to be variable (*arrowhead*). At decompression, the histological study confirmed myeloma

There remains a small group of troublesome cases in which the imaging appearances of malignancy or infection overlap, especially those cases where a single vertebral body is affected (Fig. 4.35). In these cases, recourse to CT-guided biopsy may be necessary before a diagnosis can be established. All biopsy samples of bone lesions should be sent for bacteriological as well as histological examination as, otherwise, unsuspected tuberculosis will be overlooked. The imaging characteristics of primary neoplasms of the axial skeleton are less likely to be confused with tuberculosis although, if vertebral-body collapse has developed, difficulties can arise. This is especially so if the radiographic appearances are of vertebra plana. In children, this may give rise to diagnostic difficulty, and appearances similar to those due to TS may be seen in vertebra plana due to eosinophilic granuloma.

Brucellar Spondylitis

Brucellosis is an infectious disease of wide distribution, caused by gram-negative bacilli of the genus *Brucella*. There are three commonly occurring strains of the bacillus: *B. melitensis* infects goats, *B. abortus* infects cattle and *B. suis* pigs.

Infection of humans occurs both through direct contact with infected animals, a hazard to veterinarians and animal-hide and meat-processing workers, and, more commonly, after ingestion of infected meat, milk or dairy products. The disease is endemic in countries where there is little control over animal products. This is so in the Mediterranean and Middle East, where goat farming is an important part of the rural economy. In recent years, better controls have been introduced in some countries but, despite this, brucellosis remains an important problem. Countries reporting more than 1000 cases a year include Greece, Iran, Italy, Mexico, Peru and Spain, while many countries where the disease is endemic pro-

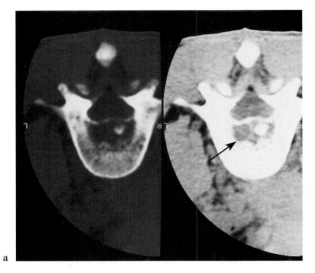

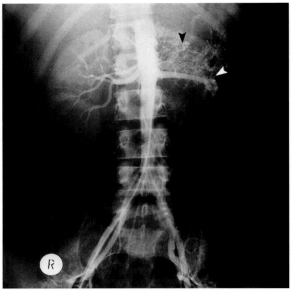

Fig. 4.35 a, b. Prone, axial computed tomography revealed a well-defined, osteolytic lesion in the posterior part of the body of L1. The patient had presented with excruciating back pain that, at first, was thought to be infective in origin (*arrow*). **b** A limited aortographic examination was possible despite the severity of the pain. This revealed extensive tumour circulation in the left supra-renal region and failure of the peripheral branches of the left renal artery to fill beyond a stretched main renal artery (*arrowheads*)

duce no statistics. In northern Europe and the USA, the disease is sporadic, with the number of cases in the low hundreds [51].

In 10% of cases, the musculoskeletal system is involved and, in 2%, there is *Brucella* spondylitis (BS). Clinically, the presentation of BS is similar to that of TS. Fever, night sweats, weight loss and back pain are common symptoms in both diseases. Brucellosis may also be accompanied by polyarthralgia.

There are two distinct types of BS: focal and diffuse. In focal BS, the infection is confined to the anterior end-plate region and is relatively slow in progress; local bone destruction is accompanied by bone sclerosis and reactive bone healing (Fig. 4.36).

In the second type (diffuse BS), the area of infection is similar to that in TS. Diffuse end-plate and disc-space infection progress with localised infection of the paravertebral tissues. With the exception of very rare cases, this soft-tissue infection is on a much more limited scale than in TS. Epidural infection with space-occupying abscesses can evolve, with resulting neurological complications (Fig. 4.37).

Spread through the vascular anastomoses to the end plate of the adjacent vertebral body occurs in both diseases. The preponderance of cases of BS occurs in males, the male:female ratio varying from 3:1 to 20:1 [1, 51]. This may reflect occupational hazards.

The area of predilection for the disease is the lower lumbar spine, although sporadic cases of cervical- and thoracic-spine infection occur. In 21 cases de-scribed by Lifeso, 6 had cervical, 8 thoracic, 13 lumbar and 2 sacro-iliac lesions. In Sharif's series of 46 patients, there were 2 cervical, 6 thoracic and 38 lumbar spine infections [1, 2, 51].

In BS, high titres of *Brucella* agglutinins are invariably present, but this may be misleading in the few cases where the two diseases co-exist. Positive blood culture for *Brucella* is present in about 30% of BS cases, and culture of fluid aspirated from any other infected joint can also be helpful in establishing the diagnosis. Histological and bacteriological studies of biopsy material tend to disappoint. Histologically, non-caseating granulomatous tissue is found in BS, and culture of biopsy material is often negative [1].

On plain-film analysis, there are a number of criteria in BS that are highly unusual in TS. In BS, the architecture of the vertebral body is preserved around the area of focal bone destruction. There is often a small collection of gas, best seen on the lateral radiograph, between the anterior margin of the vertebral body and the disc; in BS, even in the late stages, spinal deformity is rare. Other points of differentiation include the minimal reduction in disc-space height in BS; although the disc is involved in the infection, it is not herniated into the partly destroyed vertebral body. This is one element producing the associated kyphosis seen in TS (Fig. 4.38).

The extensive paravertebral infection in TS, often containing calcification, is another differentiating

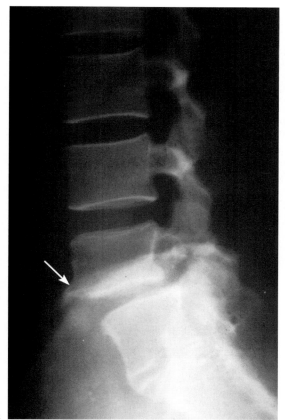

a

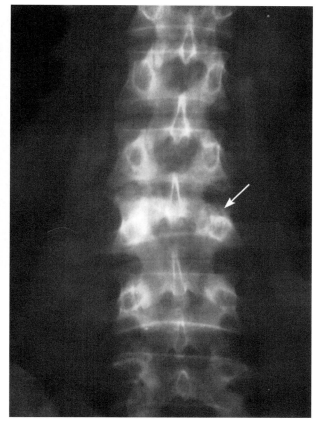

b

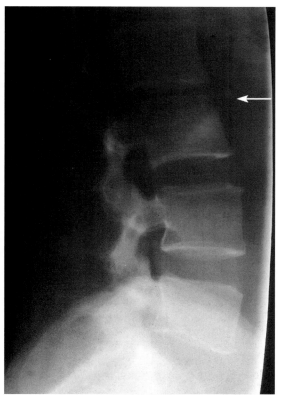

c

Fig. 4.36. a Plain radiograph of a *Brucella* lesion localised to the lower end plate of L4. An anterior osteophyte developed early in the disease (*arrow*). The appearances are complicated by the presence of a spondylolisthesis. **b, c** A case of brucellosis of L2 and L3. There is partial destruction of the upper part of the body of L3. Note the lack of kyphosis (*arrows*)

characteristic. Epidural and subligamentous infection in BS is common, but changes in the paravertebral musculature are confined to loss of fat planes resulting from oedema, rather than abscess formation. In BS, the bone infection is confined to the vertebral body, and the posterior elements are not involved. In the focal type of BS, the presence of simultaneous bone destruction and repair leads to characteristic, early anterior osteophyte formation; this may be misleading if there are osteophytes present at other levels due to degenerative disc disease (Fig. 4.39).

Isotope studies of the spine are only of help in defining the extent of the disease and in determining if there is focal *Brucella* infection in another part of the body. The poor spatial definition of bone-scan studies means that it is impossible to differentiate between BS and TS by this method of examination (Fig. 4.40).

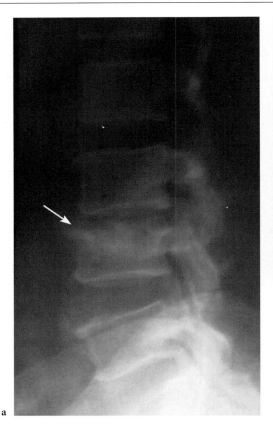

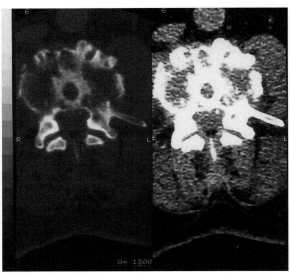

a

b

Fig. 4.37 a, b. Plain radiograph of a brucellar spondylitis of L4. A diffuse lesion with extensive bone destruction, confined to the body of L4. There is an extensive, anterior osteophyte and gas in the disc space (*arrow*). **b** computed tomography study on bone and soft-tissue windows. Extensive, patchy destruction of bone in the vertebral body. In general, the anatomy is preserved

MRI studies with contrast enhancement readily underline the differences between pathological spread in BS and that in TS. The presence of intra-osseous abscesses, extensive subligamentous spread, kyphosis and large paravertebral collections favour the diagnosis of TS (Fig. 4.41).

Fungal Infections

Fungal infections of the soft tissues and bone are rare entities, but their imaging characteristics have many similarities to more common bone infections (PS, TS and BS). In a healthy individual in an endemic area, the initial site of infection is commonly through a skin wound and is confined to the soft tissues. Extension to underlying bone develops secondarily at a later stage of the disease, either by direct invasion of bone or by local haematogenous spread. In the immunosuppressed, and especially in drug abusers, the first pathway is often haematogenous and, in the case of a spinal site of infection, both tuberculosis and spinal neoplasm are often considered as the primary diagnosis.

In the Middle East and East Africa, the most common fungal infection is mycetoma, caused by either *S. somaliensis* or *M. mycetomi*. Both of these fungi commonly present as soft-tissue and bone infections in the foot but, exceptionally, the site of entrance will be a thorn or cactus prick in the back, and vertebral infection may follow. Outside the tropical areas, fungal infections of the spine are rare but, when a patient develops an apparent granulomatous infection of the vertebrae, aspergillosis, *Nocardia*, cryptoccosis, candidiasis and actinomycosis should all be considered in the diagnosis [46].

Plain radiographic examination lacks the soft-tissue definition required to define the extent of the disease, and spondylitic changes may be absent in the early stages. Destruction of the vertebral end plate and bone cortex is accompanied by loss of disc-space height. Marginal erosion of the vertebral body is also sometimes present due to paravertebral fungal growth (Fig. 4.42).

CT and MRI are helpful, in that the soft-tissue abnormalities in the chest or abdominal wall are clearly seen, as is any bone change due either to spondylitic lesions or local bone erosion. When vertebral-body infection is established, the appearances are indistinguishable from pyogenic or tuberculous infection in the majority of cases (Fig. 4.43).

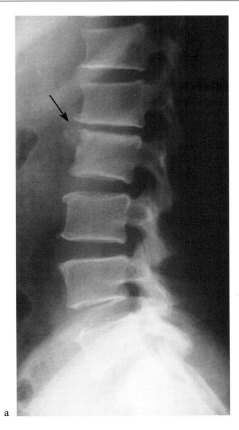

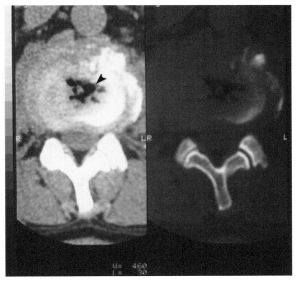

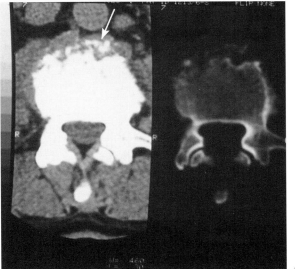

Fig. 4.38 a – c. Plain radiography of classic *Brucella* spondylitis. Shows disc-space-narrowing, anterior osteophyte development linked with marginal destruction of the upper plate of L2 (*arrow*). **b** Computed tomography through the disc space demonstrates both gas in the disc and the soft-tissue and bone lesion (*arrowhead*). **c** Another case of *Brucella* spondylitis, showing the anterior-marginal bone destruction (*arrow*)

Loss of marrow signal on T1 and heterogeneous increase in signal on T2 imaging is similar to that seen in TS. Subligamentous spread and epidural involvement with neurological complications also occur in both TS and fungal spondylitic disease [1, 2, 52]. CT-guided needle biopsy is required to differentiate between the two conditions and demonstrate the presence of fungal elements in the tissues.

Other Granulomatous Diseases

Sarcoidosis

Sarcoidosis is a multi-system, granulomatous condition that most commonly affects the lungs, skin, lymphatic system and visceral organs. Histological non-caseating granulomas are present in this condition. Skeletal sarcoid occurs in 1–13% of cases and is usually confined to the tubular bones of the hands and feet. In these cases, cutaneous sarcoid lesions are almost invariably seen. Spondylitis in sarcoid is rare, a very small number of cases having been described in the literature [53, 54]. The thoraco-lumbar region is the usual site, and the changes are accompanied by back pain and are often mistakenly attributed to disc disease. Plain radiographs of the region are often normal, although both lytic and osteosclerotic appearances have been described [52, 55].

On CT examination, the appearances are non-specific; end-plate fragmentation, with preservation

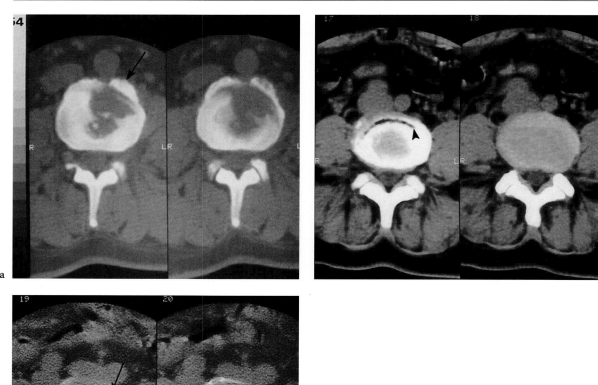

a

b

c

Fig. 4.39 a – c. Computed tomography studies of three different cases of focal brucellosis. Anterior-marginal and sub-perio-steal infection is seen (*arrows*). Also seen is gas in the disc space (*arrowhead*)

of the disc space, and the presence of paravertebral soft-tissue masses have been seen. Lytic lesions of the subcortical region may be surrounded by a rim of osteosclerosis. Lesions at multiple levels occur, although involvement of the posterior vertebral elements is unusual.

In the lesions, MRI studies reveal T1 values similar to those of other granulomatous diseases. There is hypointensity on non-enhanced T1 images and intense enhancement after Gd injection. These images appear similar to those of neoplastic, fungal, pyogenic and tuberculous osteomyelitis.

Signs and symptoms of sarcoidosis in other organs are helpful in making the diagnosis, which may be overlooked because of its rarity. Conjunctival or liver biopsy may reveal non-caseating granulomas but, often, biopsy of the involved vertebral body or paravertebral soft-tissue mass will be needed to establish the diagnosis. The preservation of the verte-bral-body architecture is an important point of dif-ferentiation from TS where, apart from very early - cases of tuberculous infection, spondylitis is ac-companied by widespread destruction in either the epiphyseal or equatorial zone of the vertebral body.

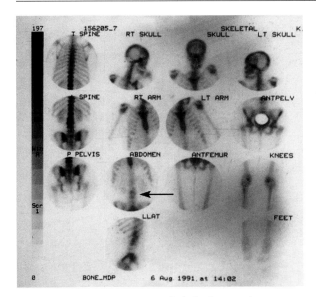

Fig. 4.40. Technetium-contrast, whole-body scan demonstrating a high uptake in the L3–L4 vertebral bodies in a case of brucellosis (*arrow*)

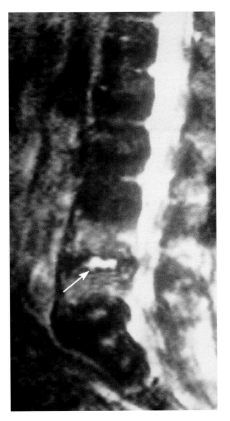

Fig. 4.41. T1-weighted magnetic resonance imaging of the lumbar spine shows a high-intensity signal throughout the bodies of L4 and L5. The infected disc also demonstrates a high-intensity signal (*arrow*). Brucellar spondylitis was confirmed

One case of sarcoid spondylodiscitis has been described [54]. The imaging characteristics were similar to those attributable to pyogenic or tuberculous infection. A narrowed disc space was accompanied by subchondral bone changes in the adjacent vertebrae, and both the disc space and the vertebral end-plate regions enhanced on T1-Gd MRI study. On CT examination, a paravertebral soft-tissue mass that contained no calcification was described. Open biopsy was necessary to confirm the diagnosis and to exclude tuberculous or pyogenic discitis.

Parasitic Disease

Hydatid Disease

Caused by the cestode *Echinococcus granulosus*, hydatid disease is usually transmitted to humans from dogs and sheep, which act as an intermediary host. Hydatid disease is common in the cattle- and sheep-breeding areas of the world. These include New Zealand, Australia, the Mediterranean and Middle East, South America and Iceland. In the United Kingdom, both shepherds and dog breeders are exposed to hydatidosis and, in Canada, the Inuit may be infected through their working dogs.

The cestode embryos enter the human portal circulation via the intestinal mucosa and are trapped either in the liver or lungs, where the developed cysts are common. Of these cysts, 75% occur in the liver and 15% in the lungs. Rarely, the ova reach the systemic circulation and are then dispersed to other organs, including bone, where 1–2.4% of mature cysts are found. In bone, the pelvis and spine are the usual sites of infestation, although the long bones are sometimes affected [32].

The developing cysts produce numerous daughter cysts, which in turn lead to bone destruction accompanied by expansion of the affected bone. In the early stages of infestation, the plain-radiographic appearances are of a diffuse osteolysis. Later, the bone surrounding the cyst becomes sclerotic, and this is visible on CT examination. Inside the rim of sclerotic bone, the fluid contents of the cyst are low in attenuation, with Hounsfield measurements of between 1 and 3 (Fig. 4.44).

The MRI appearances are of importance in demonstrating the cystic nature of the lesions, showing low T1 and high T2 excitation values. Involvement of vertebral bodies is usually caused by bone erosion from without, caused by enlargement of a mediastinal or retroperitoneal cyst.

In these cases, bone destruction due to external pressure is seen, with preservation of the intervertebral discs. Extensive scalloping of the vertebral

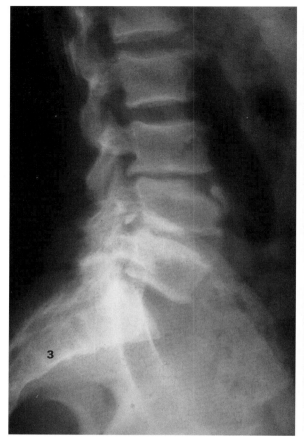

a

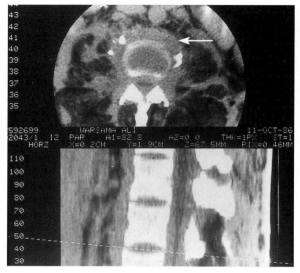

b

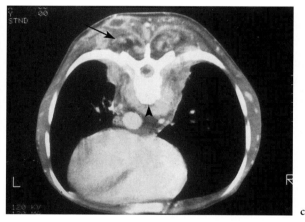

c

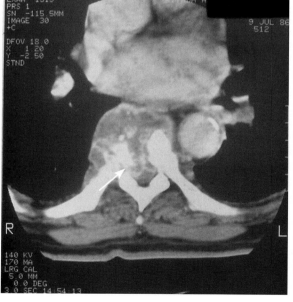

d

Fig. 4.42. a Plain radiographs of a case of *Candida* spondylitis, revealing narrow disc spaces, osteophyte formation and an anterior-marginal lesion. In general, the bony anatomy is well preserved. **b** Computed tomography demonstrates paravertebral mycetoma tissue (*arrow*) without any evidence of bone destruction. **c** Extensive posterior-muscle and soft-tissue involvement in mycetoma (*arrow*). Anteriorly, there is extensive paravertebral disease, but without bone destruction (*arrowhead*). **d** Fungal disease rarely produces a true spondylitis. In this case, the infection is confined to a thoracic vertebral body and the nearby soft tissues. The spinal canal has been invaded (*arrow*)

bodies, due to the slow rate of growth of the cysts, is evident. Pedicle destruction has been reported, as has invasion of the spinal canal through a widened intervertebral foramen [56]. This subgroup may be confused with subligamentous tuberculosis, and the paravertebral mass may be confused with a tuberculous abscess. Spinal invasion leads to extradural compression syndromes and paresis. This slow development of a spinal lesion is clinically similar to both TS and neurofibroma.

Serological tests are positive for hydatid disease in 70% of cases, and the presence of multiple cysts

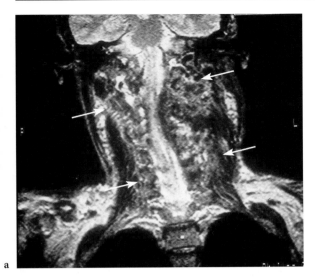

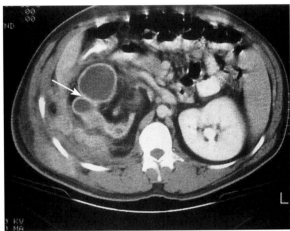

Fig. 4.43 a, b. Coronal magnetic resonance imaging demonstrating severe soft-tissue and cervical-spine destruction in a case of mycetoma (*arrows*). **b** Actinomycosis rarely affects the spine. In this case, the right kidney is destroyed, but the spine and paraspinal soft tissues are spared (*arrow*)

in other organs (the liver, lung or kidneys) will be helpful in making the diagnosis. Death of the cyst leads to calcification of the fibrotic endocyst. In a retroperitoneal lesion, this calcification has similar appearances to a calcified, tuberculous psoas abscess.

Fine-needle aspiration of the cyst, with subsequent injection of hypertonic saline, confirms the diagnosis histologically and, in selected cases, is showing considerable effect as a form of treatment. In those cysts causing vertebral destruction but no neurological complications, injection with alcohol has also produced good clinical results [56. 57].

Degenerative Disc Disease and Compression Fractures

Changes in signal on MRI images adjacent to degenerative discs result from either bone sclerosis in the end plates or from the conversion of normal, haemopoietic marrow to fatty marrow [58–60]. If bone sclerosis abutting on a degenerative disc is evident in plain radiographs, then a low signal will be seen in the end-plate region on both T1- and T2-weighted MRI images. More commonly, an increased focus or band-like signal will be present in both T1 and T2 acquisitions, due to an increase in the bone-marrow fat.

A third possibility is a relatively low-intensity signal in T1 images and an increased signal in T2 images; this signal may be confused with infective, pyogenic or TS. In this sub-group, the signal from the degenerative disc remains low in T2 images despite the absence of the nuclear cleft. This is in contrast to the high-intensity T2 signal and morphological changes that characterise discitis.

CT studies, in these cases, will show no destructive changes in the bone of the vertebral body and may reveal a vacuum effect, with gas in the degenerative disc. This gas is also often present in focal brucellosis of the vertebral end plate and has also been described in pyogenic infection [1, 2, 61]. Radionuclear examination with isotopes is of value in differentiating between infective and degenerative spondylitis, as there will be little uptake of the tracer in uncomplicated, degenerative spondylosis.

Benign compression fractures in patients with osteoporosis, and pathological fractures secondary to malignant disease, may show imaging characteristics similar to those to those of TS. Plain-film studies provide little help in differentiating the three conditions.

Isotope studies are also non-specific but show an increase in uptake of the isotope at the site of the fracture, and the intensity of the uptake will depend on the age of the lesion and the degree of bone healing that is occurring. [67]Ga citrate examinations will be negative in both benign and pathological fractures and will demonstrate the infectivity of TS lesions. With ^{99}Tc scans, multiple areas of uptake are noted in malignancy and in both brucellosis and tuberculosis if the disease is multi-focal.

CT is helpful in demonstrating both the bone destruction and paravertebral abscesses of TS, but paravertebral lesions may be present in both pyogenic and malignant disease. The presence of calcification in the paravertebral collections of TS are important in differentiating TS from other causes of paravertebral deposits.

On MRI examination, the vertebral-body-marrow signal changes due to malignant vertebral-body col-

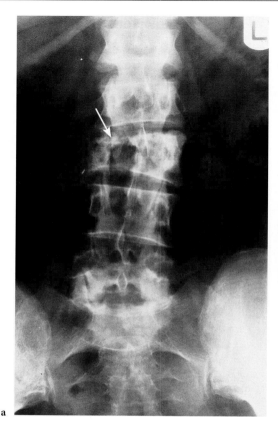

a

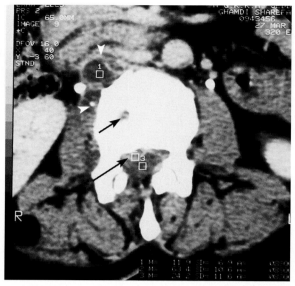

b

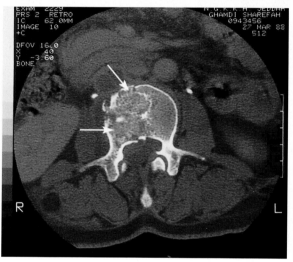

c

Fig. 4.44 a – c. Plain radiography demonstrating partial destruction of the right side of the body of L3. The disc spaces are preserved, and there is some bone sclerosis of the upper end plate (*arrow*). **b** Computed tomography (CT) of a soft-tissue window shows a destructive focus in the vertebral body on the right side (*arrow*) and two low-density, paraspinal collections (*arrowhead*). The dural sac is displaced by isodense material (*long arrow*). **c** CT scan of a bone-window setting outlines the cortical destruction and two annular hydatid cysts on the right (*arrows*). The margins of the lesions show calcification, but the contents of the cysts are isodense. In both scans the margins of the paravertebral lesions show ring enhancement. The displacement of the dural sac is related to hydatid material that has broken through the cortex of the vertebral body. Hydatid disease was confirmed, and the patient improved on therapy

lapse; these changes tend to be homogeneously present throughout the vertebra. Due to the replacement of normal marrow by malignant tissue, the signal is low on T1-weighted and high on T2-weighted acquisitions. In benign fractures, the marrow signal tends to be isointense with normal tissues. In fractures due to malignancies, the replacement of normal haemopoietic bone marrow by malignant deposits is often almost complete before fracture occurs [59].

The pattern of signal change is more likely to be confined to adjacent end-plate zones. The collapse of the vertebral body is usually angular, with a marked degree of kyphosis, as the destructive changes are often confined to the anterior components of the end plates. There will, however, be overlapping appearances in some cases, and the similar radiological findings can then only be differentiated by aspiration biopsy and bacterial culture. As TS becomes more widespread in the ageing Western population, it should be considered as a possible underlying cause of vertebral-body collapse even in the presence of extensive osteoporosis on plain radiography of the spine (Fig. 4.17).

Less Common Disorders

Amyloidosis

Primary or secondary amyloid deposits are found in vertebral bodies and must be differentiated from TS. Secondary amyloidosis occurs most frequently in those chronically afflicted by rheumatoid arthritis, neoplasms (such as multiple myelomatosis) and in chronic infections of bone and lung. The latter group are of interest, in that secondary infection of tuberculous pulmonary cavities may become chronic and lead to secondary amyloidosis.

Amyloid deposits manifest as amyloid fibrils in many organs. In the primary type of amyloid, the heart, kidneys, tongue, gastrointestinal tract, blood-vessel walls, nerves and skin are the usual sites of deposition. Secondary amyloidosis favours the spleen, liver, kidneys and gastrointestinal tract, although there may be overlap in the structures involved in the two types of the disease. The skeleton may be involved in both forms, and plain radiography initially shows osteoporosis, followed by the development of discrete, radiolucent defects. The deposits may be diffuse.

On CT examination, the vertebral architecture is well preserved, although vertebral-body collapse may be the presenting feature [62]. The type of collapse is commonly different from that seen in TS. However, when the two diseases are present simultaneously with chronic TB, paravertebral abscesses and amyloid deposits in other organs, difficulties in diagnosis may arise.

Amyloidosis tends to occur in TB patients who have been non-compliant with their regimes of anti-tuberculosis therapy. As amyloid deposits affect the haemopoietic areas of bone more than the bone cortex, MRI studies demonstrate a diffuse, homogeneous signal. The diagnosis can usually be made by gastrointestinal-mucosal biopsy, which shows the characteristic fibrils when Congo Red staining is employed.

Cervical Spondyloarthropathy

Patients undergoing long-term haemodialysis during end-stage renal disease have been shown to develop imaging changes in the cervical spine similar to changes caused by pyogenic discitis or TS. In these cases, no infection is present despite the fact that many of the patients are immunosuppressed [63, 64].

The narrowing of disc spaces associated with vertebral end-plate irregularity is the usual finding. Associated loss of vertebral-body height may occur. There is no evidence, in these cases, of paravertebral soft-tissue deposits. In T1 images, MRI shows a decrease in signal in the end plates on both sides of the disc but, in T2 sequences, the increase in signal seen in pyogenic and tuberculous infection is not present.

■ References

1. Sharif HS, Osarugue AA, Clark DC, et al. (1989) Brucellar and tuberculous spondylitis: comparative imaging features. Radiology 171:419–425
2. Sharif HS, Clark DC, Aabed MY, et al. (1990) Granulomatous spinal infections: MR imaging. Radiology 177:101–107
3. Weaver P, Lifeso RM (1984) The radiological diagnosis of tuberculosis of the adult spine. Skeletal Radiol 12:178–186
4. Whelan MA, Naidich DP, Post JD, Chase NE (1983) Computed tomography of spinal tuberculosis. J Comput Assist Tomogr 7:25–30
5. Yao DC, Sartoris DJ (1995) Musculoskeletal tuberculosis. Rad Clin North Am 33:679–689
6. Sharif HS, Morgan JL, Al Shahed, Aabed al Thagafi MY (1993) Role of CT and MR imaging in the management of tuberculous spondylitis. Radiol Clin North Am 33:787–804
7. Naim-Ur-Rahman (1980) Atypical forms of spinal tuberculosis. J Bone Joint Surg Br 62:162–165
8. Gero B, Sze G, Sharif HS (1991) MR imaging of intradural inflammatory diseases of the spine. AJNR Am J Neuroradiol 12:1009–1019
9. Hoffman EB, Crosier JH, Cremin BJ (1993) Imaging in children with spinal tuberculosis. J Bone Joint Surg Br 75: 233–239
10. Cremin BJ, Jamieson DH, Hoffman EB (1993) CT and MR in the management of advanced spinal tuberculosis. Pediatr Radiol 23:298–300
11. Jain R, Sawhney S, Berry M (1993) Computer tomography of vertebral tuberculosis: patterns of bone destruction. Clin Radiol 47:196–199
12. Liu GC, Chou MS, Tsai TC, et al. (1993) MR evaluation of tuberculous spondylitis. Acta Radiol 34:554–558
13. Omari B, Robertson JM, Nelson RJ, Chiu LC (1989) Pott's disease: a resurgent challenge to the thoracic surgeon. Chest 95:145–154
14. Jacobs P (1964) Osteo-articular tuberculosis in coloured immigrants: a radiological study. Clin Radiol 15:59–69
15. Shanley DJ (1995) Tuberculosis of the spine: imaging features. AJR Am J Roentgenol 164:659–664
16. American Thoracic Society (1992) Control of tuberculosis in USA. Am Rev Respir Dis 146:1623–1633
17. Starke JR, Jacobs RF, Jereb J (1992) Resurgence of tuberculosis in children. J Paeds 120:839–855
18. Reider HL, Snider DE, Cauthen GM (1990) Extra pulmonary tuberculosis in USA. Am Rev Respir Dis 141:347–351
19. Bell GR, Stearns KL, Bonutti PM, Boumphrey FR (1990) MRI diagnosis of tuberculous vertebral osteomyelitis. Spine 15:462
20. Ahmadi J, Bajaj A, Destian S, et al. (1993) Spinal tuberculosis: atypical observations at MR imaging. Radiology 189:489–493

21. Lifeso R (1987) Atlanto-axial tuberculosis in adults. J Bone Joint Surg Br 69:183–187
22. Lin-Greenberg A, Cholankeril J (1990) Vertebral arch destruction in tuberculosis. J Comput Assist Tomogr 14:300–302
23. Murray RO, Jacobson HG, Stoker DJ (1990) The radiology of skeletal disorders, 3rd edn, Vol. 1. Churchill Livingstone, UK, pp 292–293
24. Sartoris DJ, Moskowitz PS, Kaufman RA, et al. (1983) Childhood diskitis: computed tomographic findings. Radiology 149:701–707
25. Smith AS, Weinstein MA, Mizushima A, et al. (1989) MR imaging characteristics of tuberculous spondylitis vs vertebral osteomyelitis. AJR Am J Roentgenol 153:399–405
26. Ratcliffe JF (1985) Anatomical basis for vertebral osteomyelitis. Acta Radiol 26:137–143
27. Batson OV (1957) The vertebral vein system: caldwell lecture 1956. AJR 78:195–212
28. Babhulkar SS, Tayade WB, Babhulkar SK (1984) Atypical spinal tuberculosis. J Bone Joint Surg Br 66:239–242
29. Wiley AM, Trueta J (1959) The vascular anatomy of the spine and it's relationship to pyogenic vertebral osteomyelitis. J Bone Joint Surg Br 41:796–809
30. Katz DS, Wolgater H, Cunha BA (1992) Mycobacterium bovis vertebral osteomyelitis and psoas abscess after intravesical BCG therapy for bladder carcinoma. Urology 40:63–66
31. Fishman JR, Walton DT, Flynn NM, et al. (1993) Tuberculous spondylitis as a complication of intravesicle bacillus Calmette-Guerin therapy. J Urol 149:584–587
32. Bell D, Cockshott WP (1971) Tuberculosis of the vertebral pedicles. Radiology 99:43–48
33. Kaufmann R (1948) Quinze observations d'attaque ganglionnaire dans le mal de Pott et autres localisations de la tuberculose. Mem Acad Chir 74:238
34. Boxer DI, Pratt C, Hine AL, McNicol M (1992) Radiological features during and following treatment of spinal tuberculosis. Br J Radiol 65:476–479
35. McHenry MC, Duchesneau PM, Keys TF (1988) Vertebral osteo-myelitis presenting as spinal compression fracture. Arch Intern Med 148:417–423
36. Travlos J, du Toit G (1990) Spinal tuberculosis: beware the posterior elements. J Bone Joint Surg Br 72:722–723
37. Ragland R, Abdelwahab IF, Braffmann B, Moss DS (1990) Posterior spinal tuberculosis: a case report. AJNR Am J Neuroradiol 11:612–613
38. Lecklitner ML, Potter JL, Growcock G (1985) Computed tomography in acquired absence of thoracic pedicle. J Comput Assist Tomogr 9:395–397
39. Thrush A, Enzmann D (1990) MR imaging of infectious spondylitis. AJNR Am J Neuroradiol 11:1171–1180
40. Tuli SM (1975) Tuberculosis of the spine. Amerind Publishing Co., New York
41. Mallolas J, Gatell JM, Rovira M, et al. (1988) Vertebral arch tuberculosis in two human immunodeficiency virus-seropositive heroin addicts. Arch Intern Med 148:1125–1127
42. Haughton VM (1988) MR imaging of the spine. Radiology 166:297–301
43. Modic MT, Feiglin DH, Piraino DW, Boumphrey F, Weinstein MA, Duchesneau PM, Rehm S (1985) Vertebral osteomyelitis: assessment using MR. Radiology 157:157–166
44. Sze G, Krol G, Zimmerman RD, Deck MF (1988) Malignant extradural spinal tumours MR imaging with Gd-DTPA. Radiology 167:217–223
45. de Roos A, van Persijn EL, Bloem JL, Bluemm RG (1986) MRI of tuberculous spondylitis. AJR Am J Roentgenol 146:79–82
46. Rich AR (1951) The pathogenisis of tuberculosis, 2nd edn. Blackwells, Oxford
47. Whelan MA, Schonfeld S, Donovan Post J, Svigals P, et al. (1985) CT of non-tuberculous spinal infection. J Comput Assist Tomogr 9:280–287
48. Lisbona R, Derbekyan V, Novales-Diaz J (1993) Gallium-67 scintigraphy in tuberculous and nontuberculous infectious spondylitis. J Nucl Med 34:853–859
49. Lifeso RM, Weaver P, Harder EH (1985) Tuberculous spondylitis in adults. J Bone Joint Surg Am 67:1405–1413
50. Price AC, Allen JH, Eggers FM, Shaff MI, Everette James A (1983) Intervertebral disk-space infection: CT changes. Radiology 149:725–729
51. Lifeso RM, Harder E, McCorkell SJ (1985) Spinal brucellosis. J Bone Joint Surg Br 67:3
52. Brodey PA, Pripstein S, Strange G, Kohout ND (1976) Vertebral sarcoidosis: cases report and review of the literature. AJR Am J Roentgenol 126:900–902
53. Ginsberg LE, Williams DW, Stanton C (1993) MRI of vertebral sarcoidosis. J Comput Assist Tomogr 17:158–162
54. Kenney CM, Goldstein SJ (1992) MRI of sarcoid spondylodiskitis. J Comput Assist Tomogr 16:660–662
55. Abdelwahab AF, Norman A (1988) Case report: osteosclerotic sarcoidosis. AJR Am J Roentgenol 150:161–162
56. Parvaresh M, Moin H, Miles JB (1996) Dumbbell hydatid cyst of the spine. Br J Neurosurg 10:211–213
57. Sanchez Lopez JD, Alcalde J, Ibarra A, et al. (1997) Retroperitoneal cystic mass. Postgrad Med J 73:185–186
58. Roos de A, Kressel H, Spritzer C, Dalinka M (1987) MR imaging of marrow changes adjacent to end plates in degenerative lumbar disc disease. AJR Am J Roentgenol 149:531–534
59. Baker LL, Goodman SB, Perkash I, et al. (1990) Benign vs pathologic compression fractures of vertebral bodies: assessment with conventional spin-echo, chemical-shift and stir MR imaging. Radiology 174:495–502
60. Modic MT, Masaryk TJ, Ross JS, Carter JR (1988) Imaging of degenerative disk disease. Radiology 168:177–186
61. Bielecki DK, Sartoris D, Resnick D, et al. (1986) Intraosseous and intradiscal gas in association with spinal infection. Report of three cases. AJR Am J Roentgenol 147:83–86
62. Ollif JFC, Hardy JR, Williams MP, Powles TJ (1989) Case report: MR imaging of spinal amyloid. Clin Radiol 40:632–633
63. Rafto SE, Daalinka MK, Schiebler ML, et al. (1988) Spondylarthropathy of the cervical spine in long term haemodialysis. Radiology 166:201–204
64. Stolpen AH (1993) Case of the season: spondyloarthropathy of renal dialysis. Semin Roentgenol 28:96–100

CHAPTER 5

Osteoarticular and Soft-Tissue Tuberculosis

■ Introduction

During the period of decline of tuberculosis (TB) in the USA from 1963 to 1986, the total number of cases decreased by 5% each year, but the number of extrapulmonary cases by less than 1% per year. In 1986, extrapulmonary disease represented 17.5% of the total cases analysed by the Centres for Disease Control in Atlanta [1].

This reflected the results from Boston hospitals during the period 1968–1977. There, the overall number of cases of TB declined annually, but the number of extrapulmonary cases remained relatively constant. As a percentage of all cases of TB, this resulted in a relative increase in extrapulmonary disease [2].

In the United Kingdom, 4172 new cases of TB were noted between 1978 and 1979. Osteoarticular lesions were present in 5% of these cases. The racial distribution of the patients was 40% white and over 55% of Indian or African origin. In these groups, there was a distinctive age distribution. For white patients the general age was above 55 years while, amongst the immigrant patients, the age tended to be 35 years or younger.

In a smaller group comprising 1233 patients with extrapulmonary TB studied over a 6-month period by the Medical Research Council in 1980, the number of bone and joint lesions was high (15%) [3]. These recent statistics from the United Kingdom are slightly higher than those usually quoted in the literature, which states that 1–3% of all cases of TB develop osteoarticular tuberculous disease [4].

Since the 1970s and 1980s, the new factors of increased immigration and the spread of both the acquired immunodeficiency syndrome (AIDS) virus and intravenous (IV) drug abuse, have compounded the situation. The ageing population, poverty and the exposure of care workers to the infection are other factors in the West. In 1991, the rate of new infections of TB in New York State had risen to 17.3 per 100,000 but, in Harlem, the rate was as high as 169 per 100,000, a rate similar to the estimates from Central and East Africa [5]. Of these cases, 20% were extrapulmonary and, in those patients also infected with AIDS, the rate of extrapulmonary disease was as high as 33% [6].

In the developing world, lack of health care, poverty, inadequate chemotherapy and the AIDS epidemic are important factors for the increasing numbers of patients with TB. The inference of these figures would seem to indicate an increased chance of radiologists being confronted with osteoarticular TB in the future.

TB of bones, joints and soft tissues may develop at any site in the body. The common site, the spine, is dealt with in the chapter entitled *Tuberculous Spondylitis*, and accounts for 50% of osteoarticular TB [7]. In children in Africa, Asia and the Indian subcontinent, percentages as high as 65–70% have been reported [8].

Of the 50% of cases occurring outside the spinal region, any bone or joint may be the site of infection and, in the soft tissues, a wide distribution of infections of bursae, tendon sheaths and muscle abscesses have been described. The common sites of bone infection are the pelvis, long bones, ribs sternum, skull, patella, phalanges, tarsals and carpals. In Martini's 652 cases from Algeria, 123 cases were of tuberculous osteomyelitis [9], but Rensnick proposes a 1% rate for tuberculous osteomyelitis without joint involvement, and a higher rate of osteomyelitis among Chinese patients [10].

Tuberculous arthritis is most common in the large weight-bearing joints and, as in the case of other infectious arthritides, is usually mono-articular (Fig. 5.1). The hip and the knee represent roughly 10% each of the total cases [3, 4, 7–13], the ankle, the joints of the upper limb and the small joints of the hands and feet are infected in 2–4% of cases (Fig. 5.2).

The usual sequence of events is spread of the infection from a metaphyseal focus through the epiphysis to involve the adjacent joint, but primary infection of the synovium of the joint does occur [10,12]. Infection of a joint from a nearby tuberculous bursitis or tendon-sheath infection may also occur but is uncommon; however, spread of a pleural lesion to a rib has been described, and multiple rib lesions

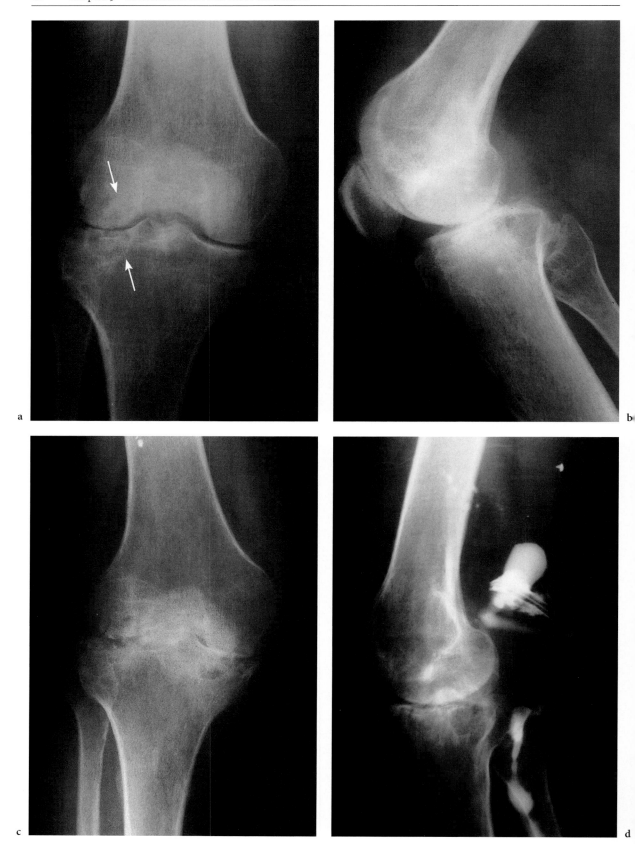

a

b

c

d

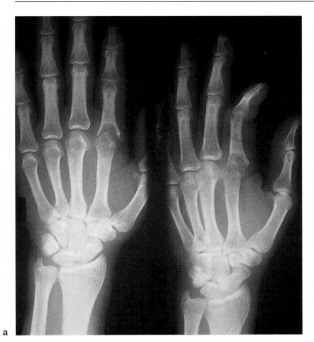

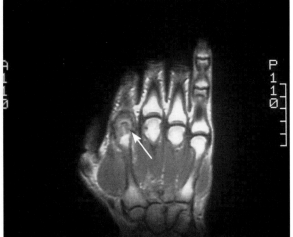

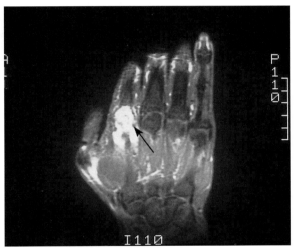

Fig. 5.2. a Plain radiography of the hand demonstrates established, destructive arthritis of the second metacarpo-phalangeal joint. **b, c** T1-weighted pre- and post-gadolinium scans show the low signal of the metacarpal head and the base of the phalanx, with marked enhancement after contrast injection (*arrows*). Alcohol acid-fast bacilli were present on synovial biopsy

are relatively frequent in multi-centric tuberculous osteomyelitis [10].

In bone, the first focus of infection is in the bone marrow, and its origin is haematogenous spread from a primary or reactivated focus in some other part of the body. There is evidence of pulmonary disease in less than 50% of cases. A granulomatous lesion develops in the bone marrow and is surrounded by polymorpholeucocytes and lymphocytes. Caseation follows and, as the lesion expands, the trabeculae of the bone are destroyed, as is the bone cortex at a later stage. The initial process is primarily lytic in nature; the development is slow, indolent and usually painless. Although the radiological presentation may be

Fig. 5.1. a, b. Anteroposterior and lateral radiographs of the knee in a middle-aged man. There is joint-space narrowing and periarticular osteoporosis. Irregular, subcortical erosions are present. The changes are more marked at the periphery and are seen on both sides of the joint space (*arrows*). No alcohol acid-fast bacilli (AAFB) were found in the joint-space aspirate. **c** Six months later, the changes were much more advanced, and a sinus had developed behind the knee joint. **d** A sinogram shows some communication with the joint, but the main sinus tract passes downward into the soft tissues of the calf. AAFB was cultured. Images by courtesy of Dr. S. Hamsa, Riyadh Military Hospital

suggestive of tuberculous infection, biopsy with histological and bacteriological confirmation is necessary. Careful biopsy from the edge of the lesion is required as, often, few tubercle mycobacteria are present, especially in the necrotic or caseous central portions of the lesion [14]. In most cases, there is a lapse of up to 18 months from the initial infection to the time of diagnosis [4, 7, 9, 13, 15]. In the vast majority of cases, the organism is *Mycobacterium tuberculosis* but, in developing countries where pasteurisation of milk is not universal, *M. bovis* infections still occur [11].

The pathological characteristics influence the radiological appearance. As the underlying lesion is granulomatous, the infection leads to hyperaemia, with resulting osteoporosis. The bone lesions are lytic, and the margins are indistinct. There is little or no bone regeneration or periosteal reaction in adults but, in children, periosteal layering is described, as is

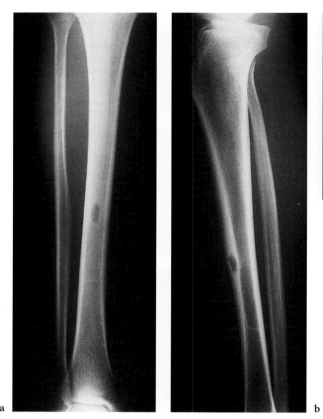
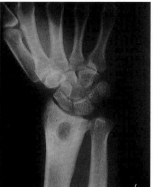

Fig. 5.3. a, b Radiographs of a tuberculous tibial cortical lesion. Characteristically, this is an oval lesion with the long axis in the vertical plane. There is some thickening of the cortex but little sclerotic reaction. **c** A tuberculous, cyst-like lesion of the lower end of the radius demonstrates similar appearances. On curettage, it was found to be filled with caseous material

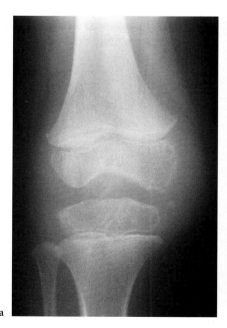
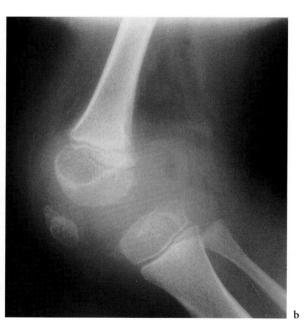

Fig. 5.4 a, b. Tuberculosis of the synovium of the knee joint in a child. There is marked synovial thickening but, apart from osteoporosis, there is no obvious bone lesion

rare, pathological fracture [8,14,16]. Sequestration is rare, and bone sclerosis is only seen in long-standing lesions or after they have become quiescent.

The bone-marrow lesion may be more extensive than revealed by plain radiographs and is better assessed by magnetic resonance imaging (MRI) or isotope studies. The common site of infection is in the metaphysis close to the epiphyseal line and, in contradistinction to pyogenic osteomyelitis, the infection commonly crosses the physis to involve the epiphysis and the adjacent joint. In children, the chronicity of the lesion linked with hyperaemia may lead to enlargement of the epiphyseal centre when compared with the normal contralateral limb. Lesions confined to the shaft of a long bone are much less common than combined bone and joint lesions (Fig. 5.3) [10].

Although cases of haematogenous tuberculous arthritis with the initial focus in the synovium or sub-articular bone occur [12], the more usual sequence is of infection of the joint secondary to a focus of infection in the adjacent metaphysis (Fig. 5.4) [17]. Both surfaces of the articular cartilage are normally affected, and the articular surface is eroded in a patchy rather than continuous manner, leaving islands of normal cartilage between areas of cartilage destruction. The subchondral regions are slowly destroyed as granulomatous tissue extends in from the periphery of the joint, leading to cartilage ischaemia and necrosis. Joint effusion follows, and the synovium becomes thickened (Fig. 5.5). Inevitably, the joint space diminishes in width, but this occurs at a much later stage than in pyogenic arthritis. Osseous erosion deep to the cartilage then occurs, with cyst-like lesions in the metaphyseal bone. In more advanced cases, the cartilage is totally destroyed, and irregular bone surfaces articulate with each other on both sides of the joint (Fig. 5.6) [9]. In the hip joint, softening of the bone may lead to protrusion of the acetabulum and to flattening of the femoral head (Fig. 5.7) [8].

If untreated, para-articular soft-tissue abscesses develop, and these may drain to the surface, with chronic sinus formation. Secondary infection of these sinuses often causes misleading bacteriological cultures to be made, as pyogenic organisms are usually found in these sinuses, and *M. tuberculosis* is rarely present. If left untreated, fibrous ankylosis of the joint eventually occurs. This is, again, a characteristic distinguishing it from pyogenic infection where early bony ankylosis is relatively common [16].

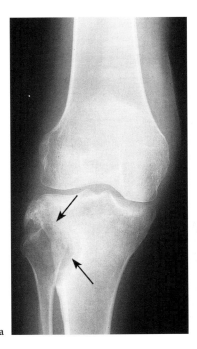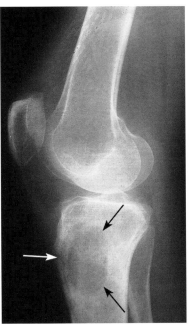

Fig. 5.5 a, b.
A large, „cystic", tuberculous lesion of the upper tibia, with erosion of the anterior cortex (*arrows*). There is some surrounding bone sclerosis

a

b

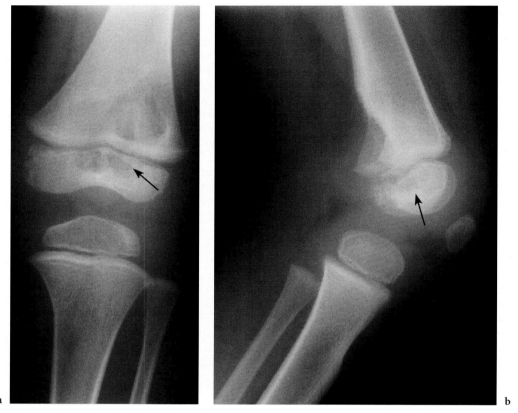

a   b

Fig. 5.6 a, b. An extensive, tuberculous bone defect in the juxta-epiphyseal region of a child's femur. The infection has crossed the physis to enter the epiphysis (*arrow*). There is associated synovial thickening and joint effusion

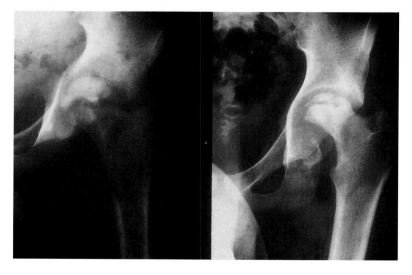

Fig. 5.7.
Two views of a tuberculous lesion of the hip joint in a child. On the first, there is loss of joint space and erosion of the femoral epiphysis. One year later. there is progressive destruction of the femoral-head epiphysis and associated widening and upward migration of the acetabulum

■ Tuberculous Osteomyelitis in Other Areas

The Skull

Calvarial lesions are rare and, apart from those seen in multi-centric tuberculous osteomyelitis and multi-cystic tuberculous bone disease in children, are usually single lesions. These focal lesions destroy the full thickness of the calvarium and are usually accompanied by an extensive soft-tissue granulomatous lesion involving the overlying scalp outside the skull (Fig. 5.8). The vernacular name for this entity is Pott's puffy tumour. They are also unusual in that the central area of bone is necrotic and forms a sequestrum. Because of their shape, these are known as button sequestra [8, 12].

There are two distinct radiological appearances. A single, well-circumscribed defect is the common form but, less commonly, the lesions may be more extensive and with less well-defined margins. These lesions are often surrounded by a zone of osteoporosis. Multiple lesions of this type are described, and these may amalgamate to form larger lesions that characteristically cross suture lines. The associated soft-tissue lesions have been noted both in the scalp and in the cranium. Large, extra-dural granulomas can develop, with extensive space occupation [18, 19]. Similar changes are reported in malignant lymphoma, in both Hodgkins and non-Hodgkins disease. Lymphomas with a considerable soft-tissue element, may be present in the calvarium. These have an appearance similar to that of Pott's puffy tumour.

Other sites of infection in the skull are less common and may be related to easy access for the mycobacterium to the adjacent bone from the nasal cavity, paranasal sinuses, outer ear or teeth. The lesions are usually osteolytic but, if secondary infection is present, they may be osteosclerotic [20]. Osteitis of the sphenoid bone is described by Cremin [8].

Infection of the temporal bone is common in children in South Africa and also occurs in adults in Europe and North America [8]. Tuberculous osteitis of the body and ramus of the mandible and overlying soft tissues of the lower jaw seems to depend on entry of the mycobacterium at the site of a dental extraction or through a carious tooth; however, in multi-centric disease, the spread is presumed to be haematogenous [21].

Heney et al. describe a case where the dentition was normal. The origin of the extensive osteomyelitic and soft-tissue lesions appears to have been haematogenous. The young patient had a positive tuberculin skin reaction as well as pulmonary hilar lymphadenopathy on chest radiography. The lesion responded well to anti-tuberculous chemotherapy [22].

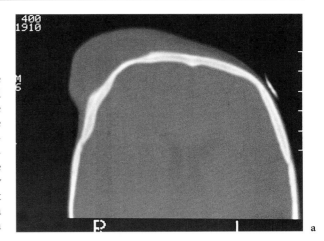

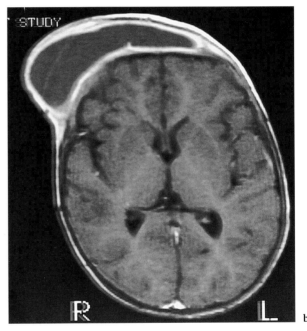

Fig. 5.8 a, b. Pott's puffy tumour. Computed tomography study of a soft-tissue lesion of the right frontal region demonstrates an extensive, isodense, soft-tissue swelling. There is thinning of the bone of the underlying calvarium. **b** Post-gadolinium magnetic resonance imaging study. This study defines the subcutaneous abscess as a low-signal collection with surrounding ring enhancement. The tuberculous osteitis of the right frontal bone is also demonstrated. Images by courtesy of Dr. B. J. Cremin, Red Cross Hospital, Cape Town

The Sacro-Iliac Joints

TB of the sacrum occurs, in most cases, by direct spread of infection from the fifth lumbar vertebra to the L5–S1 disc space and onwards to the body or ala of the sacrum. Isolated tuberculous sacroiliitis is less common and presents with localised pain radiating into the buttock and hip region. Reduced mobility of the local musculature is present. Often, constitutional symptoms of weight loss and fever are minimal, and the onset is insidious [23].

The condition is difficult to diagnose, as the initial radiographic changes are subtle, and it must be distinguished from a number of other conditions. Mono-articular sacroiliitis of infective origin is more common and is due to pyogenic organisms or gonococcal infection, both of which occur much more frequently than TB [24, 25]. Fungal infection is another possibility, while the non-infective arthritides, rheumatoid arthritis and Reiter's disease are common, but more often in a polyarthritic form. Immunosuppressed patients, drug abusers and human immunodeficiency virus (HIV) patients are susceptible to all of these conditions.

Sacroiliitis, from whatever cause, initially manifests itself in the lower third of the joint, which contains a synovium. The early radiographic changes are often confined to the iliac side of the joint. Isotope scanning with ^{99m}Tc methylene diphosphonate (MDP), ^{67}Ga citrate or ^{111}In-labelled leucocytes is positive before radiographic changes develop. Computed tomography (CT) and MRI examination are more sensitive than plain radiography, with MRI demonstrating fluid collections in the joint and surrounding soft tissues in T2-weighted images [26]. The appearances are not specific, and the diagnosis must be confirmed by aspiration and bacterial culture in order to differentiate between various organisms [27].

Tuberculous Dactylitis

An infection of the short tubular bones of the hands and feet, tuberculous dactylitis is associated with painless swelling in the surrounding soft tissues. This condition mainly affects children under the age of 5 years, but a less florid type is seen, rarely, in adults [8, 28].

Figures for the incidence of this type of osteitis vary from 0.5% to 14% of all cases of osteoarticular TB [10]. The soft tissue changes usually precede visible bone lesions and, in a few cases, may be the only manifestation of the disease. The initial insult is a granulomatous focus in the bone marrow of a digital bone, often a proximal phalanx, metacarpal or metatarsal. The fingers are more usually affected than the feet, and the lesions tend to develop consecutively rather than simultaneously. The common sites are the proximal phalanx of the index and middle fingers and the metacarpals of the middle and ring fingers [4, 12, 29].

Expansion of the granulomatous tissue in the bone-marrow cavity leads to ballooning of the bone. As the inner cortex is broken down, new bone is

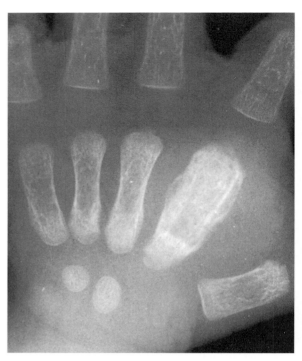

Fig. 5.9. A classical spina ventosa lesion in a young child. Expansion of the medullary cavity of the metacarpal, with a layered periosteal reaction. Image by courtesy of Dr. B.J. Cremin, Red Cross Hospital, Cape Town

created on the outer surface of the phalanx or metacarpal and is visible as periostitis along the diaphysis. Further expansion follows, and the affected bone widens to a marked degree. The resulting appearance is termed "spina ventosa" – literally, a small bone blown out like a sail (Fig. 5.9) [29].

If the metaphysis is involved, the infection may break through the epiphysis to the joint, giving rise to tuberculous arthritis. When this happens, sequestration sometimes follows and, if untreated, growth deformities of the finger and multiple sinus formation are often seen [10]. The adult form is less exuberant and, often, only a single bone is involved; arthritis and sinus formation are unusual [28]. In children, both hands are commonly affected. Rarely, similar changes have been reported in the radius, ulna and humerus [10].

Cystic TB of Bone

Although an unusual form of TB osteitis, cystic TB is troublesome in that the chief differential diagnosis is tumour of bone. Cystic TB is, in general, a disease of children and young adults and, if multiple, the lesions develop simultaneously [12]. In children, the peripheral skeleton is the usual site of the infection, predominately the long bones, but the skull and flat bones may also show lesions [30].

The foci of infection tend to be in the metaphysis and, less commonly, the diaphysis. The symptoms often refer to the nearby joint and include joint pain and reduced mobility. The cysts are clear cut and usually show no bone sclerosis, although both marginal sclerosis and periosteal reaction have been reported, as have lesions in the pelvis and the tarsal bones [10, 12]. In children, they may become large enough to expand the metaphysis, and occasional passage through the physis to involve the epiphysis is seen. The cystic lesions may be single or multiple and, if single, are likely to be confused with the more common, benign, simple or aneurysmal cystic lesions of bone. They may be comprised of a single round or oval defect or may be multi-locular [21].

In adults, the flat bones are more commonly involved, with lesions of the scapula, pelvis and skull predominating. Cystic expansion of the bone due to accumulation of granulation tissue in the medullary cavity is a feature, with minimal surrounding bone reaction (Figs. 5.10, 5.11).

In the long bones, the cystic lesions in adults are usually small and, unless subperiosteal, do not expand the bone. These lesions show a sclerotic margin and are orientated along the long axis of the limb.

In the skull, the initial lesion is in the diploic space and, as osteolysis of the inner and outer tables develops, the osteitic areas tend to be less well defined than the lesions in other areas. Cystic TB is the preferred term in this condition, rather than pseudocystic TB. As Cremin points out, the term cystic does not necessitate the presence of a fluid-filled lesion [8].

Progression of the infection is the normal clinical pattern, although spontaneous resolution can occur in the very young. As the cystic changes are usually painless and constitutional symptoms are unusual, the condition is often quite extensive by the time it is discovered [30].

Multi-Focal Osteoarticular TB

In Europe and North America, the usual pattern of tuberculous osteitis has generally been that of a disease of the elderly. This presents as a single region of infection and, in 50% of cases, affects the axial skeleton. The patients, in addition to being elderly, are often debilitated by other diseases.

In the areas of the developing world where tuberculous disease is endemic, other patterns of tuberculous osteitis are seen. Multi-centric cystic TB of bone is seen in children and young adults, and multi-centric tuberculous osteitis is found.

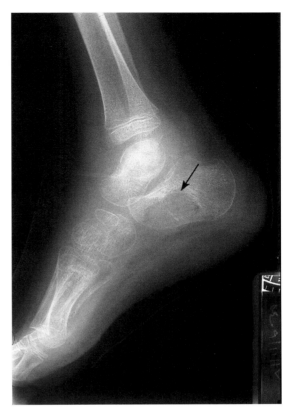

Fig. 5.10. The foot of a young man. An ill-defined, tuberculous, "cystic" lesion of the anterior calcaneum (*arrow*) There is no surrounding bone reaction

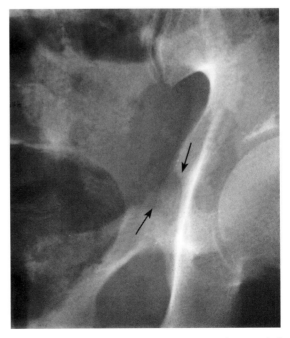

Fig. 5.11. A localised, osteolytic, tuberculous lesion of the ischium, confined to the acetabular roof (*arrows*)

Kuma and Saxema reported 48 cases of children and adults with multi-focal skeletal TB and, earlier, McTammany et al. estimated that 4.6 % of osteitic TB was multi-focal [21]. Until today, this type of infection has been a rarity in the Northern Hemisphere. However, in this decade, more and more cases are being reported in those countries where immigration rates from endemic areas are high (Fig. 5.12) [31, 32].

As early as 1964, Jacobs noted the differing patterns of infection between Caucasians and immigrants from the Caribbean and the Indian sub-continent [33]. In the ten cases reported in the recent literature, two cases each were Ethiopian, Filipino and American Negroid, one was Somalian and another Ghanaian. The timing of onset of the disease was often unrelated to their time of arrival in the new countries, with, in some cases, a lapse of some years before the manifestation of the infection [34 – 38].

Because of the increasing number of immigrants from Eastern Europe, Asia, Africa and Latin America,

the physician must be alert to this changing pattern of disease. It is now quite clear that, in any disorder presenting with recent onset of multiple osteoarticular lesions, TB should be included in the differential diagnosis in both Caucasians and immigrants. A normal chest radiograph or a negative Mantoux reaction do not exclude TB. Although the increase in the number of cases of TB in recent years has been linked to the AIDS epidemic, none of the cases described in the recent papers was HIV positive [34 – 39]. Because the working diagnosis in most of these cases was multiple bone metastases or lymphoma, they demonstrate the importance of isotope studies, as many of the lesions are asymptomatic.

Lymph-node TB, as well as axial and peripheral lesions, featured prominently, as did rib lesions. In one case, extensive calvarial TB was a feature. Other flat bones (the sternum, ribs, ileum and pubis) were affected, as were the clavicle, sterno-clavicular joint, sacro-iliac joints and acetabulum.

A number of patients exhibited paradoxical changes, in that their lesions continued to progress despite accepted anti-tuberculous therapy. This phenomenon has been previously described, in intracranial tuberculoma and tuberculous lymphadenopathy, by Chalmers, Campbell and Teoh [35, 40 – 42]. Teoh's patients required increased doses of anti-tuberculous therapy, as well as steroids, before their tuberculomas began to resolve [42].

TB of the Ribs

The usual cause of tuberculous osteitis of the ribs is by extension of tuberculous spondylitis and associated paravertebral abscesses to involve the posterior ends of the ribs and their costo-vertebral articulations. Occasionally, para-vertebral TB without vertebral involvement produces the same effect [43].

Tuberculous soft-tissue masses in the parietal pleura of the thoracic cavity are described and can be associated with osteitic changes in the adjacent ribs. These lesions are often seen in cases of multi-focal osteoarticular TB [34 – 38, 44].

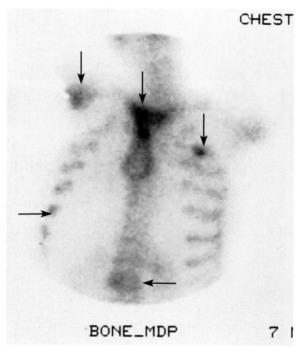

a

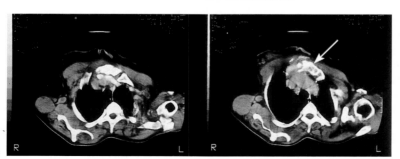

b

Fig. 5.12 a, b.
Multi-focal osteoarticular tuberculosis in an elderly woman whose symptoms were thought to indicate bone metastases.
a Technetium-contrast bone scanning demonstrates lesions in the sternum, left third rib, right shoulder, right seventh rib and the lumbar spine (*arrows*). b Computed tomography of the upper thorax demonstrates fragmentation of the sternum, with an associated bone abscess (*arrow*). Alcohol acid-fast bacilli were cultured

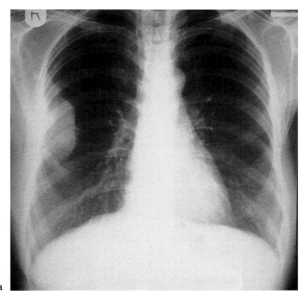 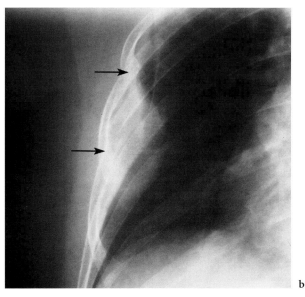

a   b

Fig. 5.13 a, b. Tuberculous osteitis of the ribs, adjacent to a pleural lesion. **a** Chest radiography demonstrates a large pleural mass in the right axillary region. **b** A detailed view shows destruction of the anterior portions of two associated ribs (*arrows*)

Rarely, chest-wall infection is the result of active pulmonary TB or the reactivation of old pulmonary disease [45]. Haematogenous spread with development of cold abscess in the chest wall and subsequent osteitis of the rib or tuberculous chondritis of the rib cartilage are also described (Fig. 5.13) [46].

Although early reports suggested that osteitis of the rib shaft was the typical presentation, later authors found a preponderance of rib-end and costo-chondral lesions. This type of lesion seems particularly common in IV-drug abusers, although the method of infection is not clearly understood [46, 47].

CT scanning is useful in defining the extent of the osteitis and its relationship to any chest-wall cold abscess or underlying pleural mass. Sung Jin Kim et al. describe a method of rib counting during CT examination to verify which rib is involved in the inflammatory process [48]. Isotope examination should be carried out in all cases, as plain radiography of the ribs has a low sensitivity for osteitic lesions (Fig. 5.14).

■ Tuberculous Infection of the Soft Tissues

By far the most common soft-tissue manifestation of TB is sinus formation, and this may develop where any bone, joint or organ infection breaks though the overlying soft tissues to the surface. In untreated infections, these sinuses become chronic and often become secondarily infected. This leads to problems of diagnosis because, although bacteriological studies will reveal the secondary organism, the mycobacterium is seldom cultured from the discharge.

The most common sites of sinus development are overlying the spine, knee joints, fingers, bursae and, occasionally, the skull [4, 8–12, 19, 34]. Empyema necessitas may develop through the chest wall where there is an underlying tuberculous empyema [45].

True soft-tissue abscesses are rare, although five cases were documented by Hugosson et al. among 30 cases of osteoarticular disease in Saudi Arabia [14]. Puncture of these abscesses revealed bacterial evidence of TB in three patients and, in the other two cases, TB at another site was present.

Less common types of tuberculous infection of muscle are focal tuberculous abscess and polymyositis due to TB. These two distinct types of lesion are increasing in incidence in cases of HIV infection. The echogenic CT and MRI findings are non-specific, and biopsy and culture is necessary to distinguish these infections from more common muscle infections. These include pyogenic abscess, tropical pyogenic myositis and AIDS polymyositis, as well as fungal disease and actinomycosis [49–52].

TB Bursitis and Tenosynovitis

Infection of bursae and tendon sheaths is a rare manifestation of TB. Osteoarticular TB affects 1–3% of all cases of TB, while disease of the tendon sheaths and bursae accounts for only 1% of osteoarticular cases. Such rarity and the characteristic indolence of

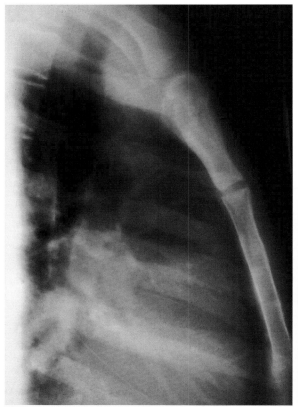

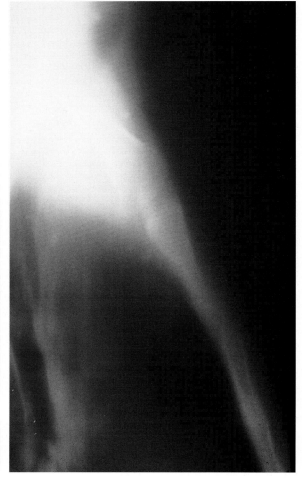

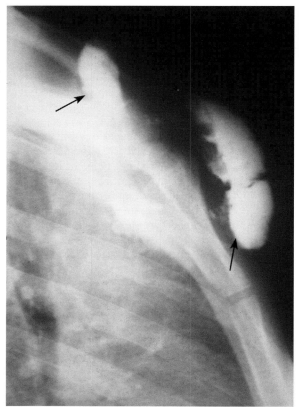

Fig. 5.14. a Plain radiography of the sternum, with some sclerosis and expansion of the manubrium sterni. **b** Plain tomography failed to demonstrate any sternal cavitation. **c** Sinogram of an overlying, discharging swelling. This defined a large, tuberculous, soft-tissue abscess anterior to the sternum and passing upwards to the region of the suprasternal notch (*arrows*). No definite communication with the manubrium is seen

the disease leads to diagnostic difficulty and, where the diagnosis is not at first considered, the condition may be overlooked for several years before the diagnosis is made. Both conditions appear to be much more common in non-Caucasians than in Caucasians.

In the majority of cases, the method of infection appears to be by haematogenous spread, and up to 30% of individuals have evidence of pulmonary TB. Local inoculation following a penetrating wound is also thought to be a factor in some cases, and trauma may also play a role [53].

Any bursa may be affected, but there is a predilection for the areas around the hips, pelvis and shoulder joints. Both primary infection of a bursa and secondary infection from a communicating, infected joint occur. Infection of the trochanteric or iliopsoas bursae is seen secondarily to tuberculous arthritis of the hip joint. Popliteal bursitis is sometimes linked with a knee-joint infection, and sub-deltoid bursitis may be secondary to shoulder-joint infection. However, primary bursitis is known to occur in all of these situations, and the spread of infection can be reversed from the bursa to a nearby joint.

Jaovisidha et al. describe nine cases of primary bursitis, five of which were around the hips, in the trochanteric, iliopsoas and ischial-gluteal bursae. Three cases were sub-deltoid and one was retrocalcaneal. The male:female ratio was 6:3, and this male preponderance is borne out in all studies of tuberculous bursitis and tenosynovitis. The caseating material within the bursa develops punctate calcification, and this and the accompanying soft-tissue mass is visible on plain radiographs. Later, the inflammatory process leads to osteoporosis and lytic bone destruction in the adjacent bone, usually the greater trochanter, the ischio-pubic ramus and the ischial tuberosity. Rupture of the bursa will lead to abscess formation in the surrounding soft tissues [54].

The soft-tissue elements of the infection are best seen on ultrasound, CT, and MRI examinations. If there is communication with a joint, then intra-articular contrast medium will pass from the joint to outline the bursa.

TB tenosynovitis is uncommon, and most of the reported cases are from the period before anti-tuberculous therapy was available, such as Kanavel (1923), Mason (1934) [55], Donovan (1940) and Briede (1945) [54]. Since MRI became available, more cases have been noted, and the anatomical details of the infection have been described in detail. However, as is the case with tuberculous infections elsewhere, the findings are non-specific, and the diagnosis depends on bacteriological and histological study of aspirate and biopsy material [53, 54, 56 – 58].

The commonly affected regions are the flexor tendons of the fingers, the palmar spaces and the radial and ulnar bursae in the wrist. The tendon sheaths become infiltrated with granulomatous tissue, leading to thickening of the tendon-sheath surface. Straw-coloured fluid containing decidual material fills the sheath space, distending it. As the contents caseates, small foci of calcific tissue known as rice bodies develop. These are often visible both on plain radiography and axial scanning and are highly suggestive of tuberculous infection. The tendons within the sheath may appear normal, thinned, or clumped and distorted, depending upon the stage of infection. In long-standing cases, tendon rupture may occur. These changes are visible on MRI examination.

Less commonly, the affected tendon sheaths are those of the foot and ankle; the extensor, peroneal, posterior tibial and Achilles sheaths can be affected [54]. The clinical manifestations are swelling of the involved fingers, palm and wrist. The condition is often painless, but movement of the infected tendons is reduced. Unlike chronic tuberculous infections elsewhere, sinus formation is uncommon. As in the case of bursitis, adjacent bone structures may be affected by erosion or, if infected, by lysis. In the region of the wrist, the flexor retinaculum narrows the infected bursae as the bursae pass beneath it; this causes bulging of the bursae distal and proximal to the retinaculum. Rarely, compression of the structures of the anterior compartment of the wrist leads to carpal tunnel syndrome [57].

Injection of therapeutic steroids in patients with an inflammatory bursitis exposes the patient to tuberculous bursal infection. The diagnosis will not made until biopsy material is examined.

■ Tuberculous Osteitis Resulting from Bacille Calmette-Guerin Vaccination

Attenuated bovine tubercle bacilli, in the form of the vaccine bacille Calmette-Guerin (BCG), very rarely give rise to generalised TB or bone and joint TB. This can occur in immunosuppressed individuals. In children, it is thought that between 1 in 5000 and 1 in 80,000 cases may develop bone or joint TB [10, 55]. To this group must be added a group of patients treated for superficial carcinomas of the bladder by instillation of BCG intravesically. Two of these patients are reported to have developed tuberculous spondylitis [55, 59, 60].

In post-vaccination osteitis, the children are usually below the age of 6 years, and the long bones are commonly affected with single lesions. Other sites include the ribs, sternum and small bones

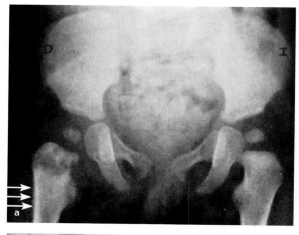

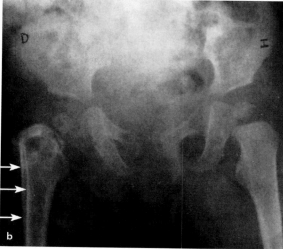

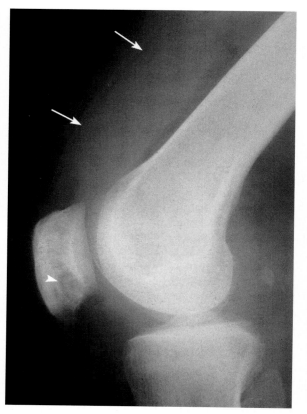

Fig. 5.16. Lateral radiograph demonstrates extensive supra-patellar swelling in a middle-aged man (*arrows*). There is an isolated osteolytic tuberculous lesion in the lower third of the patella (*arrowhead*)

Fig. 5.15 a, b. Post-bacille Calmette-Guerin tuberculous osteitis in a 6-month-old girl. **a** An extensive metaphyseal lesion of the right upper femoral shaft. There was an associated periosteal reaction (*arrows*). Histology confirmed tuberculosis, with granulomas, multinucleated giant cells and epitheloid cells. **b** Follow-up study after one month of anti-tuberculosis treatment. The metaphyseal lesion was reduced in size, with developing bone sclerosis. The periosteal reaction was unchanged (*arrows*). Images by courtesy of Dr. F.G. Arias, Hospital San Agustin, Aviles, Spain

of the hands and feet (Fig. 5.15). An idiosyncrasy is that lesions of the tubular bones are often confined of the same side of the body as the site of vaccination.

The infection commonly develops within the first year after inoculation, but longer delays have been noted [10, 14]. In infants, the metaphyseal lesions are lytic but may show accompanying periostitis. Histological studies show granuloma, but the bacillus is very difficult to culture, and response to anti-tuberculous therapy may be the only way of confirming the nature of the infection [55].

■ Imaging Methods

Plain Radiography and Tomography

The mainstay of imaging investigation of osteo-articular TB is the plain radiograph. The characteristics of tuberculous bone lesions are suggestive of the disease, but a broad differential diagnosis remains. In most instances, the lack of bone sclerosis, reactive periostitis and sequestration, associated with hyperaemic osteoporosis, indistinct outline of the lesions and indolence, points in the direction of TB as the diagnosis. In all cases, study of biopsy material is mandatory and, as mycobacteria are scarce in the lesions, direct staining techniques are usually unsuccessful. Culture, however, is positive in a large proportion of cases (Fig. 5.16).

Plain radiographs of affected joints are often suggestive of the disease, especially in the presence of Phemister's triad. This comprises juxta-articular osteoporosis, peripheral osseous erosions and gradual narrowing of the joint space (Fig. 5.17). The

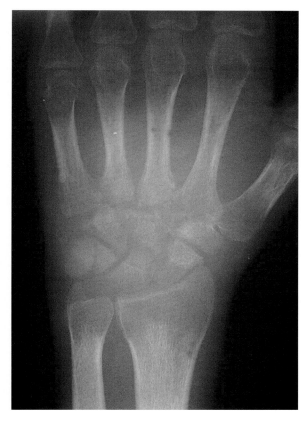

Fig. 5.17. Severe juxta-articular osteoporosis in a wrist joint, with tuberculous arthritis of the small joints of the wrist

differential diagnosis remains wide, although, in many other mono-articular lesions, the radiological changes develop rapidly, as opposed to the insidious nature of tuberculous infection (Fig. 5.18) [6, 10, 12]. In the adult hip joint, destruction of articular cartilage is an early sign of infection. This is combined with periarticular osteoporosis. Sub-articular, cystic destruction then develops on both sides of the joint space. The femoral head is usually more severely involved in the destruction than the acetabular aspect (Figs. 5.19, 5.20). In children, the immaturity of the skeleton allows protrusio acetabulae to develop at an early stage. Later, upward migration of the acetabular roof continues and, eventually, the hip may dislocate posteriorly. Flattening of the femoral head epiphysis may also be a feature in childhood [8, 14].

In the shoulder joint, there is often absence of a joint effusion, and the infection is characterised by punched-out areas of cortical and sub-cortical bone in the humeral head. This is the usual appearance on plain film and CT examination in classic caries sicca of the shoulder joint (Fig. 5.21) [8, 13, 15]. Biopsy of any adjacent bone lesion, culture of any sparse synovial fluid or synovial biopsy will be necessary to pinpoint the diagnosis [14, 61]. Search for tuberculous foci in other parts of the body yields positive results in less than 50 % of cases.

In the knee joint, the initial, sub-cortical bone defect in the metaphysis of the femur or tibia is recognisable. Later, spread of infection through the epi-

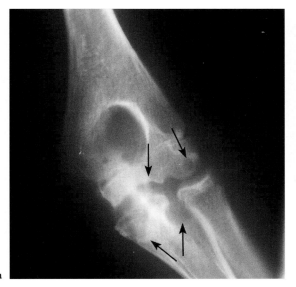

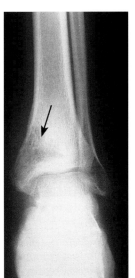

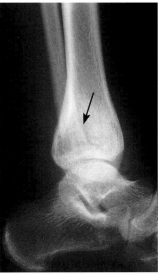

a
b, c

Fig. 5.18 a – g. A young man presenting with persistent pain in the left elbow and left ankle. **a** A plain radiograph of the elbow demonstrated subcortical, epiphyseal bone destruction on both sides of the joint space, with osteolysis in the ulnar and extensive changes in the humeral epiphysis. There is also loss of articular cartilage and irregularity of the articular surface (*arrows*). **b, c** Plain radiographs of the left ankle revealed an ill-defined, osteolytic lesion of the lower tibia, involving the medial malleolus (*arrow*). **d – g** *s. p. 96*

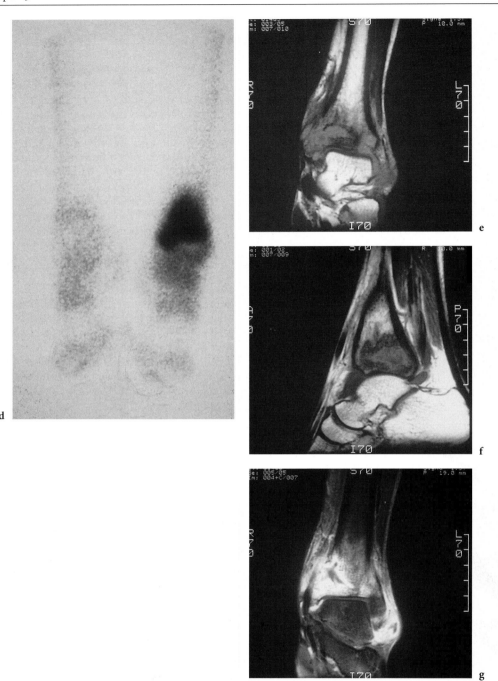

Fig. 5.18 d–g (*continued*). **d** Blood-pool image of a three-phase, technetium-contrast bone scan demonstrates a much more extensive area of increased uptake of the tracer than expected. **e, f** Coronal and sagittal T1-weighted magnetic resonance imaging scans define the extent of bone and bone-marrow involvement and extension into the joint space, giving rise to areas of low signal. **g** A post-gadolinium-injection T1 scan confirms the bone and joint-space infection and indicates the extent of soft-tissue and tendon-sheath infection on both the lateral and medial aspects of the joint. Alcohol acid-fast bacilli was found in the joint aspirate

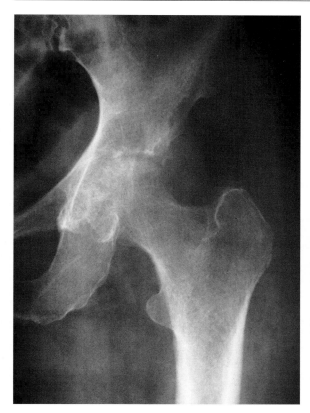

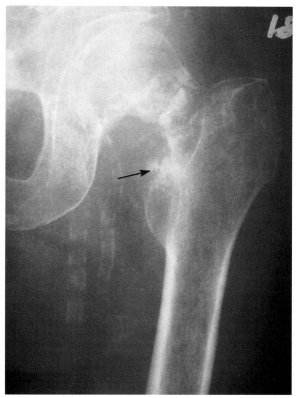

Fig. 5.19. Left hip of a middle-aged man. Early joint tuberculosis. There is some loss of joint space and reduction in definition of the cortex of both the acetabulum and the femoral head. There is periarticular osteoporosis

Fig. 5.20. Advanced tuberculosis in an elderly diabetic. Destruction of the medial aspect of the femoral neck, with a pathological fracture of the subcapital region. There is punctate calcification in the soft tissues (*arrow*). Alcohol-acid-fast-bacilli culture was positive

physis, involvement of the peripheral sub-articular areas and development of a joint effusion is the usual sequence of development.

Isotope Scanning

Although positive findings of both ^{99}Tc and ^{67}Ga scanning are non-specific and, in some stages of the disease, prove negative, bone scans are of great assistance in documenting osteoarticular TB. The uptake of ^{99m}Tc MDP in a tuberculous bone lesion is dependent upon a degree of hyperaemia in the bone (Fig. 5.22). Ga scans help to differentiate between infective and non-infective lesions and reveal associated soft-tissue lesions. ^{111}In-labelled-leucocyte scans are reported to be more sensitive than other isotope scans

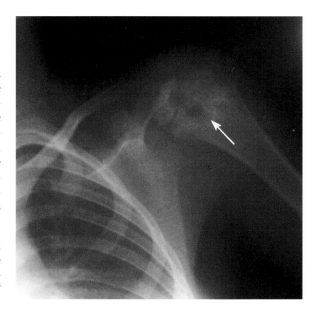

Fig. 5.21. Plain radiograph of the shoulder in a case of tuberculous arthritis "sicca". There is partial destruction of the humeral head epiphysis, with cloaca formation in the humeral metaphysis (*arrow*). Upward migration of the humerus is similar to that seen in tuberculosis of the hip joint

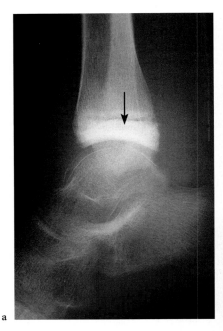

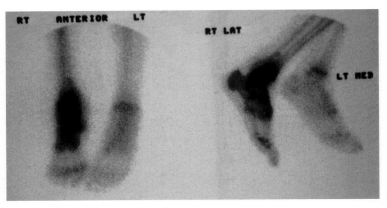

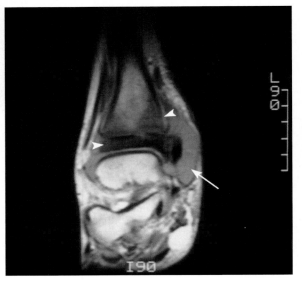

Fig. 5.22. a Plain radiographs of the ankle in a twelve year old girl revealed osteosclerosis confined to the epiphysis and metaphyseal line (*arrow*). There was a fluctuant swelling over the medial malleolus, and tuberculosis was suspected. **b** Technetium-contrast bone scans of the ankle raised suspicions of an extensive infection. **c** T1-weighted magnetic resonance imaging scan confirmed the mixed-signal abscess overlying the medial malleolus and extending into the joint (*arrow*). The sclerotic bone of the tibial epiphysis is also seen, as well as reduced-signal areas in the tibial bone marrow (*arrowheads*). At incision of the abscess, thick pus was drained, but no alcohol acid-fast bacilli were found. Histological specimens revealed metastatic disease arising from an unexpected retinoblastoma. Images by courtesy of Dr. Mona Shahed, Riyadh Military Hospital

in imaging infective lesions, but false positives are reported. Both Ga and Tc scans are also of importance in the demonstration of multiple lesions, many of which are clinically silent.

Ultrasound

Ultrasound examination is of value in defining infected bursae, as well as soft-tissue masses and abscesses close to bone lesions and infected joints [8]. In general, ultrasound search for abdominal lymph nodes and psoas abscess masses is helpful. In tuberculous sacroiliitis, the presence of both pelvic ilio-

psoas and sub-gluteal abscesses can be detected. Periarticular bursitis is also apparent on ultrasound. In particular, it is of use in the presence of iliopsoas bursitis in hip-joint infections and in differentiating the bursa from other mass lesions in the region of the neurovascular bundle. Although the findings are non-specific, ultrasound can be used to direct diagnostic bursa aspiration.

Arthrography

Injection of the joint capsule with iodinated contrast material reveals thickening and nodulation of

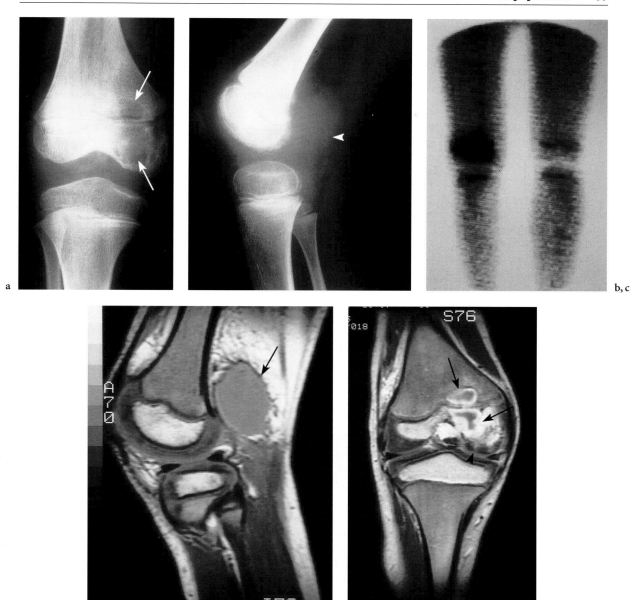

Fig. 5.23 a–e. Childhood tuberculosis. Plain radiographs demonstrating osteolysis in the femoral epiphysis and the metaphysis, with irregularity of the medial articular surface (*arrows*). There is a marked soft-tissue swelling behind the knee (*arrowhead*). **c** The blood-pool phase of a technetium-contrast bone scan defines the extent of the lesion. **d** Sagittal, T1-weighted scan demonstrates the intermediate signal in the large posterior collection (*arrow*). The destructive changes in the metaphysis and epiphysis are less well seen. **e** Coronal, post-gadolinium-injection T1 scan defines the intra-osseous abscesses (*arrows*) and the destruction of the articular cartilage (*arrowhead*)

the synovium as well as filling defects due to caseating material, but similar changes are seen in other conditions. It is of value in outlining both communication with adjacent bursae and the pathway of any sinus tracks arising from the joint [62].

CT Scanning

CT scanning is used to study both bone lesions and any surrounding soft-tissue masses. CT is especially useful in defining the presence of soft-tissue calcification, which may be of insufficient density to be defined on plain radiographs. In joint infections, early bone erosions are well seen, as are joint effusions, but the application is limited due to the axial nature of the scans.

MRI Scanning

With the possibility of multiplanar scanning, MRI is of great value in defining the extent of tuberculous infection. This is especially so in synovial disease. The extent of joint effusion, surrounding soft-tissue reaction, bone-marrow oedema, bone erosion and cartilage destruction are all well demonstrated. Images obtained on T1 after administration of intravenous gadolinium (Gd) outline any abscess formation. In tendon-sheath infections, effusion and the presence of caseation and calcification, such as rice bodies, can be seen (Fig. 5.23) [54, 57, 58]. In long-bone lesions, both the bone defect and the extent of bone-marrow and soft-tissue infection is demonstrated.

Recent studies using Gd enhancement are promising in documenting the extent of inflammatory tissue. Again, the changes are non-specific and require bacteriological confirmation. However, the examination is of great value, in assessing not only the extent of the disease but also the progress of healing on follow-up examination (Fig. 5.24).

■ Differential Diagnosis

In the USA, extra-pulmonary TB is less likely to infect Caucasians than American Indians, Inuit, Afro-Caribbeans, Pacific Islanders, immigrants from the Indian sub-continent and Africa, and people of American Hispanic origin. Among these latter patients, it is a disease of relatively young people, usually below the age of 30 years.

To these groups may be added patients showing a low resistance to the mycobacterium. These include the elderly, diabetics, those using steroids, post-transplant patients, ethanol and IV-drug abusers and AIDS-infected patients. People in overcrowded accommodations or of low socio-economic classes are at increased risk, as are prisoners and prison officers; health-care workers are also exposed to the disease. In these groups, TB should be borne in mind when an indolent lesion of a bone joint or bursa is being considered for diagnosis.

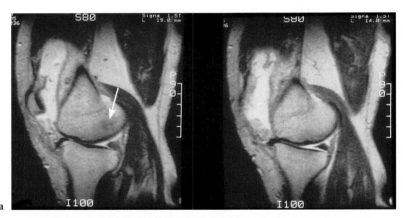

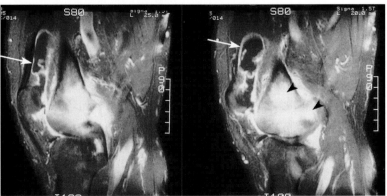

Fig. 5.24 a, b.
Pre- and post-gadolinium scans of the knee. T1 scanning demonstrates the extent of a large, supra-patellar bursal effusion. There is also a low-signal nidus in the femoral epiphysis (*arrow*). **b** A post-gadolinium-injection scan shows the effusion to be a tuberculous synovial abscess (*arrows*). There is also extensive uptake of the contrast in the bone marrow of the femur (*arrowheads*)

Pyogenic Osteitis

Tuberculous osteitis is usually monostotic and must be differentiated from acute pyogenic ostemyelitis. The acute, florid presentation of the pyogenic form, accompanied by constitutional symptoms of fever, toxicity and leucocytosis is a very different picture from the insidious onset of TB. Fever is uncommon, as is pain, although local swelling may be present.

Metaphyseal pyogenic lesions rarely involve the physis or adjacent joint. They are usually accompanied by reactive bone changes and periostitis, which is unusual in tuberculous infection, apart from in the very young [8, 14]. Blood culture and cultures from the lesion itself may be needed to make the diagnosis of pyogenic infection. Chronic pyogenic infections, such as Brodie's abscess, usually are distinguished by the presence of reactive bone changes and surrounding bone sclerosis.

Pyogenic osteomyelitis of the calvarium must be distinguished from Pott's puffy tumour, and both show well-defined osteolytic lesions involving both the inner and outer tables of the skull. Both lesions demonstrate marginal enhancement on computer-enhanced CT and, usually, biopsy is required to differentiate between the two conditions.

In endemic regions, Brucellar osteitis is rare in the long bones. When it occurs, the femur and the area around the hip joint are the usual sites of infection. Lesions of the upper limb and the flat bones have been reported but are less common. It appears overwhelmingly to be a disease of the vertebrae and, to a lesser extent, the joints [63].

Focal fungal disease of bone occurs in endemic areas. Inoculated fungal disease, such as madura foot, is unlikely to be confused with TB and is usually confined to the soft tissues and bones of the foot, with occasional secondary lesions of the tibia due to sitting in the cross-legged position, which causes local inoculation of infected material (Fig. 5.25).

Fungal lesions are either punched-out lytic lesions with a surrounding thin sclerotic rim, or permeative lesions with surrounding osteoporosis. These latter are difficult to differentiate from tuberculous lesions. Biopsy and histology are necessary to differentiate the disease from other fungal infections and TB. Pyogenic infection of the fingers of a polyostotic type is rare, and tuberculous dactylitis has to be differentiated from syphilitic dactylitis, which is congenital (and, therefore, affects a younger age group) and tends to produce symmetrical lesions. Other conditions giving rise to expansile lesions of the small bones are sickle cell disease and other congenital anaemias. In these cases, unless the bones are secondarily infected, there is usually little difficulty in making the correct diagnosis. In adults, sarcoidosis may produce similar expansile lesions in the metacarpals, but the subchondral erosions in the phalanges are an important pointer to sarcoidosis, as are manifestations of the disease in other organs. Isotope examination of the affected area will be positive before changes are visible on plain radiography.

Tumours of Bone

Tumours of the diaphysis tend to be accompanied by significant reactive change at the time of presentation, including periosteal new-bone formation

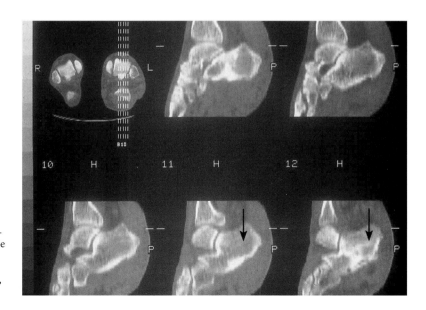

Fig. 5.25.
Computed tomography scan with sagittal reconstructions of the ankle in a case of mycetoma. The pathological change lies mainly in the soft tissues. There is some patchy osteolysis in the calcaneus, with areas of bone sclerosis (*arrows*)

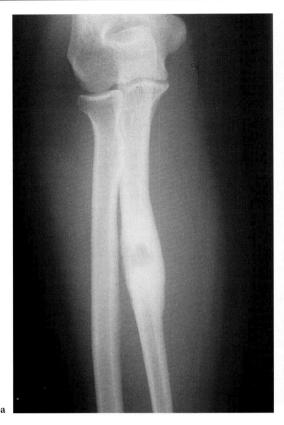

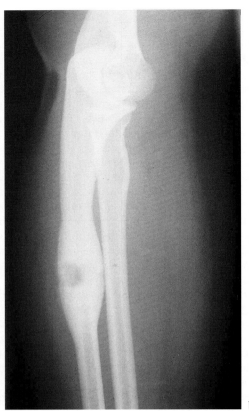

a

b

Fig. 5.26. Tuberculosis in the shaft of the ulna. A cavity is surrounded by exuberant new bone formation and bone sclerosis. It is not possible to distinguish this lesion from any other form of chronic bone infection

(Fig. 5.26). Metastatic bone tumours are more difficult to differentiate from tuberculous osteitis, as single lytic lesions lacking bone sclerosis often occur in both conditions. Diaphyseal tuberculous foci are usually more regular in outline and are often orientated along the long axis of the bone shaft. In many cases, the primary malignant tumour will already have manifested itself in the lung, breast, thyroid, kidney or gastrointestinal tract by the time metastasis occurs.

Tumours confined to the epiphysis, such as chondroblastoma, are usually proliferative as well as lytic. Sarcomas often show a soft-tissue element, but the accompanying destruction of the cortex and typical periosteal reaction are rare in tuberculous osteitis apart from in the very young [14]. Lack of pain and slower development is also a characteristic not shared by metastasis and sarcoma.

Isotope bone scanning including the tracer ^{67}Ga citrate is very helpful, where available, showing the inflammatory nature of TB and revealing any distant occult lesions. Multiple myeloma is difficult to differentiate unless the typical changes in the vertebral column and skull are present. Serum protein studies are diagnostic. In the case of solitary plasmocytoma of bone, difficulties arise, although the lesions are often multilocular, which is unusual in isolated TB foci. In the skull, although the plain radiographic changes may be similar to TB, the physical feel of the hard, subcutaneous mass accompanying a plasmocytoma is different from the soft Pott's puffy tumour [18, 19, 64]. Another point of differentiation is that isotope studies of myeloma and plasmocytoma are usually photopenic on Tc-contrast bone scans. Other lesions of the calvarium to be considered are syphilitic osteitis, eosinophilic granuloma, histiocytosis X and sarcoidosis.

Other Forms of Arthritis

Phemister's triad of juxta-articular osteoporosis, marginal erosions and narrowing of the joint space, although suggestive in the appropriate clinical setting, is non-specific. Tuberculous arthritis is usually mono-articular. The hip joint and the knee are the two most common sites [65]. In the case of the knee, tuberculous arthritis has been described, accompanied by osteitis, confined to the patella. Both lytic and osteosclerotic changes may be present, and sequestration in the patella is described [66]. In the hip and knee, joint communication of the infected joint space with surrounding bursae is not unusual (Fig. 5.27) [62]. Rheumatoid arthritis is usually poly-arthritic, and the small joints of the hands and feet are almost invariably affected. The destruction of articular cartilage, bone erosion and joint effusion with accompanying synovial thickening parallels the changes of tuberculous disease. The loss of joint space in rheumatoid disease is more rapid, and the arthritic changes are commonly painful. Blood serology is helpful in differentiating rheumatic disease.

The most common mono-articular arthritis in the last 10 years has been gonococcal arthritis. The arthritis is painful, and the knee is the most common site, followed by the wrists, hands and ankles. Tenosynovitis often accompanies the arthritis. The hip joint is rarely affected. In one type, the accompanying joint effusion is purulent and contains the micro-organism, in contrast to the usual straw-coloured effusion of TB. A second type of this arthritis has a sparse effusion with a negative culture but, in this second type of infection, blood culture is often positive. The radiological changes include early osteoporosis but, if untreated, the condition progresses to a destructive arthritis.

In secondary syphilis, the arthritis is usually poly-arthritic, but unilateral sacroiliitis occurs. The associated soft-tissue lesion of tuberculous sacroiliitis may be aspirated and cultured.

Late-stage neuropathic changes in syphilis are accompanied by the characteristic serum reactions. In endemic regions, late presentation of the patient may lead to advanced radiological appearances in tuberculous arthritis. This is also the case in advanced diabetic, neuropathic arthropathy, where diabetes and TB may co-exist.

Lyme disease, in addition to leading to a meningopolyneuritic syndrome, similar to neurotuberculosis, may develop arthritis. This is usually a poly-arthritis involving the larger joints, with transient joint effusions. Fungal arthritides are impossible to differentiate on imaging grounds alone.

Candidal arthritis is becoming more common with the spread of IV-drug abuse but may also develop as a complication in systemic candidal infection affecting immunosuppressed individuals. A relationship between addiction to brown (Iranian) heroin (which, because of its relative insolubility in water, is dissolved in lemon juice before intravenous injection) and systemic candidal infection has been described in Europe. Cutaneous, ophthalmic and musculoskeletal lesions are common. The common skeletal lesion is multiple *Candida* abscesses at the costo-chondral junctions; these lesions must be differentiated from tuberculous lesions by aspiration biopsy [67].

Disseminated coccidioidomycosis leads to a chronic mono-arthritis, usually affecting the knee joint. The initial focus is in the bone, and the joint infection develops secondarily to this. The infection cannot be differentiated from TB by imaging techniques alone [68, 69]. Multicentric disease is usual, and the spine is the most common site, but the long bones may also be affected, and the ribs may demonstrate multiple lesions with punched-out areas described as "moth-eaten" ribs. Biopsy and a search for the fungus or its derivatives is necessary to confirm the diagnosis [68, 69].

Mono-articular arthritis also occurs in blastomycosis and histoplasmosis in endemic areas. The arthritis is acute, in contrast to TB, and the joint effusion is purulent. Sinus formation is common. The commonly affected joints are the knee, ankle, elbow and wrist. Osteitis changes are often present in the vertebrae, ribs, skull and long bones. Biopsy and culture are necessary to confirm the diagnosis.

Cryptococcus neoformans has become a common secondary infection in AIDS patients. The region of the knee is commonly affected, but characteristically with a destructive lesion of the tibial plateau, which only rarely proceeds to arthritis.

Non-Infectious Arthritides

Conditions of the large joints, such as pigmented villous synovitis, is usually differentiated from tuberculous arthritis by lack of osteoporosis, preservation of the joint space and the presence of haemosiderosis, demonstrated as an imaging void on MRI examination. In gout, osteoporosis is usually absent, and the presence of tophi in the soft tissues is a helpful sign. Transient osteoporosis of the neck of the femur is usually differentiated by the clinical course of the disease and the lack of joint destruction.

Tenosynovitis and Bursitis

By far the most common causes of tenosynovitis and bursitis are inflammatory, often low-grade infections [54, 70]. Penetrating injuries play a part in the infection of flexor sheaths in pyogenic, mycobacterial and fungal lesions. Rheumatic disease is a common cause of tenosynovitis and of various bursal inflammations; inflammatory bowel disease complicated by tenosynovitis is less common. Calcification is often present in the contents of bursae and tendon sheaths infected by TB, and this appearance is highly suggestive of the disease.

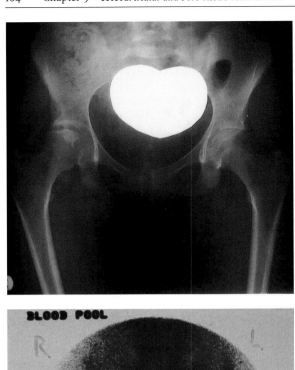

a

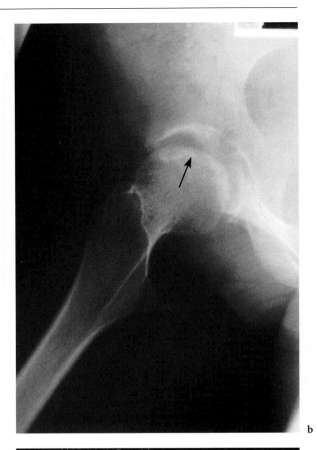

b

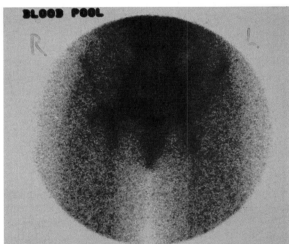

c

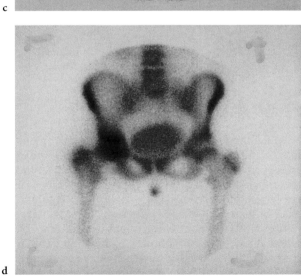

d

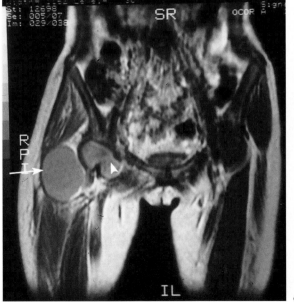

e

Fig. 5.27 a–e. *f–h s. p. 105*

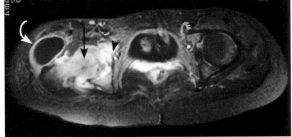

g

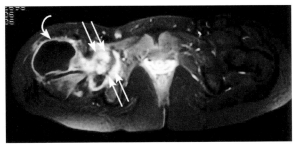

h

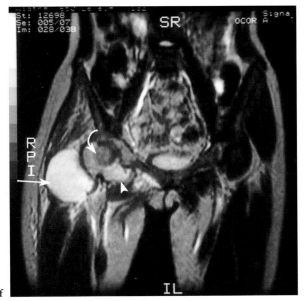

f

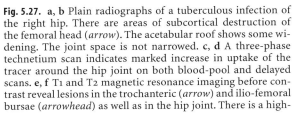

Fig. 5.27. a, b Plain radiographs of a tuberculous infection of the right hip. There are areas of subcortical destruction of the femoral head (*arrow*). The acetabular roof shows some widening. The joint space is not narrowed. **c, d** A three-phase technetium scan indicates marked increase in uptake of the tracer around the hip joint on both blood-pool and delayed scans. **e, f** T1 and T2 magnetic resonance imaging before contrast reveal lesions in the trochanteric (*arrow*) and ilio-femoral bursae (*arrowhead*) as well as in the hip joint. There is a high-

intensity signal in the femoral head in the T2 image (*curved arrow*). **g, h** Post-gadolinium-injection T1 scanning reveals an enhancement of the femoral head and neck (*arrow*), and enhancement of the ilio-femoral bursa (*arrowhead*) in **g**. In both illustrations, the enhancement of the trochanteric bursa is peripheral only (*curved arrows*) This indicates necrotic caseating material in the trochanteric bursa. In **h**, there is also intense enhancement in the joint space and in the marrow of the femoral head (*double arrows*)

■ References

1. Rieder HL, Dixie E, Cauthen GM (1990) Extrapulmonary tuberculosis in the United States. Am Rev Respir Dis 141:347–351
2. Alvarez S, McCabe WR (1984) Extra pulmonary tuberculosis revisited: a review of experience in Boston City and other hospitals. Medicine 63:25–55
3. Davies PDO, Humphries MJ, Byfield SP, et al. (1984) Bone and joint tuberculosis. J Bone Joint Surg Br 66:326–330
4. Yao DC, Sartorius DJ (1995) Musculoskeletal tuberculosis. Radiol Clin North Am 33:679–689
5. Brudney K, Dobkin J (1991) Resurgent tuberculosis in New York City. HIV, homelessness and the decline of tuberculosis control programs. Am Rev Respir Dis 144:745–749
6. Onorato IM, McCray E (1992) Prevelence of HIV infection among patients attending tuberculosis clinics in the USA. J Infect Dis 165:87–92
7. Thyn CJP, Steensma JT (eds) (1990) TB of the skeleton. In: Focus on radiology. Springer, Berlin Heidelberg New York
8. Cremin BJ, Jamieson DH (1995) Imaging of skeletal tuberculosis. In: Childhood tuberculosis: modern imaging and clinical concepts. Springer, Berlin Heidelberg New York
9. Martini M, Ouahes M (1988) Bone and joint tuberculosis: a review of 625 cases. Orthopedics 11:861–866
10. Resnick D, Niwayama G (1988) Diagnosis of bone and joint disorders, 2nd edn, vol 4. Saunders, Philadelphia, pp 2661–2686
11. Watts HG, Lifeso RM (1996) Tuberculosis of bones and joints. J Bone Joint Surg Am 78:288–298
12. Murray RO, Jacobson HG, Stoker DJ (1990) The radiology of skeletal disorders, 3rd edn, Vol 1. Churchill Livingstone, London, pp 282–289
13. Autzen B, Elberg JJ (1988) Bone and joint tuberculosis in Denmark. Acta Orthop Scand 59:50–52
14. Hugosson C, Nyman, Brismar J, et al. (1996) Imaging of tuberculosis (V). Peripheral osteoarticular and soft tissue tuberculosis. Acta Radiol 37:512–516
15. Antti-Poika I, Vankaa E, Santavirta S, Vastamaki M (1991) Two cases of shoulder joint tuberculosis. Acta Orthop Scand 62:81–83
16. Shanmugasundaram TK (1987) Bone and joint tuberculosis. Surgery Medical Education (International) Ltd., pp 1060–1066
17. Abdelwahab IM, Present DA, Gould E, Klein MJ, Nelson J (1988) Tuberculosis of the distal metaphysis of the femur. Case report 473. Skeletal Radiol 17:199–202
18. Gupta PK, Kolluri VR, Chandramouli BA (1989) Calvarial tuberculosis: a report of two cases. Neurosurgery 25:830
19. Campi de Castro C, Garcia de Barros N, de Sousa Campos ZM (1995) CT scans of cranial tuberculosis. Radiol Clin North Am 33:753–769
20. Nemir RL, Branom-Genieser N, Balasubramanyam P (1979) Extensive sclerosis of the base of the skull due to primary nasal tuberculosis. Pediatr Radiol 8:42
21. Lachenauer CS, Consentino S, Wood RS, Yousefzadeh DK, McCarthy CA (1991) Multifocal skeletal tuberculosis presenting as osteomyelitis of the jaw. Pediatr Infect Dis J 10:940–944

22. Heney C, Baise T (1988) Tuberculosis of the mandible: a case report. Pediatr Infect Dis J 7:74–76

23. Thuan-Phuong Nguyen, Burk DL (1995) Musculoskeletal case of the day: tuberculous sacroiliitis. AJR Am J Roentgenol 165:205–206

24. Guyot DR, Manoli A, King GA (1987) Pyogenic sacroiliitis in IV drug abusers. AJR Am J Roentgenol 149:1209–1211

25. Klein MA, Winalski CS, Wax MR, Piwnica-Worms DR (1991) MR imaging of septic sacroiliitis. J Comput Assist Tomogr 15:126–132

26. Bittini A, Dominguez PL, Martinez Pueyo ML, Lopez Longo FJ, Monteagudo I, Carreno L (1985) Comparison of bone and gallium-67 imaging in heroin users arthritis. J Nucl Med 26:1377–1381

27. Pouchot J, Vinceneux P, Barge J, et al. (1988) Tuberculosis of the sacroiliac joint: clinical features, outcome, and evaluation of closed needle biopsy in 11 cases. Am J Med 84:622–628

28. Abdelwahab IF, Lewis MM, Klein MJ, Hermann G (1989) Tuberculous dactylitis (right great toe). Case report 528. Skeletal Radiol 18:133–135

29. Clarke JA (1990) Tuberculous dactylitis in childhood, the need for continued vigilance. Clin Radiol 42:287–288

30. Rasool M, Govender S, Naidoo K (1994) Cystic tuberculosis of bone in children. J Bone Joint Surg Br 76:113–117

31. Shannon FB, Moore M, Houkom JA (1990) Multifocal cystic tuberculosis of bone. J Bone Joint Surg Am 72:1089–1092

32. Nielsen FF, Helmig O, de Carvalho A (1989) Tuberculosis of calcaneus and talus with negative tuberculin skin test. Case report 533. Skeletal Radiol 18:153–155

33. Jacobs P (1964) Osteoarticular tuberculosis in coloured immigrants: a radiological study. Clin Radiol 15:59–69

34. Muradali D, Gold WL, Vellend H, Beker E (1993) Multifocal osteoarticular tuberculosis: report of four cases and a review of management. Clin Infect Dis 17:204–209

35. Ip M, Tsui E, Wong KL, Jones B, Pung CF, Ngan H (1993) Disseminated skeletal tuberculosis with skull involvement. Tuber Lung Dis 74:211–214

36. Hardoff R, Efrat M, Gips S (1995) Multifocal osteoarticular tuberculosis resembling skeletal metastatic disease. Clin Nucl Med 20:279–281

37. Marom EM, Porter A, Gornish M, Cohen M, Russo I (1995) Atypical skeletal tuberculosis. Skeletal Radiol 24:620–622

38. Frankel DG, Daffner RH, Wang SE (1991) Case report 654: disseminated tuberculosis. Skeletal Radiol 20:130–133

39. Abdelwahab IF, Kenan S, Hermann G, et al. (1991) Atypical skeletal tuberculosis mimicking neoplasm. Br J Radiol 64:551–555

40. Chambers ST, Hendrickse WA, Record C, et al. (1984) Paradoxical expansion of intracranial tuberculomas during chemotherapy. Lancet 28:181–184

41. Campbell IA, Dyson AJ (1977) Lymph node tuberculosis: a comparison of various methods of treatment. Tubercule 58:171–179

42. Teoh R, Humphries MJ, O'Mahony G (1987) Symptomatic intracranial tuberculoma developing during the treatment of tuberculoma: a report of 10 patients with a review of the literature. QJM 63 241:449–460

43. Ip M, Nai-kwai Chen, Shun-Yang So, Shui-Wah Chiu, Wah-Kit Lam (1989) Unusual rib destruction in pleuropulmonary tuberculosis. Chest 95:242–244

44. Adler BD, Padley SPG, Muller NL (1993) Tuberculosis of the chest wall: CT findings. J Comput Assist Tomogr 17:271–273

45. Bhatt GM, Austin HM (1985) CT demonstration of empyema necessitatis. J Comput Assist Tomogr 9:1108–1109

46. Lee G, Jung-Gi Im, Kim JS, et al. (1993) Tuberculosis of the ribs: CT appearance. J Comput Assist Tomogr 17:363–366

47. Firooznia H, Seliger G, Abrams RA, et al. (1973) Disseminated extrapulmonary tuberculosis in association with heroin addiction. Radiology 109:291–296

48. Kim SJ, Jung-Gi Im, Sung-Tae Cho, et al. (1993) Rib counting on CT using the sternal approach. J Comput Assist Tomogr 17:358–362

49. Beltran J, Noto AM, McGhee RB, et al. (1987) Infections of the musculoskeletal system: high-field strength MR imaging. Radiology 164:449–454

50. Fleckenstein JL, Burns DK, Murphy FK, et al. (1991) Differential diagnosis of bacterial myositis in AIDS: evalution with MRI imaging. Radiology 179:653–658

51. Wilbur AC, Gorodetsky AA, Hibbeln JF (1995) Tuberculous myositis: CT and sonographic findings in two cases. J Clin Ultrasound 23:495–499

52. Pouchot J, Vinceneux P, Barge J, et al. (1990) Tuberculous polymyositis in HIV infection. Am J Med 89:250

53. Jackson RH, King JW (1989) Tenosynovitis of the hand: a forgotten manifestation of tuberculosis. Rev Infect Dis 11:616–618

54. Jaovisidha S, Chen C, Ryu KN, et al. (1996) Tuberculous tenosynovitis and bursitis: imaging findings in 21 cases. Radiology 201:507–513

55. Arias FG, Rodriguez M, Hernandez JG (1987) Osteomyelitis deriving from BCG-vaccination. Pediatr Radiol 17:166–167

56. Abdelwahab IF, Kenan S, Hermann G (1993) Tuberculous peroneal tenosynovitis. J Bone Joint Surg Am 75:1687–1690

57. Sueyoshi E, Uetani M, Hayashi K (1996) Tuberculous tenosynovitis of the wrist: MRI findings in three patients. Skeletal Radiol 25:569–572

58. Hoffman KL, Bergman AG, Hoffman DK, Harris DP (1996) Tuberculous tenosynovitis of the flexor tendons of the wrist: MR imaging with pathological correlation. Skeletal Radiol 25:186–188

59. Katz DS, Wolgater H, Cuhna BA (1992) Mycobacterium bovis vertebral osteitis and psoas abscess after intervesical BCG therapy for bladder carcinoma. Urology 40:63–66

60. Fishman JR, Walton DT, Flynn NM, et al. (1993) Tuberculous spondylitis as a complication of intravesicle bacillus Calmette-Geurin therapy. J Urol 149:584–587

61. Forrester DM, Feske WI (1996) Imaging of infectious arthritis. Semin Roentgenol 31:239–249

62. Steinbach LS, Schneider R, Goldman AB, et al. (1985) Bursae and abscess cavities communicating with the hip. Radiology 156:303–307

63. Madkour MM (1989) Brucellosis. Butterworths, London, pp 99–103

64. Wilson P, Chumas P, van der Walt JD (1990) Case report: solitary plasmocytoma of the frontal bone. Clin Radiol 42:289–290

65. Araki Y, Tsukaguchi I, Shino K (1993) Tuberculous arthritis of the knee: MR findings. AJR Am J Roentgenol 160:664

66. Hernandez Gimenez M, Tovar Beltran JV, Segui MIF, Gomez EP (1987) Tuberculosis of the patella. Pediatr Radiol 17:328–329

67. Bisbe J, Miro JM, Latorre X, et al. (1992) Disseminated candidiasis in addicts who use brown heroin: report of 83 cases and review. Clin Infect Dis 15:910–923

68. Zeppa MA, Laorr A, Greenspan A, et al. (1996) Skeletal coccidioidomycosis: imaging findings in 19 patients. Skeletal Radiol 25:337–343

69. Lund PJ, Chan KM, Unger EC, Galgiani TN, Pitt MJ (1996) Magnetic resonance imaging in coccidioidal arthritis. Skeletal Radiol 25:661–665

70. Zeiss J, Coombs RJ, Booth RL, Saddemi SR (1993) Chronic bursitis presenting as a mass in the pes anserine bursa: MR diagnosis. J Comput Assist Tomogr 17:137–140

CHAPTER 6

Tuberculosis of the Gastrointestinal Tract and Peritoneum

■ Introduction

In the past decade, two distinct patterns of intra-abdominal tuberculosis (TB) have emerged. First, the classical disease, affecting the peritoneum, gastrointestinal tract, lymphatic system and solid organs and, second, the disease as an acquired immunodeficiency syndrome (AIDS)-related condition. AIDS-related abdominal TB has a different pattern of symptoms, signs and pathology and is dealt with in a later chapter. In the years 1963–1986, 132 cases of peritoneal TB were reported in the USA, out of a total of 3942 records of extrapulmonary disease [1]. Of these, 71.2% of the 3942 cases fell amongst the racial minorities and the foreign born. In some studies, peritoneal TB occurred as a complicating illness in those patients already known to have hepatic cirrhosis or alcohol addiction [2, 3].

In the late 1970s and early 1980s, the annual number of cases of extrapulmonary TB in England and Wales was much higher, at approximately 2500 per annum. In one district general hospital, 109 new cases of gastrointestinal TB were treated between 1970 and 1985. This was in an area where 70% of all TB cases were in the immigrant population [4].

In a 10-year study at a London hospital, the number of gastrointestinal-TB patients was 90 and, during the same period, 102 cases of Crohn's disease were treated. Eighty-two per cent of the tuberculous patients were of Asian origin [5]. Similar patterns of abdominal TB are reported from two other English centres where there are large immigrant communities [3, 6]. In Leicester, 146 cases of abdominal TB were in Asian migrants and six were amongst Europeans.

In these four centres, a total of 415 cases are reported over a 15-year period, compared with 132 cases in a similar period in the larger population of the USA. Whether a marked increase in cases among susceptible groups in the USA will occur in the near future remains to be seen. In the meantime, it would be prudent for the physician to consider TB as the diagnosis in instances of unusual abdominal pain, malaise and weight loss. In a series of 81 cases from British Columbia over a period of 11 years, Jakubowski et al. noted drug abuse or alcoholism in roughly 25% of their cases; they also noted a high proportion of minority groups. An unusual feature was that 16 of the patients presented with an anorectal lesion. In this group of patients, the average age was higher, at 51 years; 81% were male, and many were Caucasians. This type of presentation appears to be linked to active pulmonary disease as a result of swallowed infectious sputum, rather than from haematogenous spread [7].

Numbers of cases reported in centres in the USA vary considerably. In a centre in Miami, an area with a high percentage of Hispanic immigrants, peritoneal TB was rightly regarded as uncommon during the period 1972–1986. Only six cases were proven (by laparoscopy) in a series of 529 examinations [8]. Guth et al. reported an increasing frequency of abdominal TB in an urban population and noted two distinct groups: native-born Americans with AIDS, and immigrants [9].

The contrast between the Northern and Southern Hemispheres is dramatic. In the South, where TB is endemic, abdominal TB is a very common disease. Both the wide occurrence of pulmonary TB and the use of non-pasteurised milk favour its development. The present Asian and African AIDS pandemic will only lead to more cases.

Marshall reviewed a number of papers from around the world [9] and emphasised the target groups of patients in the USA. There, the major increases in case numbers are amongst Hispanics, Afro-Americans, immigrants and refugees. He emphasised the increase of the disease in the younger age groups amongst the urban poor, minority groups on reservations, the prison population and, particularly, those with drug or alcohol abuse or AIDS.

However, a further group of the elderly, particularly those in nursing homes, and their care givers, present a special problem. The wider extent of the problem is reflected in the number of papers recently published, which compare the value of sonography, computed tomography (CT) and magnetic resonance imaging (MRI) as diagnostic methods (in India

[10–13], the Middle East [14–22], the Far East [23], South Africa [24–26], Europe and the USA [27–30]).

■ Clinical Features

Abdominal TB develops in between 2% and 4% of patients with pulmonary TB [25]. The infection may affect any organ or space within the abdominal cavity and, indeed, cold abscesses also occur in the abdominal wall. Because of these varying sites of infection, a broad spectrum of signs, symptoms and complications is encountered. The common sites of infection are the abdominal lymph nodes, the peritoneal cavity and the gastrointestinal tract. Less commonly, the solid organs and the female adnexa are infected. Overlap between infections of the various systems also causes variations in the clinical presentation. Lymph nodes are usually affected to some extent, in both peritoneal and gastrointestinal infection.

The disease is generally one of young adults or the middle aged and, in a number of large studies, infects men and women in almost equal numbers [10–12, 17, 21, 23]. In a small number of studies, there is a preponderance of men [16, 18, 23, 29] and, in two studies, of women [14, 25].

In a high proportion of individuals, the disorder runs an insidious course, and what symptoms there are may be present for one or two years. In others, acceleration of symptoms may occur, and an acute presentation leads to intestinal obstruction, or perforation or, rarely, rectal blood loss or haematemesis [31].

In a series of 300 cases of abdominal TB, Bhansali recorded 76 cases requiring emergency surgery; however, this was at a time when clinical examination and barium contrast studies were the main diagnostic tools available [32]. In countries where more sophisticated methods of investigation are generally available, and where there is early recourse of the patient to the doctor, then an acute presentation is less usual and, in those cases with an acute presentation, tuberculous appendicitis is often the underlying cause [20].

The most common symptoms are varying degrees of abdominal pain, loss of weight, abdominal distension, low-grade fever or night sweats, anorexia, vomiting and diarrhoea. Less commonly, bleeding per rectum or dysphagia are symptoms.

Presenting signs include abdominal distension, ascites, abdominal tenderness and abdominal masses, often in the right iliac fossa. Less commonly, masses are present in the midline, due to either lymph-node enlargement, matted loops of bowel or thickened omentum. These are all findings that have to be considered when choosing the method of imaging investigation. Hepato-splenomegaly is a less common presentation and, in a few cases, fistula to the surface or fissure in ano may be a presenting feature. As anaemia often accompanies the disease, pallor is often a physical sign. The anaemia is of a normocytic, normochromic type and is often accompanied by thrombocytosis. Cervical lymphadenopathy is present in some cases, as are other foci of extrapulmonary TB, but pulmonary TB is present in less than 30% of cases. Mantoux reaction is positive in between 50% and 70% of cases, although it is negative in anergic patients. Many patients who present after months or years of tuberculous gastrointestinal disease are malnourished and have hypoalbuminaemia. The erythrocyte sedimentation rate is often raised but, being a non-specific sign, is of little value in differentiating TB from other common conditions, such as malignant disease or lymphoma.

■ Pathogenesis

TB reaches the abdomen by three main mechanisms. The ingestion of either *Mycobacterium Bovis* or *M. Tuberculosis* from infected milk is still widespread in those areas where milk is not pasteurised and in countries where nomadic people ingest milk taken from their animals. Another method of infection is in those patients with active pulmonary TB who ingest infected sputum, which gains entry through the mucosa of the intestine.

These two mechanisms lead initially to infection of the gastrointestinal tract. Later, the peritoneum is involved as, with penetration to deeper layers of the bowel wall, serosal TB develops. By the same method, lymphatic spread leads to regional lymph-node infection. The third main pathway is haematogenous spread from a tuberculous focus elsewhere in the body, or miliary infection. In these cases, the peritoneum, lymph nodes and solid abdominal organs are involved [17, 20, 29, 33]. The onset of progressive abdominal TB does not always begin at the time of haematogenous spread. Foci of latent infection may lay dormant for some years before reactivation. Less commonly, peritonitis develops by direct spread from TB of the fallopian tubes or adnexa [17, 29, 30]. Rarely, direct spread to the peritoneum from a psoas abscess, secondary to tuberculous spondylitis, is seen.

■ Histopathology

In the gastrointestinal tract, tuberculous enteritis gives rise to three main types of pathological change. In the most common form, mucosal ulceration develops. The ulcers are secondary to infection of the sub-mucosal lymphatic tissue, leading to the development of granulomatous tubercles, with subsequent caseation, necrosis and the formation of multiple ulcers [31, 33 – 35]. Fibrotic healing results in narrowing of the intestinal lumen and stricture formation. Regional lymph nodes are infected at an early stage and show varying degrees of enlargement, caseation and necrosis. Inflammatory involvement of the mesentery by granulomatous tissue and local lymph-node enlargement leads to contraction of the mesenteric root and mesocolon, with displacement of bowel loops and the colon flexures. Serosal tubercles result in exudative peritoneal effusion. Pockets of ascites and adhesive bowel loops are common. The omentum becomes inflamed, thickened and often adherent to the bowel or abdominal wall. These last three mechanisms result in the formation of palpable abdominal masses. Serosal tubercles are characteristic of the disease and, when these white to yellow tubercles are recognised at laparoscopic examination, these alone are highly suggestive of TB. Histological presence of epithelioid and Langerhans' giant cells, coupled with caseation, is further evidence. Mycobacteria may also be present, either on direct histology or on culture [10]. The second type of gastrointestinal lesion is a hypertrophic enteritis or colitis. Marked thickening of the bowel wall results, and mucosal and sub-mucosal lesions encroach on the bowel lumen, forming a cobblestone-like surface. Masses may reach a considerable size and can be confused with tumours. Hypertrophic change in the bowel wall often extends over several centimetres and leads to symptoms of obstruction.

Acute perforation of tuberculous ulcers into the general peritoneal cavity leads to peritonitis. More usually, the perforation is enclosed by local adhesions, causing a localised peritoneal reaction and, eventually, a cold abscess. Rupture, into the peritoneal cavity, of enlarged, caseating lymph nodes also gives rise to an acute abdominal syndrome [32], while bowel stricture, adhesive-peritoneal disease and hypertrophic stenosis lead to symptoms of sub-acute or acute intestinal obstruction [32, 33, 35 – 37].

The third type of histopathology is a hybrid mixture of both ulcerative and hypertrophic pathologies. In haematogenous spread, the liver, spleen, pancreas and adrenals are more likely to be affected than the gastrointestinal tract. This type of spreading may also promote the development of the wet type of ascites. In this condition, there is a high proportion of associated infections of solid organs [17, 23]. Hulnick also cites a case where ascites was an isolated condition, with no other evident focus of infection [29]. Singh et al. also describe 47 patients where peritonitis was the presenting feature, and extensive barium studies of the gastrointestinal tract and hystero-

salpingography were negative for TB. This, again, suggests haematological dissemination as the source of isolated peritoneal TB.

■ Abdominal TB

The subdivision of abdominal TB into the categories of peritoneal, lymphatic, gastrointestinal and solid-organ TB is arbitrary, as these are all part of one disease process and, in practice, there is usually considerable overlap between the conditions, and there is a potential for more than one of these systems to be infected. Isolated solid-organ or peritoneal TB occurs rarely. The number of centres of infection depends on the stage of the disease. For example, in established gastrointestinal TB, the regional lymph nodes will be infected and, in all probability, the peritoneum as well [17, 20, 21, 32].

Although spread of infection from the bowel to the peritoneum is common, the reverse is not true. In both renal-tract TB and TB of the peritoneal cavity, spread to the gastrointestinal tract is very rare [33]. Many studies describe peritoneal infection arising from an infected, tuberculous, tubovarian mass, the incidence being 2 – 5 % [11, 17, 20, 21, 29, 30].

The symptoms of abdominal TB at the time of diagnosis are very similar, whether the site of infection is peritoneal or gastrointestinal. The spectrum of abdominal pain, distension, anorexia, weight loss, fever and night sweats is typically found and is described in a number of papers, reporting on some hundreds of patients [11 – 14, 16, 18, 20, 30, 32 – 34].

The symptom of abdominal distension is more pronounced in those cases with "wet" ascites. The pain in solid-organ TB often differs in its pattern, in that it is focal to the organ involved but, even in these cases, secondary spread of the infection to lymph nodes produces symptoms associated with more widespread disease

■ Tuberculous Peritonitis

Since the descriptions of Frank (1937) and Auerbach (1950) [24], tuberculous peritonitis (TBP) has been divided into three groups. The term "wet peritonitis" is applied where large quantities of ascitic fluid accumulate free in the peritoneal cavity or where there are large pockets of ascites. This fluid is of high protein content (2.5 g/100 ml) and contains many lymphocytes. Bacteriological studies and culture of this fluid have a very low rate of positive results. Singh et al., using a technique of centrifuging a litre of ascitic fluid, report a positive culture rate of 83 %, but direct microscopy and culture of small amounts

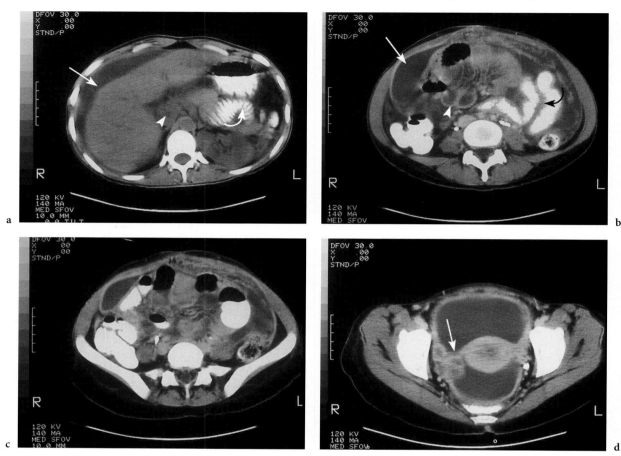

Fig. 6.1. a A young woman with tuberculous ascites. Pre-contrast computed tomography (CT) demonstrates high-density ascites (*arrow*), para-aortic and retroperitoneal lymphadenopathy (*arrowhead*) and an abnormal jejunal loop (*curved arrow*). **b** Post-contrast CT shows peritoneal enhancement with encysted ascites (*arrow*). There are enlarged lymph nodes with ring enhancement (*arrowhead*) and thickening of the bowel wall (*curved arrow*). **c** Image at a lower level showing similar changes. **d** Extensive pelvic ascites is present with peritoneal enhancement. There are fallopian-tube changes on the right (*arrow*)

of ascitic fluid are disappointing [25, 38]. However, microscopy and culture of biopsy material from tubercles visualised by peritoneoscopy show a high return of positive results [10, 18, 20, 25].

On sonographic examination, bowel loops are seen to float in the ascitic fluid, and fibrous strands of proteinaceous tissue pass between bowel loops and between the various peritoneal surfaces. In more advanced cases, these strands may develop to produce a latticework appearance. Although the wet type of ascites may be found with minimal changes in intra-abdominal structures, lymphadenopathy, mesenteric thickening and adherent bowel loops are often present. The echographic appearance of the fluid varies from "clear" to "complex". In the latter, floating or sedimentary, hyperechoic elements are apparent. It is in these complex cases that floating membranes and fixed septa are seen, due to organisation of the protein content of the ascitic fluid.

In the clear type, reliance on clinical signs and other sonographic findings is necessary to differentiate from ascites due to cirrhosis, heart failure and renal failure. It must be remembered that cirrhosis is present in up to 20% of TBP cases. Both sonography and CT scanning have roles to play in the diagnosis of TBP.

Sonographic studies are reduced in value in the presence of excess bowel gas, which may obscure important pathological change. In the presence of frank ascites, this problem is minimised, and the ascitic fluid itself and the mesentery are usually clearly visible. As peritonitis progresses, thickening of the mesentery develops, and sonographic measurements of a thickness of above 1.5 cm are abnormal. This thickening is often coupled with both hyper-reflective and hypo-reflective areas within it, which are thought to represent areas of caseating material and enlarged intra-mesenteric lymph nodes, respectively [10–13, 15, 22, 23, 27].

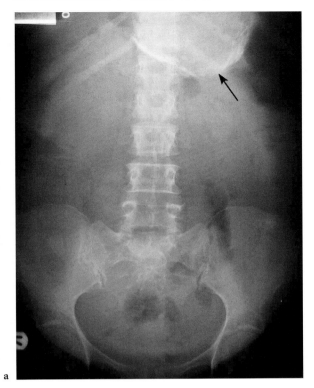

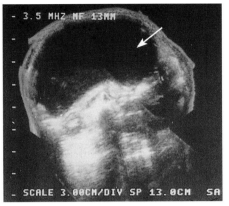

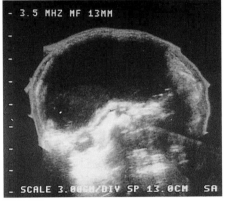

Fig. 6.2. a Abdominal radiography with a calcified lesion in the left upper quadrant (*arrow*). **b** Abdominal ultrasound shows this to be a partially fluid-filled lesion (*arrow*). **c** *s. page 112*

CT examination confirms these findings, and the density of the ascites can be documented. The formation of septa is well demonstrated [22]. Loculation of ascites is also seen, and administration of intravenous contrast demonstrates enhancement of the parietal peritoneum (Fig. 6.1). This, also, may be thickened, and lacks the nodularity and irregular thickening associated with the changes seen in malignant disease [27, 35] (Fig. 6.2).

Lymphadenopathy is also well demonstrated by CT examination and, as well as the characteristic distribution of the lymph nodes, often shows rim enhancement after intravenous contrast injection. Although these peritoneal and lymph-node changes are not specific to TB, their appearance, in the right clinical context, is highly suggestive of abdominal TB [17, 29, 39, 40].

Plastic or dry peritonitis is the type likely to be the result of a more general intra-abdominal TB, involving the mesentery, lymph nodes and the bowel wall. The amount of ascitic fluid is, characteristically, more limited than in the wet type, and it is often trapped between bowel loops or encysted in the peritoneal cavity. In this type of peritonitis, there is mesenteric thickening due to the infection, with mesenteric lymph-node enlargement on a greater scale as well as regional lymph-node masses. As the mesenteric nodes drain primarily into the cisterna chyli and, subsequently, the thoracic duct, retroperitoneal lymph-node enlargement is relatively uncommon [3, 17, 19, 22, 28, 29, 40], although it does occur [21, 24]. Fibrous peritonitis almost certainly represents a later stage of the disease. The peritoneum is markedly thickened and rigid. The omentum presents as a midline mass stretching from the mesocolon down to the pelvis. Adhesions of bowel loops and the mesentery to the abdominal wall are often present, making laparoscopy impossible or dangerous. Very little fluid is present, and sonography is also of limited value. CT examination is the examination of choice in these cases.

Tuberculous Peritonitis as a Complication of Peritoneal Dialysis

In areas of the world where TB is endemic, there is a risk of tuberculous peritonitis in patients undergoing peritoneal dialysis. Due to an impaired cellular immunity, end-stage renal failure carries with it a lowered resistance to infection. Many patients on dialysis are diabetics or belong to other high-risk groups,

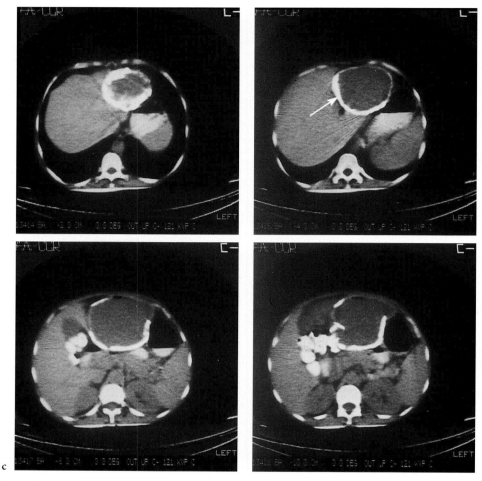

Fig. 6.2 (*continued*). **c** Computed tomography examination revealed an irregularly thickened, calcified wall (*arrow*). At first, this was thought to be hydatid disease, but the aspirate contained alcohol acid-fast bacilli

such as post-renal transplant patients, who have undergone immunosuppressive regimes. In both intermittent and continuous peritoneal dialysis (IPD, CPD), bacterial, fungal and eosinophilic peritonitis are not uncommon causes of peritonitis. TB should be considered the cause where symptoms of peritonitis occur in the presence of a cloudy dialysate but in the absence of an immediate pathogenic growth on smear or culture.

As in other forms of TBP, immediate smears and microscopy for alcohol acid-fast bacilli (AAFB) are usually negative. Also, in these dialysis cases, the peritoneal fluid is not lymphocytic. As there is a high mortality, anti-tuberculous chemotherapy should be established if the patient shows no response to systemic or intraperitoneal antibiotic regimes. Cultures of the peritoneal fluid show high rates of growth of AAFB. Early treatment preserves the perfusion integrity of the peritoneal membrane, and transfer to haemodialysis can be avoided. Ultrasound findings

have, so far, not been reported, but the window provided by the dialysate should, in theory, provide access for examination of the peritoneum. Future studies should be carried out to test the presence or absence of the characteristic changes of TBP. So far, no laparoscopic studies have been reported [41].

Adenosine Deaminase Activity in Tuberculous Peritonitis

Adenosine deaminase is an enzyme active in the proliferation and differentiation of lymphocytes. The measurement of adenosine deaminase activity is of value in patients with tuberculous ascites. It has been shown to be raised in the cerebrospinal fluid, pleural effusions and ascites of tuberculous patients. It is of value in differentiating the ascites of TB from other conditions, such as cirrhotic, malignant and septic ascites. One great advantage is the rapidity of the investigation when compared with the long wait required for the results of culture samples. In Voight's two studies, the sensitivity of the test varied between 95% and 100% and the specificity from 96% to 98%. Where available, it is a quick and useful method in pointing towards TB as the cause of ascites [42].

Gastrointestinal TB

Tuberculous infection of the bowel is a common form of abdominal TB. In Bhansali's 300 cases of abdominal TB, 196 affected the gastrointestinal tract. In 1977, when his paper was published, the imaging facilities in India were even more limited than they are now, and barium studies linked to elective or emergency laparotomy were the only available means of making the diagnosis. The high morbidity and mortality figures of this study, where toxaemia, intestinal obstruction, peritonitis and hypo-proteinaemia played important roles, has led to a constant search for less invasive methods of investigation. For those in the developed world, the luxury of CT scanning, sonography, laparoscopy and endoscopy is readily available. In the developing world, examination of ascitic fluid and blind peritoneal biopsy are often still the only diagnostic tools available to the physician.

Barium studies are still necessary to confirm the diagnosis in areas of the gastrointestinal tract that lie beyond the reach of the endoscope. They are also of considerable value in the ileocaecal region and the colon, where tuberculous enteritis or colitis commonly occurs [7, 12, 16–18, 20, 21, 32, 33, 36, 37, 43, 44].

In a series of 21 cases, Makanjuola et al. pointed out that cases of abdominal TB often present with unexpected complications, the most common of these being small-bowel intestinal obstruction, which was the presenting factor in 6 of her 21 cases. Small-bowel enema was a rewarding method of investigation. Haemorrhages severe enough to require blood transfusion were present in three cases. Endoscopy or barium enema may be inconclusive due to large quantities of blood in the bowel lumen. Angiography or isotope studies are often of value in these cases [31].

Cases presenting as malabsorption syndrome are the result of two types of complications. Tuberculous internal fistulas can short circuit the small bowel, leading to a state of malabsorption, but sub-mucosal infiltration by macrophages in cases of enteric TB leads to a Whipple-like state of malabsorption. The presentation of gastrointestinal TB as malabsorption appears to be common on the Indian sub-continent. Fistula formation is particularly common in the dual AIDS–TB infection. Changes in the mucosal pattern, the presence of ulceration and variations in the lumen of the bowel are all important indicators of tuberculous disease. Unfortunately, these changes are non-specific, as is demonstration of changes in the spacing of bowel loops, resulting from ascites, cold abscess formation or mesenteric, inflammatory thickening. These symptoms, as well as fistula formation, are also found in a great number of infectious, inflammatory, benign and malignant diseases.

TB of the gastrointestinal tract is not confined to the bowel wall and, although demonstrating intrinsic lesions, barium studies convey little or no information about the complex patterns of tuberculous disease affecting the mesentery, peritoneum and lymphatic system. The combination of CT scanning, sonography and separate barium studies reveals the true extent of the disease. Combined with endoscopic, laparoscopic, sonographic or CT-guided biopsy, the diagnosis can be made in a high proportion of cases. These investigations, linked with the investigation of the ascitic fluid, are the armamentarium of today's physician. In particular, CT diagnosis of gastrointestinal TB has evolved since the first papers describing findings in abdominal TB. High-density ascites, low-density lymph nodes with rim enhancement, irregular soft-tissue densities in the omentum, and ascitic fluid and bowel forming poorly defined masses were described [24, 28, 29, 45]. A good outline of the bowel lumen using oral contrast agents enables accurate measurement of bowel-wall thickening and often outlines the extent of ileocaecal disease [21, 28, 29, 35, 39, 46]. A limitation of CT and ultrasound examination is their failure to accurately define stenosis in the bowel in patients with threatened obstruction. Thickening of the ileocaecal valve and the caecal wall around it, as well as local lymph-node enlargement, are highly suggestive patterns. Serial studies of enlarged lymph nodes after intravenous contrast injection define patterns of enhancement characteristic – but not specific – for TB, and enhancement of the peritoneum helps to differentiate between TB and the more irregular and nodular pattern common in peritoneal malignancy [22, 39, 40]. In the ileocaecal region, sonography has been shown to document characteristic changes. An empty right iliac fossa results from contracture and upward displacement of the caecum (Fig. 6.3). Bowel-wall thickening reveals itself as the "third-kidney sign", and caecal ulceration may be seen [12]. Associated mesenteric inflammatory changes linked with localised ascitic collections held between bowel loops are responsible for a pattern of linear, alternating high and low echoes, known as the "club-sandwich sign" [11, 12, 15, 19]. Although small lymph nodes localised to the ileocaecal region are rarely seen with ultrasound, the larger, distal enlarged nodes are readily visible.

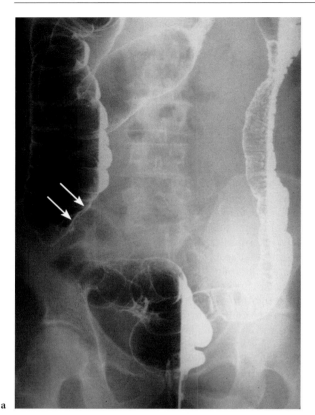

a

Fig. 6.3. a Barium enema in the left-side-down decubitus position. The patient presented with a right iliac fossa mass. The caecal tip fails to fill on this horizontal-beam study (*arrows*). **b** Ultrasound examination demonstrates the „third kidney sign", due to the thickened caecal wall (*arrows*), and the thickened wall of the terminal ileum (*arrowheads*). A common appearance in ileocaecal tuberculosis

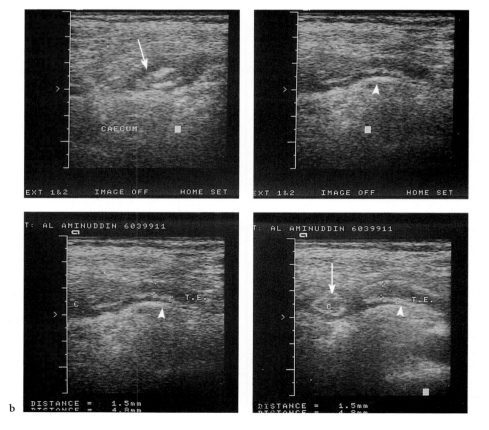

b

■ Tuberculous Enteritis and Enterocolitis

The ileocaecal region is by far the most common area of infection in tuberculous enteritis, but any part of the jejunum or ileum can be affected [17, 19, 20, 21, 31, 32, 36, 37, 43, 44]. After colonisation of the submucosal lymphatic tissue by the mycobacterium, resulting in granulomatous tubercle formation, ulceration in the overlying mucosa develops. These ulcers multiply and may become circumferential; characteristically, they are linear and transverse. Short or long segments of small bowel are involved, with superficial or deep ulceration, mucosal oedema, spasms and thickening of the bowel wall. In the hypertrophic type, luminal narrowing may be severe. Acute or sub-acute intestinal obstruction may develop in the ulcerative type due to cicatrisation and fibrotic healing. All of the intraluminal lesions are visible in barium studies; the changes in the bowel wall, mesenteric inflammation, lymphadenopathy and ascites are seen in sonographic and CT examinations.

Skip lesions with intervening normal segments are common, and dilated loops between narrow segments and stenoses are a feature. Other causes of obstruction are the result of matted, kinked bowel loops, fibrotic healing of mesenteric lesions and, more rarely, obstruction due to outside pressure from lymphoid masses (Figs. 6.4, 6.5).

Ultrasound examination of the small bowel is often limited by the presence of gas in overlying intestinal loops. Visualisation of bowel loops enables measurements of the thickness of the wall to be made. CT also demonstrates the presence of wall thickening. Kedar et al. identified a thickness of 5 mm to be abnormal; in dilated bowel loops, 3 mm was abnormal [12]. Internal fistulas are seen, and may lead to the formation of blind loops with malabsorption syndromes [32]. Rarely, in the case of the small bowel, external fistulas occur. Perforation is also a complication and is often closed off by local peritoneal adhesions [21, 32] (Fig. 6.6).

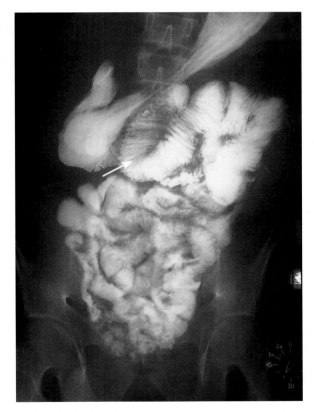

Fig. 6.4. On barium follow-through examination, there is a mass of dilated, matted jejunal loops (*arrow*). This mass displaces the stomach. This was a young woman who experienced considerable weight loss. Peritoneal endoscopy revealed tubercles

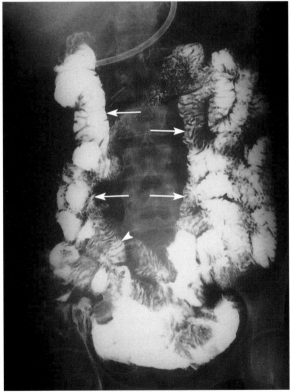

Fig. 6.5. Small-bowel enema in a young woman with a central abdominal mass, which proved to be thickened tuberculous mesentery. The small bowel is displaced from the midline (*arrows*), and there is thickening of the ileal mucosal folds (*arrowhead*)

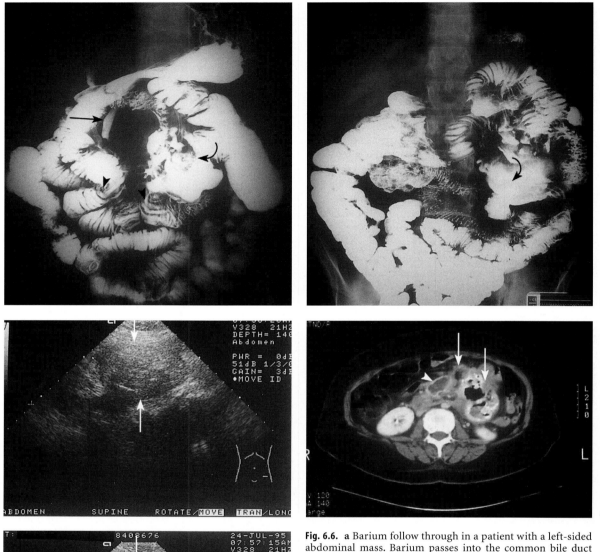

Fig. 6.6. **a** Barium follow through in a patient with a left-sided abdominal mass. Barium passes into the common bile duct through a fistula (*arrow*). There is displacement of midline bowel loops, which show dilatation and thickened mucosa (*arrowheads*). There is a collection of barium pooled in the region of the left-sided mass (*curved arrow*). **b** Later in the study, there are thick-walled loops of jejunum seen, and there is a collection of barium outside the bowel lumen (*curved arrow*). **c** Ultrasound of the area of the mass revealed an apparently homogeneous solid lesion (*arrows*). **d** Post-contrast computed-tomography examination demonstrated a complex mass of bowel loops and an abscess cavity containing oral contrast medium and air (*arrows*). Anterior to the aorta is a group of enlarged lymph nodes showing rim enhancement (*arrowhead*). These nodes probably represent the lesion demonstrated by ultrasound. The patient responded to anti-tuberculosis chemotherapy

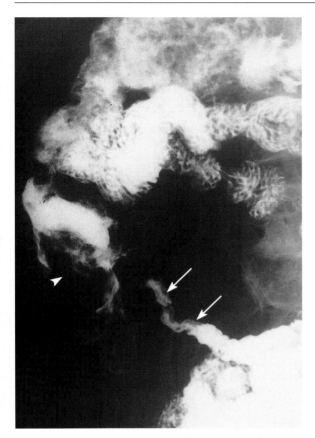

Fig. 6.7. Ilio-caecal tuberculosis. The terminal ileum is narrowed, ulcerated and demonstrated reduced motility (*arrows*). The tip of the caecum failed to fill (*arrowhead*). There was a mass present in the right iliac fossa. Colonoscopy and caecal biopsy is often fruitful in these cases

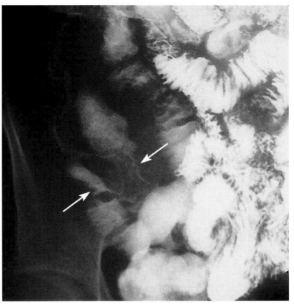

Fig. 6.8. Small-bowel enema shows oedema and thickening of the terminal ileal loops. The caecum fails to fill (*arrows*)

Despite imaging techniques, without biopsy material, the diagnosis can only be inferred. Laparoscopic visualisation of serosal tubercles and the histology of biopsy specimens is a valuable diagnostic tool and, even where erythaemic serosal lesions (as opposed to serosal tubercles) are biopsied, the bacteriological and histological picture is diagnostic in a high proportion of cases [25]. Laparotomy should be avoided wherever possible and a trial of anti-tuberculous chemotherapy instigated. Even severe stenotic lesions have been seen to resolve with conservative treatment. Surgical intervention should be reserved for either emergency situations or for elective operations in cases of intestinal obstruction.

The appearances of the terminal ileum and its relationship to the caecum are of great importance in both small-bowel and barium-enema studies. In TB, the caecum is often shortened due to fibrotic contraction, and this, in turn, straightens the terminal ileum. The distal part of the caecum may develop a conical appearance or, in advanced cases, fail to fill with barium [44] (Figs. 6.7, 6.8). The terminal ileum, in some cases, appears to empty directly into the ascending colon (Stierlin's sign). In other cases, the inflexible, gaping ileocaecal valve is associated with narrowing and ulceration of the terminal ileum (Fleischner's sign) [35]. Differentiation from Crohn's ileocolitis, other infectious lesions, carcinoma and amoeboma on barium studies alone is not possible, and the application of other diagnostic methods, including CT scanning, laparoscopy and endoscopy, along with histological and bacterial study of biopsy material, is necessary to make the diagnosis [35, 37, 43, 44, 47–52] (Fig. 6.9).

■ Tuberculous Colitis

By far the most common form of tuberculous colitis (TBC) is the combined ileocaecal infection, which accounts for up to 90% of cases [35, 47] (Figs. 6.10, 6.11). Less common is segmental colitis, affecting the ascending, transverse or descending colon. Unusually, a pan-colitis occurs in 1–2% of cases and is difficult to differentiate from ulcerative colitis. Clinically, the patient complains of abdominal pain, weight loss and diarrhoea. Rectal blood loss may be a feature, as may fever and anorexia (Fig. 6.12).

The abdomen is usually tender to palpation and, when the ileocaecal segment is affected, a palpable mass is usually present. Ascites is detectable in up to 10% of cases. Hepatomegaly, if present, may yield

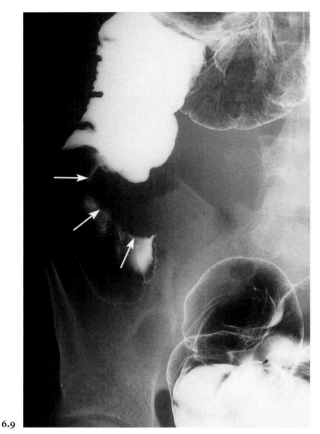

Fig. 6.9. Barium-enema-demonstrated space occupation around the ileocaecal valve and the mesenteric wall of the caecum (*arrows*). This was thought to be due to a tumour. Endoscopic biopsy produced tissue containing granulomas and alcohol acid-fast bacilli

evidence of hepatic granuloma on biopsy. Only 30% of cases show evidence of TB on chest radiographs. The imaging appearances are governed by histological changes, and double-contrast barium enemas reveal the intra-luminal changes.

The mucosa is ulcerated by clean-cut transverse lesions. These give rise to local spasms, and healing changes lead to short-stricture formation. Sub-mucosal nodules are seen, as are polypoid mucosal changes and, rarely, filiform polyposis [51] (Fig. 6.13).

Rarely, aphthous ulceration or cobblestone-like mucosal patterns raise the possibility of Crohn's disease. Usually, the changes are segmental, and ileocaecal TB may coexist with segmental TB in other areas of the colon. CT examination is helpful in defining lymphadenopathy, the nodes showing rim enhancement, and the characteristic changes in the ileocaecal valve and the medial caecal wall may also be demonstrated. Ascites, if present will be seen, as will enhancement of the parietal peritoneum.

Ultrasound is generally only of value in ileocaecal lesions, as the presence of intraluminal gas often diminishes the value of the images. The endoscopic appearances and biopsy material, together, differentiate TBC from other inflammatory colitides [50], ulcerative colitis, benign and malignant polyps, amoebiasis and Crohn's disease. The results on barium studies and CT are not characteristic (Fig. 6.14). Shah et al. diagnosed TBC on the basis of biopsy findings in 40 of 50 patients. Histological appearances were helpful, but the results of bacteriological studies were disappointing, the results of microscopy and culture being positive in 6% of cases [47]. Tandon et al. had a higher positive culture rate of four out of eleven cases (Fig. 6.15) [52].

Gastrointestinal TB in Less Common Sites

Oesophageal TB

In immunocompetent patients, oesophageal TB is a rare occurrence. Recent reports indicate that it is not uncommon amongst patients with AIDS [34, 53] (Chap. 8).

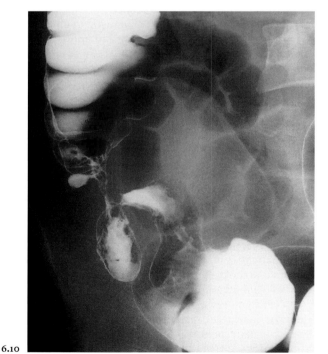

Fig. 6.10. Classical appearances of the contracted caecal tip, stenosis of the caecum and abnormal terminal ileum in ileocaecal tuberculosis

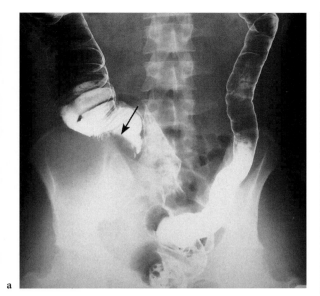

a

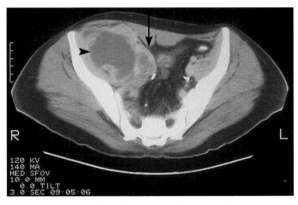

b

Fig. 6.11. a A right-iliac-fossa mass displaces the caecum upwards and medially. The caecal tip fails to fill (*arrow*). **b** Computed tomography of the same patient demonstrates an abscess in the caecal tip (*arrow*) and a large, tuberculous iliopsoas collection (*arrowhead*)

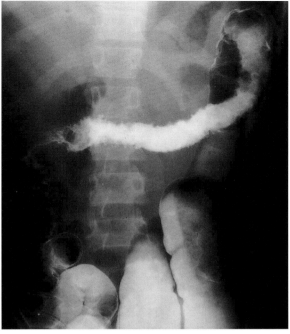

Fig. 6.12. Barium enema in a case of tuberculous colitis, with many deep mucosal ulcers. Indistinguishable from ulcerative colitis or Crohn's colitis. Endoscopy and biopsy is necessary to make the diagnosis

The rarity of the disease may be due to the physical structure and function of the oesophagus. Lack of stasis due to peristalsis, and the stratified epithelium, which is coated with saliva, are thought to provide protection from the mycobacterium. Rubenstein suggested four mechanisms leading to oesophageal tuberculous infection:

1. Infection of a pre-existing, non-tuberculous mucosal lesion
2. Direct extension from infection in the larynx and pharynx
3. Direct extension from structures outside the oesophagus, usually lymph nodes, rarely from tuberculous spondylitis
4. Haematogenous spread [54]

Most reported cases arise as a result of spread from infected, contiguous mediastinal, lymph nodes. Enlarged nodes often compress and displace the oesophagus (Fig. 6.16). The lesion is most often in the plane of the bifurcation of the trachea. Perihilar or subcarinal lymphogenous tissue is usually involved [55, 56].

Dysphagia is the common symptom and may be accompanied by epigastric or substernal pain (Fig. 6.17). Fever is sometimes present. A history of past tuberculous lymphadenopathy or pulmonary TB may be forthcoming. Concurrent mediastinal lymphadenopathy or active pulmonary TB is usual. Broncho-oesophageal fistulas are a common complication and, in such cases, coughing attacks after swallowing are characteristic (Fig. 6.18). Laryngitis and cervical and supraclavicular lymph-node enlargement have been reported as precursors of oesophageal lesions [55, 57, 58]. Primary oesophageal TB is unusual. Marshal et al. describe a case presenting with dysphagia due to a single, deep oesophageal ulcer. There was no evidence of any other tuberculous focus. Penetration of the ulcer through the oesophageal wall and multiple sinuses in the ulcer bed led to a small mediastinal abscess. Whether or not this represented an initial focus in a necrotic lymph node was not clear [59]. Mucosal ulceration is

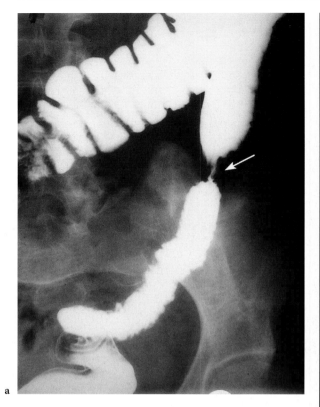

a

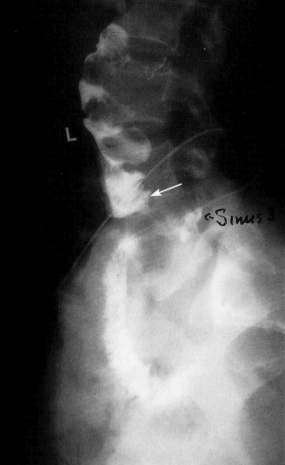

c

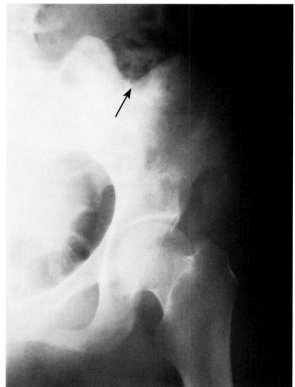

b

Fig. 6.13. a Barium enema in a woman complaining of abdominal pain and a chronic discharging sinus in the left flank. A short, stenotic segment of colon is seen, related to a defect in the iliac crest (*arrow*). **b** Radiograph of the pelvis demonstrates a "V"-shaped bone defect with some surrounding bone sclerosis. **c** A sinogram. The injected contrast passes through the area of defective bone and enters the stenotic region of the colon through a fistula (*arrow*)

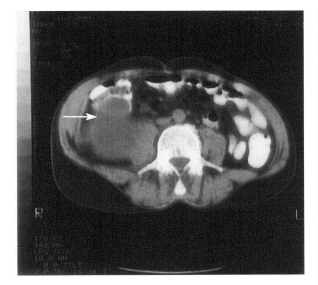

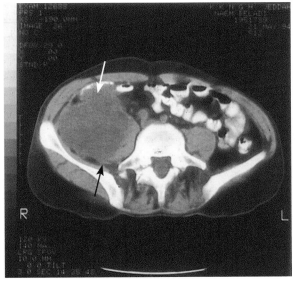

Fig. 6.14. A psoas sheath collection thought, initially, to be tuberculous (*arrows*). Fine-needle-aspiration biopsy produced mucin from a mucin-producing carcinoma of the caecal tip

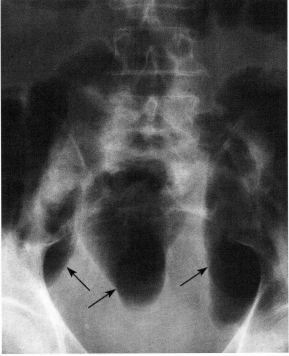

a

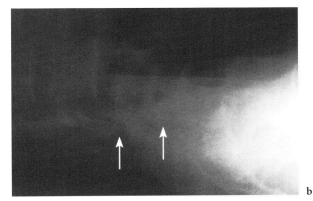

b

Fig. 6.15 a, b. A very obese 60-year-old man presented with severe lower-abdominal and back pain. He had been constipated for some days. He could not sit or lie on his side. Plain radiographs appeared to indicate low intestinal obstruction. Dilated colonic loops were noted (*arrows*). On the horizontal-beam lateral image (b), the fluid levels were thought to be in the bowel (*arrows*). **c** s. page 122

the usual lesion. The ulcers are linear and clear cut. They are surrounded by normal mucosa, in contrast to colonic ulcers, which demonstrate surrounding mucosal erythema and friability [47, 52]. Biopsy samples reveal caseating granulomas, and AAFB may be seen on staining or culture [58, 59]. A second type of lesion is hypertrophic [57] or encephaloid and may be combined with ulceration. Barium studies reveal compression and displacement of the oesophagus by

mediastinal lymph nodes. Mucosal irregularity is due to ulceration, which may lead to sinus formation. As broncho-oesophageal fistula may be present, water soluble contrast medium should be used initially, and barium should be employed with caution.

CT scanning delineates thickening of the oesophageal wall, the extent of mediastinal lymph-node infection and any associated abscess formation. Oesophagoscopy presents difficulties when the oeso-

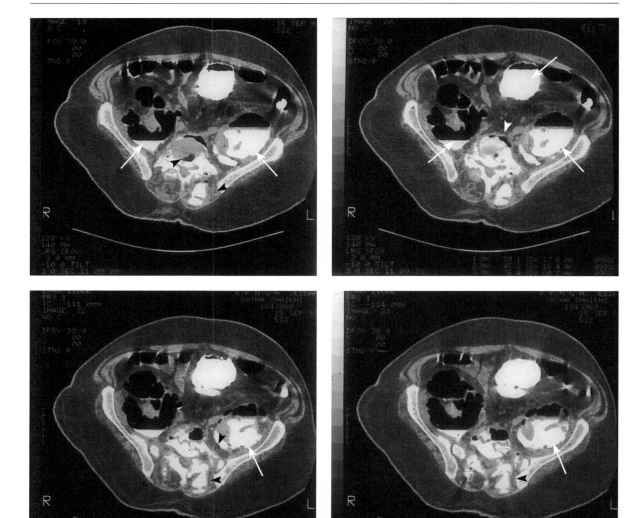

c

Fig. 6.15 (*continued*). **c** A limited barium-enema examination was begun, but the barium passed immediately into the cavity of a pelvic abscess, so the examination was abandoned. Computed-tomography examination demonstrated a number of abscess cavities containing air and barium (*arrows*). The body and left ala of the first sacral segment has been destroyed by tuberculous osteitis, and barium has passed through the bone abscess into the muscles of the back (*arrowheads*)

phagus is compressed or displaced. True stenosis does not occur. ^{67}Ga-citrate scanning has a place in investigation. The isotope is taken up in the infected oesophagus itself and in the involved lymph nodes [58]. The response to anti-tuberculosis chemotherapy is satisfactory but, in cases complicated by fistula formation, surgery may be required. In the case of chronic broncho-oesophageal fistula, pulmonary lobectomy may be required to close the fistula and remove bronchiectatic lung.

Gastric TB

Gastric TB is rare in developed countries. With the increase in numbers of the susceptible patient groups, one must expect an increase in incidence in the coming years [1,33]. In the pre-chemotherapy era, Good reported a gastric TB frequency of between 0.3% and 2.3% in autopsies of patients with pulmonary TB [54].

In areas where TB is endemic, gastric TB is still uncommon. Bhansali reported one partial gastrectomy among 300 patients [32]. In a series of 100 cases of

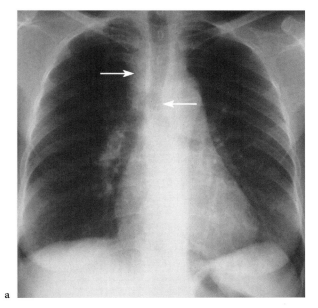

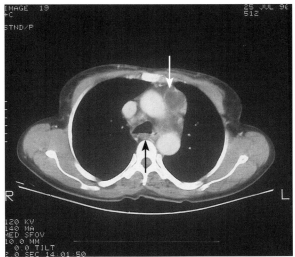

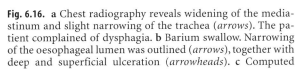

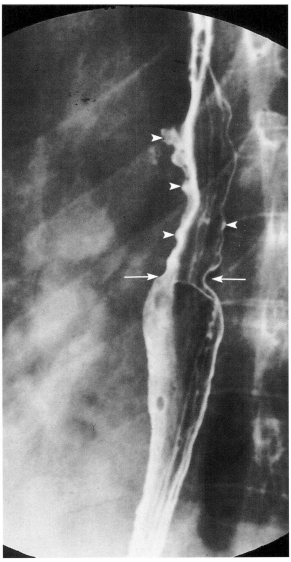

Fig. 6.16. **a** Chest radiography reveals widening of the mediastinum and slight narrowing of the trachea (*arrows*). The patient complained of dysphagia. **b** Barium swallow. Narrowing of the oesophageal lumen was outlined (*arrows*), together with deep and superficial ulceration (*arrowheads*). **c** Computed tomography after contrast defined an extensive, tuberculous, mediastinal abscess surrounding the trachea and oesophagus and extending anteriorly to involve ring-enhancing, enlarged lymph nodes in the para-aortic area (*arrows*)

gastrointestinal TB in Saudi Arabia, there were five cases of gastric TB. Of these, three were apparent primary cases, and two had simultaneous infection elsewhere in the gastrointestinal tract. One case had concomitant supraclavicular lymphadenopathy, and another both hepatic and colonic TB (Al Karawi and Yasawi, personal communication).

As in the case of the oesophagus, physical reasons are postulated for the rarity of gastric involvement. The low pH of the stomach contents, the relatively rapid emptying of the stomach and the sparse pre-sence of gastric lymphoid tissue may be factors. In comparison, in the caecum there is stasis of the contents and a relatively high sub-mucosal lymphatic-tissue content.

The presence of a pre-existing mucosal lesion seems to be a factor characteristic of this disease and, in one of Karawi's patients, a signet cell carcinoma with tuberculous supra-infection was found at operation. Other associations include non-Hodgkins lymphoma [17] and gastric adenocarcinoma [16].

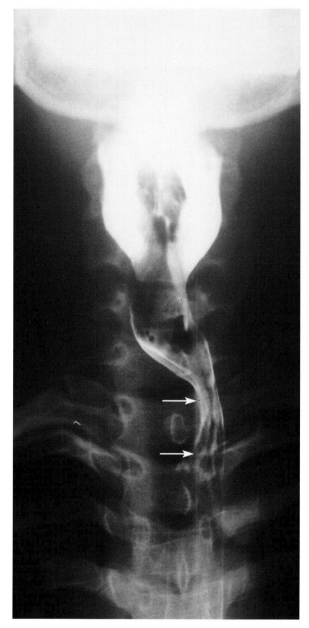

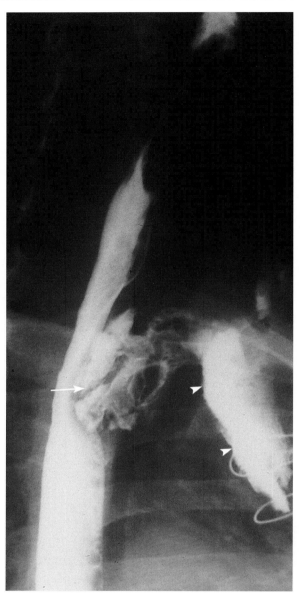

Fig. 6.17. Barium swallow. The more usual type of oesophageal involvement is obstruction due to external pressure from enlarged tuberculous lymph nodes (*arrows*)

Fig. 6.18. Perforation of the oesophagus by a para-tracheal abscess (*arrow*). The abscess extends retro-sternally (*arrowheads*). It was the result of a mass of tuberculous lymph nodes in the para-tracheal group. The patient had had coronary artery surgery in the past

Spread from adjacent lymph nodes can be the origin of infection, as can haematogenous spread. The role of pulmonary TB is unclear. Although, at the time of introduction of chemotherapy, Mitchell and Bristol [54] demonstrated a link between the severity of pulmonary TB and associated gastric TB, recent studies have reported other findings. Pettengell et al., in a study of 50 patients with active cavitating TB, found 23 cases of gastrointestinal TB, but the oeso-

phagus, stomach and duodenum were not affected in this series [26].

Gastric TB affects a young age group; the average age in Karawi's series was 27 years, excluding the patient with simultaneous carcinoma of the stomach, who was 65 years old. Abdominal pain and weight loss are the usual presenting symptoms, but haematemesis and melaena may be present, and symptoms of pyloric obstruction may intervene. The chest ra-

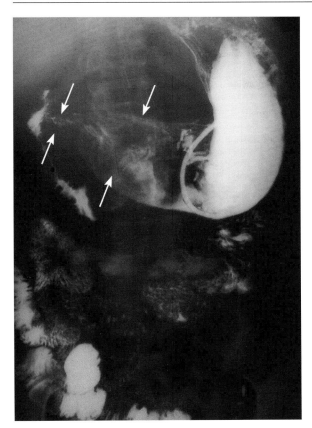

Fig. 6.19. Pyloric stenosis and obstruction resulting from hypertrophic tuberculosis of the pyloric antrum (*arrows*)

diograph is normal in over 50% of cases, but tuberculin skin testing is rewarding. As in TB at other gastrointestinal sites, ulcerative lesions predominate. Hypertrophic and ulcero-hypertrophic lesions are less frequent. Pyloric obstruction may arise from both pyloric deformity, due to ulceration, oedema, inflammatory changes and fibrosis, or to a combination of gastric-wall changes combined with lymphadenopathy in the gastric-outlet region. Four of five of Karawi's cases had gastric-outlet obstruction (Fig. 6.19).

Sub-mucosal granulomas with caseation and giant cells are histological pointers to the diagnosis and, although the tests for the presence of AAFB on direct smear in biopsy material are disappointing, mycobacterial culture has a high rate of success. Barium studies reveal non-specific findings, similar to those seen in peptic ulcers, gastric lymphoma, carcinoma and the granulomatous diseases syphilis and sarcoidosis. Eosinophilic gastroenteritis must also be considered in the differential diagnosis, but the common disease that must be excluded is Crohn's disease, for which the radiological appearances are

similar. Treatment with steroids for presumed Crohn's disease in cases of TB can have dire effects [35].

CT examination is of value in showing the extent of associated lymphadenopathy and in follow-up studies. Endoscopy is of great value. The gastric mucosa appears erythematous and inflamed, and submucosal nodules may be present [20]. Clean-cut ulcers or hypertrophic lesions provide biopsy material. In addition to biopsy, for both histology and culture, a search should be made for other sites of systemic and gastrointestinal infection. In particular, peritoneal, ileocaecal, hepatic or colonic TB may be present [16,17,20]. Anti-tuberculous chemotherapy is the treatment of choice, but those cases with pyloric obstruction will require surgical relief.

Duodenal TB

Primary TB of the duodenum is rare, occurring in 1–3% of patients with gastrointestinal TB [37]. In three recently published studies from Saudi Arabia, it was found in 1/65 [18], 3/130 [20] and 1/112 [21] of cases of abdominal TB.

Duodenal obstruction due to involvement with a lymph-node mass is a much more likely presentation. This was the case in 15 of Bhansali's 300 cases [32], in 22 of Gupta's 30 cases [60] and in two out of 23 cases in Denton's study [17]. The clinical picture is of epigastric pain, often over a long period, which is sometimes worsened by food. Accompanying anorexia, nausea, vomiting and weight loss are, in some ways, similar to the symptoms of peptic ulcer, but night pain and relief by food are not a feature.

As the disease progresses, these symptoms are overlain by those of high intestinal obstruction. Vomiting becomes more of a feature and weight loss may be dramatic. Low-grade fever and haematemesis are also described [31, 61]. Patients with obstruction due to lymphadenopathy present with an upper abdominal mass, recognisable on sonography or CT examination.

In intrinsic tuberculous duodenitis, the symptoms and signs are those of proximal duodenal disease or gastric-outlet obstruction, and both the pylorus and the duodenal bulb are often simultaneously involved by the infection. Barium examination demonstrates pyloric-wall thickening and narrowing to the lumen. The duodenal bulb is often deformed, and the deformity leads to obstruction at the level of the bulb or in the post-bulbar duodenum.

In these cases, endoscopy is difficult, and passage of the endoscope beyond a distal obstruction impossible. The mucosa proximal to the lesion will often only show the signs of non-specific duodenitis or a normal mucosa. As the degree of obstruction is often advanced at the time of presentation, laparotomy with surgical relief is, in many cases, the treatment of choice [62].

In those cases where endoscopic visualisation of the duodenum is possible, the ulcerative form of TB is usual. Ulcers are small and multiple. Biopsy reveals submucosal, caseating granulomas, but initial bacteriological studies are often unrewarding.

As the site of lymphadenopathy is, in most cases, in the prepancreatic and superior mesenteric artery regions, duodenal obstruction due to extrinsic pressure affects the distal duodenum. On barium examination, the first and second divisions of the duodenum are distended and show thickening of the mucosal folds. There is often a sharp cut-off of the lumen at the site of the superior mesenteric artery. Sonography and CT examination demonstrate a matted mass of lymph nodes and inflammatory tissue in the mesenteric root, compressing the third and fourth parts of the duodenum, often at the ligament of Treitz [17, 60].

Internal fistula formation is not uncommon. Duodenal communication with the right renal pyelum leads to a non-functioning right kidney [62, 63]. Duodeno-enteric and duodeno-colonic fistulae also occur (Al Karawi and Yasawy, personal communication). Duodenal-aortic fistula is an exceedingly rare complication [64].

In cases of primary duodenal TB, the lesion is usually isolated. In cases of disease resulting from para-aortic lymph-node enlargement, tuberculous enteritis is likely to be present in the small bowel or colon, and there is a high incidence of hepatic and splenic TB.

TB of the Appendix

There are two main types of TB infection of the appendix. The most common form is where the appendix is infected by direct extension of an ileocaecal lesion. In these cases, the signs and symptoms are those of the dormant ileocaecal infection. Appendicular TB with a normal ileocaecum is much less common. There is usually TB elsewhere in the gastrointestinal tract. In both types of appendicitis, both acute and chronic inflammation occurs. Often, acute appendicitis, as a result of obstruction of the appendix lumen, is the presenting symptom of ileocaecal disease and, in suspected cases, sonographic assessment is mandatory before appendicular surgery. Acute appendicitis occurred in six of 100 cases of abdominal TB recently treated in Saudi Arabia (Al Karawi and Yasawy, personal communication); emergency laparotomy was necessary in all of these cases.

In chronic appendicitis, intermittent right iliac fossa pain is a feature, and periappendicular abscess with a mass lesion is a common presentation. Sonography is helpful in defining the appendicular abscess. Singh reported two cases of acute inflammation in 17 cases of proven tuberculous appendicitis [65], Bhansali reported one case in 300 [32] and Al Karawi five cases of appendicitis in 130 instances of abdominal TB [20].

Anal TB

In the last few decades of the post-chemotherapy era, anal TB became a rarity. With the emergence of the "new tuberculosis" [66], anal TB is reappearing. Jakubowski reported 16 cases in a series of 81 cases of abdominal TB. Many of these were alcoholic or drug-dependent patients, and eight of the 16 had active pulmonary TB [7]. Anal TB has remained a common disease in the developing world and, as in the West, is characterised by an anal ulcer, fissure, fistula or as a hypertrophic, often warty growth. Crohn's disease is a much more common cause of such lesions in the West, and this, as well as carcinoma and venereal disease, must be considered in the diagnosis. Despite the high proportion of active TB in Jakubowski's cases, the chest radiograph may be normal and the Mantoux reaction negative. Biopsy and bacteriological investigation should be carried out on all anal lesions.

■ Solid-Organ Abdominal TB

Hepatosplenic TB

In patients with AIDS, both *M. Tuberculosis* and atypical mycobacteria infect the liver and spleen. These infections in AIDS sufferers have a different imaging spectrum from that seen in immunocompetent patients, and are dealt with separately in the section on AIDS and TB.

There are two chief types of hepatosplenic TB in non-AIDS patients. The common form is a widespread infection of the hepatic or splenic tissues or of both simultaneously. This is the result of haematogenous spread of infection, often from pulmonary or miliary TB, but in some cases spread occurs through the portal venous system from gastrointestinal lesions. The usual manifestation is hepatosplenomegaly; either the liver or spleen is clinically palpable or measures 20 cm and 13 cm, respectively, on CT or sonography in adults. In two recent studies of reported gastrointestinal TB, 24 of 65 patients had hepatic and 15 of 65 splenic manifestations [18], and 19 of

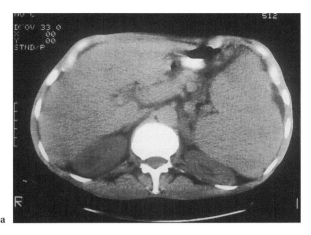

a

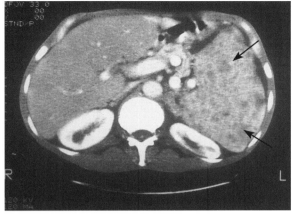

b

Fig. 6.20 a, b. Pre- and post-contrast computed-tomography examination in splenic tuberculosis. The spleen is enlarged and contains numerous non-enhancing granulomas (*arrows*)

130 cases exhibited hepatic TB [20]. These cases were part of two groups with proven peritoneal, small-bowel or colonic infection.

Much less common is the macronodular form of hepatic or splenic disease. In the rare primary type, no other intra-abdominal lesion is seen, and there is no obvious focus elsewhere in the body [67–72]. This type of macronodular disease is also reported in small numbers in patients presenting with tuber-

Fig. 6.21. Hepato-splenic tuberculosis. Post-contrast comput-ed-tomography examination. There are multiple, hypodense granulomas in the liver and spleen (*arrows*). One in the liver contains a focus that enhances centrally (*arrowheads*). Those in the spleen fail to enhance

culous gastrointestinal or abdominal lymph-node lesions [9, 17, 19, 21, 29, 30, 73] (Figs. 6.20, 6.21).

In the miliary type of infection, either the liver or the spleen – or, in some cases, both organs – may be infected. It has been suggested that, in addition to the systemic haematogenous route, the pathway of infection may include spread by way of the portal venous system or by lymphatic spread via porta-hepatis lymphatics.

Low-grade fever, weight loss and localised pain are presenting features. Disturbed hepatic function is a common laboratory finding, but TB is often un-suspected, although the Mantoux reaction is positive in a high proportion of cases. Hepatic or splenic tenderness and enlargement are often the only ab-normal findings on clinical examination.

Histologically, tissue acquired by fine-needle-aspiration biopsy, reveals widespread microscopic granulomas. These show both caseating and non-caseating qualities, and epithelioid cells and giant

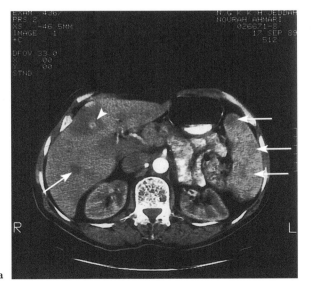

a

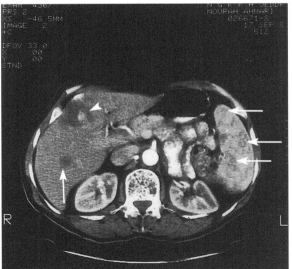

b

cells may be present. Immediate staining for AAFB has poor results, but cultures are positive in about 60 % of cases. The granulomas are too small to be visualised on CT or sonography but, collectively, produce a "bright" echogenic picture of the liver or spleen.

In endemic areas, other causes of granulomatous disease must be considered, and *Brucella*, bilharzia, fungal disease, biliary cirrhosis and sarcoidosis must all be excluded, as well as less common conditions, such as typhoid, familial granulomatous hepatitis and drug-induced granulomatosis [74]. The presence of tuberculous lymphadenopathy or gastrointestinal lesions points towards TB as the diagnosis, and examination of any ascitic fluid for the level of adenosine deaminase is useful.

Relatively few cases of primary macronodular hepato-splenic lesions have been reported. Macronodular lesions in the spleen have become relatively common in AIDS cases but remain uncommon in the general population.

The clinical presentation of macronodular disease is similar to that of the diffuse condition. In some cases, the presence of calcification in the lesions suggests chronicity before presentation and makes plain radiography of the abdomen worthwhile [69, 73]. Macronodular lesions may be single or multiple, and their relative rarity means that pyogenic, fungal or amoebic abscesses are usually the considered diagnosis, as well as primary or metastatic neoplasms and lymphoma, which are much more common conditions (Fig. 6.22).

The imaging appearances are in no way characteristic, and there is a wide range of sonographic and CT findings. Although, echographically, the lesions are usually homogeneously hypoechoic, echogenic appearances have been reported, and calcification

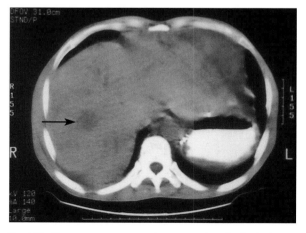

Fig. 6.22. Pre-contrast computed tomography of a single, hypodense, tuberculous granuloma in the right lobe of the liver (*arrow*). Diagnosis was made by fine-needle biopsy

may lead to acoustic shadowing [17, 67–70]. CT scanning reveals widespread, rounded, low-attenuation lesions similar to those seen in pyogenic and fungal abscess [75] (Fig. 6.23)

Metastatic foci from intra-abdominal adenocarcinoma produce confusingly similar lesions and must be distinguished by fine-needle biopsy. The hepatic metastases of mucus-producing tumours of the colon are known to contain variable amounts of calcification and may also show similar appearances.

The "cluster sign", seen in pyogenic lesions, where multiple small abscesses appear to coalesce to form a larger abscess, is also reported [73, 76]. The changes seen in CT images after intravenous contrast injection are also varied.

Some lesions are hypodense and non-enhancing. A second common manifestation is hypodensity with rim enhancement. The inner, non-enhancing core represents caseation, but echoes the appearances of central necroses seen in both metastases and pyogenic lesions. MRI is also non-specific in defining hepatic tuberculomas, but there are a number of features helping to differentiate them from other hepatic ring lesions. Primary hepatocellular carcinoma, haematomas, inflammatory cysts, amoebic abscesses and the various types of haemangiomas all come into consideration. Despite some differences in appearance on sonograms, CT and MRI, biopsy for histology and culture will be needed where there is an overlap in imaging appearances. This is almost always so in the case of hepatic metastatic disease [72, 77, 78].

Large, single hepatic or splenic lesions are usually similar in appearance to smaller, widespread tuberculomas. Large tuberculomas have been described as having an internal 'honeycomb' appearance and little enhancement centrally or peripherally [68].

Varying degrees of calcification have been reported, both in tuberculomas and in liver or splenic tissue. Some calcifications indicate spontaneous healing, but active tuberculomas and calcified foci occur simultaneously in a number of cases [75].

Splenic tuberculomas are often single and, on CT examination, are large, low-attenuating lesions. Rim enhancement is not universally present and may depend on the age or maturity of the tuberculoma [68, 70, 71].

In the immunosuppressed non-AIDS patient, widespread, hypoechoic, low-attenuating lesions may be due to either TB or to fungal abscesses, and ^{67}Ga-citrate scans are helpful in confirming the inflammatory nature of the disease. Echo-guided biopsy will be necessary to distinguish between fungal and tubercular infection [79].

Splenic lesions can occur without apparent hepatic involvement and without evidence of TB elsewhere. In these cases, lymphoma will usually be

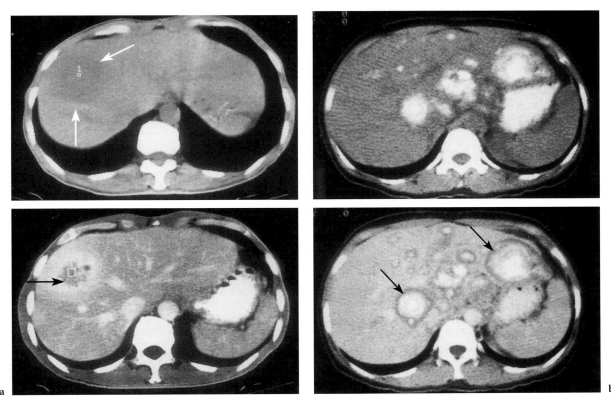

a

b

Fig. 6.23. a Pre- and post-contrast computed-tomography scans of the liver. The pre-contrast image shows a single, large, hypodense lesion in the right hepatic lobe (*arrows*). Post-contrast, the hepatic abscess enhances intensely peripherally. The central area remains hypodense due to the presence of caseating material (*arrow*). **b** Pre- and post-contrast CT scans of the liver. There is extensive focal, hepatic calcification in hepatic tuberculous granulomas. After contrast injection, the calcified foci show a halo of non-enhancing granulomatous tissue (*arrows*). Images by courtesy of Dr. J. Pang, Department of Medicine, Prince of Wales Hospital, Shatin, Hong Kong

the presumptive diagnosis, imaging findings may be similar in the two conditions, and scintigraphic studies will be of little value, as lymphoma tissue takes up the Ga isotope. Aspiration biopsy will be necessary to make the diagnosis. Recently, numerous cases of isolated splenic TB have been reported in AIDS patients [80–82].

Although uptake of gallium is seen in a number of other conditions, such as lymphoma, septic abscess and sarcoidosis, isotope scanning is still of considerable value in abdominal TB. Focal uptake in lesions in the liver or spleen can be confirmed by sonographic or CT examination, when the infection can be characterised. A great advantage of isotope study is that, as it is a whole-body study, infection in other organs can be visualised [83–85].

Pancreatic TB

Pancreatic TB is, historically, extremely rare. The pancreas is infected in the miliary spread of TB in a small number of patients. Cho quotes Auerbach (1944), reporting only 4.7% of pancreatic lesions in 297 autopsies of patients with miliary TB [86]. Pancreatic lesions in miliary disease are unlikely to be diagnosed unless accompanied by laboratory findings suggesting pancreatic dysfunction [87]. Focal pancreatic TB, or tuberculous abscess, has until recently been very seldom reported but, during the last 15 years, a number of cases have been described in the literature.

Two factors seem to be at play here. First, the increased accessibility of the pancreas to imaging by ultrasonography and axial imaging methods has lead to the diagnosis in unsuspected cases. A second factor is the predilection of TB to infect the pancreas in patients with AIDS [86, 88]. In 1982, Stambler could find no report of the condition over the previous 15 years. Since then, 12 cases have been reported in the literature [17, 21, 86–92].

Being a relatively common condition, adenocarcinoma of the pancreas is the usual presumptive diagnosis in mass lesions of the pancreas. It is a con-

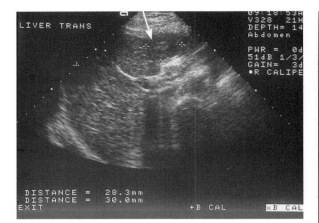

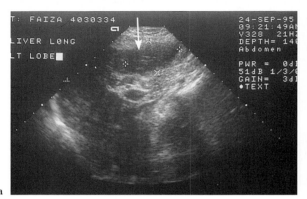

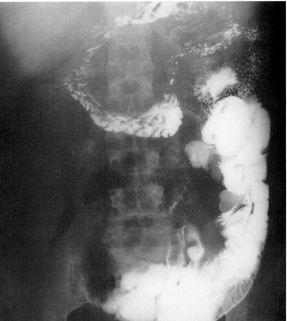

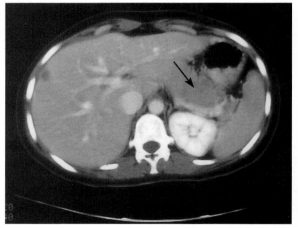

Fig. 6.24. a Transverse and sagittal ultrasound demonstrates a hypoechoic mass in the head and body of the pancreas (*arrows*). **b** Barium meal with expansion of the duodenal loop due to the mass lesion. Fine-needle biopsy obtained pus containing alcohol acid-fast bacilli (AAFB). **c** In another patient, there is a non-enhancing mass in the pancreatic tail (*arrow*). Fine-needle aspiration produced granulomatous tissue, and AAFB was cultured

dition that requires confirmation by histological diagnosis. Both malignant disease of the pancreas and pancreatic abscess in chronic pancreatitis have appearances similar to those of focal TB of the pancreas.

At aspiration or operative biopsy of a pancreatic abscess, the infecting organisms are commonly *Escherichia coli*, *Klebsiella*, *Proteus*, *Streptococcus* and *Staphylococcus aureus*. Less commonly, *Pseudomonas* or *Areobacter* are found. Uncomplicated tuberculous abscesses will yield none of these organisms, and direct staining for *M. Tuberculosis* and atypical mycobacteria, with samples for culture, is mandatory in all cases of pancreatic abscess. This is so even when pus is aspirated, as opposed to caseating tissue.

Failure of a pancreatic abscess to respond to antibiotic therapy is also a pointer towards TB being the infecting organism [87]. The histopathology of the lesion is of caseating granuloma formation, with epithelioid and giant cells aggregating into a larger lesion. Eventually, a large granuloma results, which develops central caseation and necrotic material. In biopsy reports, fibrotic and non-tuberculous inflammatory tissue has been prominent [17]. It is essential to biopsy at the edge of the lesion to successfully retrieve granulomatous tissue and mycobacteria. In patients with advanced necrosis of the focus, pus may be aspirated, with a good chance of a positive bacteriological study [17, 87, 88]. The tuberculous lesion is often in the head or neck of the pancreas, although lesions in the tail have also been described [21]. Local groups of lymph nodes are often enlarged and, on CT examination, show the characteristic appearance of hypodense nodes with rim enhancement. They may be absent during the acute stage of the infection [90].

The pancreas is often the sole site of infection, and normal chest radiography, barium studies and Mantoux reaction in no way exclude the diagnosis [86, 87]. However, a positive Mantoux reaction is reported in the majority of cases and, in some, a previous history of TB was elicited. In one case, an associated erythematous skin lesion showing caseating granulomas on biopsy, proved to be tubercular [91]. Despite a predilection of the pancreatic head, and in contrast to pancreatic carcinoma, tuberculous abscess is rarely a cause of obstructive jaundice [89].

The clinical presentation is of weight loss, low-grade fever, anorexia and upper abdominal pain. The constant back pain of pancreatic carcinoma is uncommon in tuberculoma. Pointers towards the diagnosis include the absence of a history of chronic pancreatitis or chronic biliary disease. Alcoholism poses a diagnostic problem, as alcoholics are susceptible to both chronic pancreatitis and TB. Sonography is the initial examination of choice and reveals a well-defined, hypoechoic lesion in the pancreas, usually in the pancreatic head, neck or, less commonly, the body or tail (Fig. 6.24).

Most tuberculomas are between two and five centimetres in diameter at the time of presentation. Pre-pancreatic lymph-node enlargement is sometimes present. Confirmation of the mass by CT scanning allows greater detail to be seen. The pancreas is expanded by the mass and may show an irregular, nodular margin. The lesion is of low attenuation, and shows some peripheral enhancement on intravenous contrast injection. After initial examination, it is of value to image the pancreas using 0.5-cm slices during dynamic injection of a contrast bolus. Appearances similar to those of tuberculoma are to be found in both primary and metastatic carcinoma of the pancreas [93]. In one case, a small quantity of gas was seen in the lesion, which is unusual in pancreatic malignancies [91]. In a second case, diffuse tiny pockets of gas were seen throughout the gland on both CT and sonographic examination. Guided aspiration biopsy elicited turbid fluid. Subsequent culture revealed both pyogenic and mycobacterial organisms. *Streptococcus sanguis* and *Bacteroides* species, cultured from the fluid, were presumably responsible for the accumulation of gas and the emphysematous appearance, while the underlying infection was due to *M. tuberculosis* [92]. Endoscopic retrograde cholangiopancreatography (ERCP) examination has demonstrated normal bile and pancreatic ducts; this finding, and the lack of duct dilatation and irregular-

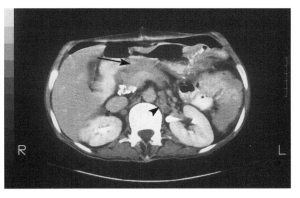

Fig. 6.25. Computed tomography reveals a non-enhancing mass of lymph nodes anterior to the pancreas (*arrow*). A group of retroperitoneal lymph nodes with ring enhancement lies medial to the left kidney (*arrowhead*). Culture of fine-needle-aspiration material was positive for alcohol acid-fast bacilli

ity on both CT and sonography, is an important difference from carcinoma and chronic pancreatitis [86, 87]. Ultrasound- or CT-guided biopsy will yield caseating material or, more commonly, creamy or yellow pus. Direct staining for AAFB has a high positive result. The results of histological examinations are less positive unless a very careful technique is employed, with multiple passes through the periphery of the lesion. Laparotomy should be avoided, as it may lead to dissemination of TB [87]. If undertaken, a hard mass will be found, similar to carcinoma. In tuberculous obstruction of the biliary system, laparotomy may be unavoidable, as stenting of the common bile duct may not be possible, and a biliary bypass surgery may be necessary to relieve biliary obstruction. In gastrointestinal TB, the pre-pancreatic lymph nodes are often enlarged, but it is usually possible to differentiate this lymph-node mass from an intrinsic lesion in the pancreas [21] (Fig. 6.25).

Pancreatic metastases, commonly secondary to carcinomas of the lung, kidney or breast or to melanoma can give rise to diagnostic problems if the metastasis is single. At the time of diagnosis of the pancreatic lesion, the primary tumour will usually have manifested itself elsewhere and, in the case of a renal primary tumour, this may have occurred a number of years before. Metastases to the pancreas often demonstrate a pancreatic mass with central necrosis and peripheral enhancement on post-contrast CT examination. They are impossible to distinguish from tuberculomas on imaging alone, and biopsy is necessary to confirm the diagnosis. Biopsy is also required to exclude other uncommon diseases of the pancreas, such as fungal abscess, benign tumour, sarcoidosis and Castelman's disease [91, 93, 94].

Pancreatic tuberculous lesions respond well to anti-tuberculous chemotherapy if an early diagnosis is made. The infection must be considered in the differential diagnosis of pancreatic lesions despite its rarity as, untreated, it is a mortal condition.

Gall-Bladder TB

TB very rarely affects the gall bladder, the normal mucosa and gall bladder wall appearing resistant to *M. Tuberculosis*. Underlying pathology, usually cholelithiasis, is present in most reported cases.

The common form of infection is an extension of abdominal TB. Laparoscopic examination reveals extensive tubercles covering the serosal surface of the bowel and tubercles on the surface of the liver and peritoneum, combined with peritoneal adhesions. Adhesions involving the gall bladder are also seen. One such case of acute cholecystitis in a gall bladder containing gallstones occurred as an acute abdominal emergency in a series of 100 cases of abdominal TB. The gall bladder was acutely inflamed and encased by multiple adhesions of tuberculous peritoneal tissue (Al Karawi and Yasawy, personal communication). In a group of 42 cases of abdominal TB from Kuwait, one case of gallbladder TB is cited, but no detailed description is given [16].

Even in endemic areas, gall-bladder TB is extremely rare. Jain et al. treated a case successfully with anti-tuberculous therapy [95]. Presentation was in conjunction with severe abdominal TB affecting the peritoneum, mesentery and lymph nodes. Echographically, the gall bladder was grossly enlarged, thick walled, and contained not only a gallstone but a soft-tissue mass.

Gall-bladder masses are more commonly due to carcinoma and, although there is absence of any evidence of invasion of any surrounding structures in TB, the two conditions are indistinguishable by imaging methods. Echo-guided biopsy is necessary to distinguish between the two conditions. In Jain's case, the intraluminal mass, which did not enhance on CT study, resolved after 7 weeks of therapy. At the same time, the gall-bladder mass reduced in size, and the wall thickness diminished. The general condition of the patient improved, as did the signs of general intra-abdominal TB.

■ Hepatobiliary TB

Hepatobiliary TB is an extremely rare condition, with few reports in recent years. However, Alvarez et al. have reported a number of cases in patients of Filipino origin [96]. Hepatobiliary TB probably occurs as a complication of miliary hepatic TB. Clinically, it presents as fever, weight loss, hepatomegaly and recurrent jaundice. The illness runs a chronic course. A high proportion of cases show a chest radiograph positive for pulmonary TB; Alvarez quotes 64%, compared with 20–30% in other studies of cases of abdominal TB. Plain radiographs often show multiple dense, chalky calcifications in the liver parenchyma and calcified lymph nodes in the porta hepatis. In most cases, it is these lymph nodes that cause biliary obstruction by compressing the bile ducts, usually high in the porta hepatis. Other features include long, distal stenoses in the common bile duct or, in some cases, a picture of cholangitis of both the distal and intrahepatic ducts. A tight hilar stricture of the common bile duct is another characteristic finding.

Examination by CT, ERCP or percutaneous transhepatic cholangioscopy is necessary to distinguish the disease from obstruction due to gallstones, cholangiocarcinoma, ampullary carcinoma or pancreatic carcinoma. In this differentiation, the presence of focal hepatic calcification in TB is a helpful finding. The cholangitis of AIDS may be problematic when concurrent abdominal TB is present.

TB in patients with hepatobiliary disease responds to anti-tuberculous chemotherapy, but the obstruction may not as, in many cases, the strictures are fibrous. This often necessitates biliary stenting or bypass surgery to relieve the condition.

■ Tuberculous Abdominal Lymphadenopathy

One of the most common forms of intra-abdominal TB infection of the lymph nodes may occur as an isolated lymph-node disease or in combination with solid-organ TB, tuberculous peritonitis or gastrointestinal TB. The percentages of cases of abdominal TB with abdominal lymphadenopathy described in the literature vary considerably. In 506 cases reported recently, the average of lymph-node involvement was between 25% and 30% [11–13, 17, 21, 32]. A much higher percentage of 55% was found by Hulnick et al. [29, 34], but his cases included a proportion of immunosuppressed patients while, in a report from Turkey, 90% of 11 patients had lymph-node involvement [22]. Lower percentages of 9% and 13% are also quoted [20, 23]. In a group of 596 patients recorded earlier, between 1975 and 1988, and reviewed by Marshall, only 48 had lymph-node disease [33]. This discrepancy probably reflects the general introduction of sonography and CT imaging in recent years. In 205 cases investigated by endoscopy and laparoscopy, lymph-node presence is not revealed [16, 18, 25, 26]. To demonstrate the full extent of abdominal TB, the ideal protocol would include sonography, CT scanning and "scopic" examination. However, none of these methods of investigation produces specific evidence unless biopsy material or peritoneal aspirate is acquired. Lymph-node involvement is usually secondary to gastrointestinal TB, and by far the most common association is with ileocaecal lesions. Less often, tuberculous peritonitis or solid-organ lesions are the primary site of infection. Isolated cases do occur without evidence of visceral disease [29]. This is often the case in tuberculous periportal lymphadenopathy [97].

The clinical presentation of lymphadenopathy is similar to that of other forms of abdominal TB, and it is unusual for a palpable lymph-node mass to be present, although hepatosplenomegaly is sometimes a finding. The nodes may be seen in any of the main compartments, but the common areas are the mesenteric, pre-pancreatic, and para-aortic groups. Pelvic nodal enlargement is seen when the pelvic organs are infected; rarely, inguinal nodes are involved (Fig. 6.26).

Histopathology

The histological changes in the lymph nodes alter as the disease progresses. Four different stages have been suggested for cervical lymph nodes, and there are similarities with the changes in abdominal nodes [39, 98, 99]:

1. Lymphoid hyperplasia with formation of tubercles and caseating granulomas
2. Caseating necrosis in the lymph-node centre
3. Capsular destruction, with periadenitis and adherence between nodes to form a lymph-node mass
4. Rupture of the lymph nodes, discharging caseous and necrotic material into the surrounding tissues, leading to formation of a cold abscess [98, 99]

CT examination demonstrates all phases of lymph-node pathology. Nodes vary considerably in size in the same patient and vary in appearance at the same time. Nodes may enhance homogeneously or heterogeneously due to mixed zones of enhancing granulomas and areas of caseation (Fig. 6.27). Nodes may show thick marginal-rim enhancement due to peri-

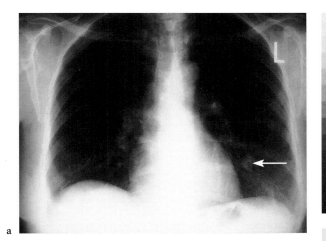

a

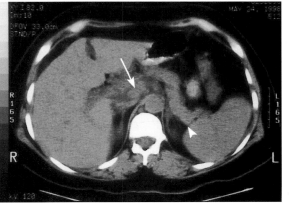

b

c

Fig. 6.26. **a** Chest radiography demonstrates a single granuloma in the left lower lobe (*arrow*). **b, c** Pre- and post-contrast computed-tomography scans demonstrate a mass in the porta hepatis behind the portal vein. This shows ring enhancement (*arrows*). The splenic vein is large due to early obstructive change, but the spleen is only slightly enlarged (*arrowhead*). Anti-tuberculosis chemotherapy was effective in this case

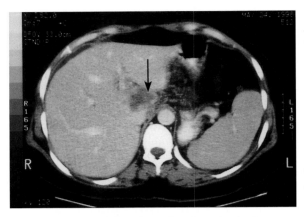

Fig. 6.27. A group of hypodense lymph nodes in the porta hepatis, with ring enhancement (*arrow*). Fine-needle aspiration revealed granulomatous tissue and cultured positive for alcohol acid-fast bacilli

pheral inflammation and neovascularity surrounding caseating or necrotic material. The thickness of the enhancing rim varies but is usually greater than 20% of the diameter of the lymph node (Figs. 6.28–6.30).

At later stages, the nodes may become matted or lose their individual identity and enhance around the margins of the group. In advanced lymph-node disease, there is loss of nodal architecture, enhancement of the margins of the mass and central low-density material, representing cold-abscess development. On imaging before contrast injection, nodes are usually hypodense or of soft-tissue density. In the healing stage of discrete nodes, fibrosis is followed by calcification, which may be intense enough to be visible on plain abdominal radiographs. The infected

nodes vary in size between 2 cm and 5 cm. Echographic imaging reveals hypoechoic nodes even in the early phases of infection. Those lying in the mesentery are accompanied by mesenteric thickening, with increased echoes in the surrounding tissues. The mesentery, in these cases, increases to between 2 cm and 4 cm in thickness [13]. Groups of hypoechoic nodes are also seen in the mesenteric root and the pre-pancreatic and para-aortic areas.

In patients with AIDS and TB, large, hyperdense, hypoechoic lymph nodes are seen. On CT, these often show minimal rim enhancement. This is presumably due to the diminished inflammatory reaction associated with the condition. They cannot be readily distinguished from those associated with Kaposi sarcoma, lymphoma or opportunistic infections [100].

The imaging patterns of lymph nodes are highly suggestive of TB in the correct clinical situation, but the patterns are not specific, and a number of conditions show similar appearances. Low-density nodes are seen in the metastasised testicular tumours, but the distribution of the nodes is usually para-aortic and retroperitoneal [101]. Although they do occur, retroperitoneal nodes are less prominent in TB than in other conditions [17, 21, 29, 30, 34, 35, 39].

Other malignant metastases in lymph nodes show distributions similar to those of tuberculous nodes, particularly metastases from carcinomas of the alimentary tract and ovaries, but the distribution of associated peritoneal lesions may help to distinguish them, as well as the nodular thickening of the peritoneum in malignant diseases [40]. A similar distribution of lymph-node enlargement is seen in the lymphomas and, after treatment, some lymphoma patients may demonstrate a similar type of rim enhancement [102].

Rarely, the lymphadenopathy of benign conditions may cause diagnostic difficulties. Rim enhancement of lymph nodes is reported in Crohn's disease, although lymph-node enlargement in this condition is

Fig. 6.28. Large, lymphoid masses in the para-aortic region in a case of abdominal tuberculosis (*arrows*). These are impossible to differentiate from lymphoma without biopsy

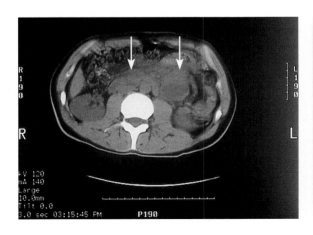

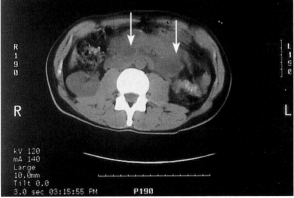

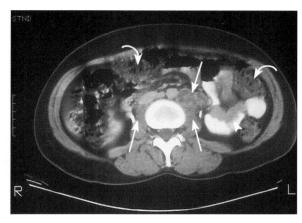

Fig. 6.29. A mass of para-aortic lymph nodes show ring enhancement. There are also retroperitoneal lymph nodes (*arrows*). The small bowel shows wall thickening (*arrowhead*), and there are lymph nodes in the mesentery (*curved arrows*). The patient responded to anti-tuberculosis therapy

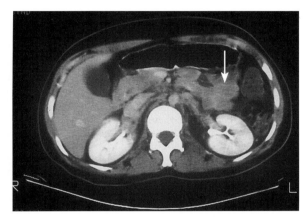

Fig. 6.30. Abdominal tuberculosis, with extensive ring enhancement of lymph nodes in the mesenteric root (*arrow*)

unusual. It is important to make the distinction, as treatment with steroids leads to rapid advance of the disease if the nodal infection is tuberculous. Sarcoidosis is another condition in which similar lymph-node changes may be seen, but the absence of other abdominal sites of involvement and the presence of bilateral hilar lymphadenopathy in sarcoidosis can help in differentiating between the two conditions [103]. In Whipple's disease, the enlarged nodes are of low density due to the presence of fatty acids and are usually retroperitoneal; the presence of weight loss and diarrhoea is similar to the presenting symptoms of gastrointestinal TB.

Abdominal Castleman's disease is responsible for extensive para-aortic and retroperitoneal lymph-node enlargement. The enhancement tends to be dense and homogeneous, and the presence of hypergammaglobulinaemia helps in distinguishing the two conditions [104]. In cases where isolated lymph-node enlargement is the only finding on imaging, TB should be considered as the possible cause, especially when the patient belongs to one of the target groups of patients [29, 105].

■ References

1. Rieder HL, Snider DE, Cauthen GM (1990) Extrapulmonary tuberculosis in the United States. Am Rev Respir Dis 141:347–351
2. Alvarez S, McCabe WR (1984) Extrapulmonary tuberculosis revisited: a reveiw of experience at Boston City and other hospitals. Medicine 63:25–55
3. Probert CSJ, Jayanthi V, Wicks AC, et al. (1992) Epidemiological study of abdominal tuberculosis among Indian migrants and the indigenous population of Leicester, 1972–1989. Gut 33:1085–1088
4. Klimach OE, Ormerod LP (1985) Gastrointestinal tuberculosis: a retrospective review of 109 cases in a district general hospital. QJM 56:569–578
5. Palmer KR, Patil DH, Basran GS, et al. (1985) Abdominal tuberculosis in urban Britain: a common disease. Gut 26:1296–1305
6. Sharp JF, Goldman M (1987) Abdominal tuberculosis in East Birmingham: a 16-year study. Postgrad Med J 63:539–542
7. Jakubowski A, Elwood RK, Enarson DA (1988) Clinical features of abdominal tuberculosis. J Infect Dis 158:687–692
8. Reddy KR, Di Prima RE, Raskin JB, et al. (1988) Tuberculous peritonitis: laparoscopic diagnosis of an uncommon disease in the United States. Gastrointest Endosc 34:422–426
9. Guth A, Kim U (1991) The reappearance of abdominal tuberculosis. Surg Gynecol Obstet 172:432–436
10. Bhargava DK, Shriniwas, Chopra P, et al. (1992) Peritoneal tuberculosis: laparoscopic patterns and its diagnostic accuracy. Am J Gastroenterol 87:109–112
11. Ramaiya LI, Walter DF (1993) Sonographic features of tuberculous peritonitis. Abdom Imaging 18:23–26
12. Kedar RP, Shah PP, Shivde RS, Malde HM (1994) Sonographic findings in gastrointestinal and peritoneal tuberculosis. Clin Radiol 49:24–29
13. Jain R, Sawhney S, Bhargava DK, Berry M (1995) Diagnosis of abdominal tuberculosis: sonographic findings in patients with early disease. AJR Am J Roentgenol 165:1391–1395
14. Bastani B, Shariatzadeh MR, Dehdashti F (1985) Tuberculous peritonitis; report of 30 cases and a review of the literature. QJM 56:549–557
15. Ozkan K, Gurses N, Gurses N (1987) Ultrasonic appearance of tuberculous peritonitis. J Clin Ultrasound 15:350–352
16. Al Hadeedi S, Walia HS, Al Sayer HM (1990) Abdominal tuberculosis. Can J Surg 33:233–237
17. Denton T, Hossain J (1993) Radiological study of abdominal tuberculosis in a Saudi population, with special reference to ultrasound and computed tomography. Clin Radiol 47:409–414
18. Al Quorain AA, Satti MB, Al Freihi HM, et al. (1993) Abdominal tuberculosis in Saudi Arabia: a clinicopathological study of 65 cases. Am J Gastroenterol 88:75–79

19. Sheikh M, Abu-Zidan F, Al Hilaly M, Benbehani A (1995) Abdominal tuberculosis: comparison of sonography and computed tonography. J Clin Ultrasound 23:413–417

20. Al Karawi MA, Mohamed AE, Yasawy MI, et al. (1995) Protean manifestation of gastrointestinal tuberculosis: Report of 130 patients. J Clin Gastroenterol 20:225–232

21. Lundstedt C, NymanR, Brismar J, et al. (1996) Imaging of tuberculosis II: abdominal manifestations in 112 patients. Acta Radiol 37:489–495

22. Demirkazik FB, Akhan O, Ozmen MN, Akata D (1996) US and CT findings in the diagnosis of tuberculous peritonitis. Acta Radiol 37:517–520

23. Lee DH, Lim JH, Ko YT, Yoon Y (1991) Sonographic findings in tuberculous peritonitis of the wet-ascitic type. Clin Radiol 44:306–310

24. Epstein BM, Mann JH (1982) CT of abdominal tuberculosis. AJR Am J Roentgenol 139:861–866

25. Manohar A, Simjee AE, Haffejee AA, Pettengell KE (1990) Symptoms and investigative findings in 145 patients with tuberculous peritonitis diagnosed by peritoneoscopy and biopsy over a five year period. Gut 31:1130–1132

26. Pettengell KE, Larsen C, Garb M, et al. (1990) Gastrointestinal tuberculosis in patients with pulmonary tuberculosis. QJM 74:303–308

27. Zirinsky K, Auh YH, Kneeland JB, et al. (1985) Computed tomography, sonography and MR imaging of abdominal tuberculosis. J Comput Assist Tomogr 9:961–963

28. Dahlene DH, Stanley RJ, Koehler RE, et al. (1984) Abdominal tuberculosis: CT findings. J Comput Assist Tomogr 8:443–445

29. Hulnick DH, Megibow AJ, Naidich DP, et al. (1985) Abdominal tuberculosis: CT evaluation. Radiology 157:199–204

30. Bankier AA, Fleischmann D, Wiesmayr MN, et al. (1995) Update: abdominal tuberculosis – unusual findings on CT. Clin Radiol 50:223–228

31. Makanjuola D, Orainy I, Al Rashid R (1998) Radiological evaluation of complications of intestinal tuberculosis. Eur J Radiol 26:261–268

32. Bhansali SK (1977) Abdominal tuberculosis. Am J Gastroenterol 67:324–337

33. Marshall JB (1993) Tuberculosis of the gastrointestinal tract and peritoneum. Am J Gastroenterol 88:989–999

34. Leder RA, Low VHS (1995) Tuberculosis of the abdomen. Radiol Clin North Am 33:698–705

35. Balthazar EJ, Gordon R, Hulnick D (1990) Ileocecal tuberculosis: CT and radiological evaluation. AJR Am J Roentgenol 154:499–503

36. Anand BS, Nanda R, Sachdev GK (1988) Response of tuberculous stricture to antituberculous treatment. Gut 29:62–69

37. Paustian FF, Marshall JB (1985) Intestinal tuberculosis. In: Berk JE (eds) Bockus gastroenterology, 4th edn. WB Saunders, Philadelphia, pp 120, 2018–2036

38. Singh MN, Bhargava AN, Jain KP (1969) Tuberculous peritonitis: an evaluation of pathogenic mechanisms, diagnostic proceedures and therapeutic measures. N Engl J Med 281:1091–1094

39. Pombo F, Rodriguez E, Mato J, et al. (1992) Patterns of enhancement of tuberculous lymph nodes demonstrated by computed tomography. Clin Radiol 46:13–17

40. Rodriguez E, Pombo F (1996) Peritoneal tuberculosis versus peritoneal carcinomatosis: distinction based on CT findings. J Comput Assist Tomogr 20:269–272

41. Cheng IKP, Chan PCK, Chan MK (1989) Tuberculous peritonitis complicating long-term peritoneal dialysis. Am J Nephrol 9:155–161

42. Voigt MD, Kalvaria I, Trey C, et al. (1989) Diagnostic value of ascites adenosine deaminase in tuberculous peritonitis. Lancet 1:751–754

43. Reeder MM, Palmer PES (1989) Inflammatory diseases. In: Margulis AR, Burhenne HJ (eds) Alimentary tract radiology. Mosby, St. Louis, pp 797–798

44. Eisenberg RL (1983) Coned caecum. In: Gastrointestinal radiology. Lippincott, Philadelphia, pp 584–594

45. Hanson RD, Hunter TB (1985) Tuberculous peritonitis: CT appearance. AJR Am J Roentgenol 144:931–932

46. Brown JH, Berman JJ, Blickman JG, Chew FS (1993) Primary ileocecal tuberculosis. AJR Am J Roentgenol 160:278

47. Shah S, Thomas V, Mathan M, et al. (1992) Colonoscopic study of 50 patients with colonic tuberculosis. Gut 33:347–351

48. Healy JC, Gorman S, Kumar PJ (1992) Case report: tuberculous colitis mimicking Crohn's disease. Clin Radiol 46:131–132

49. Downey DB, Nakielny RA (1985) Aphthoid ulcers in colonic tuberculosis. Br J Radiol 58:561–562

50. Collins MA, Peh WCG, Evans NS (1992) Aphthous ulcers in salmonella colitis. AJR Am J Roentgenol 158:918

51. Peh WCG (1988) Filiform polyposis in tuberculosis of the colon. Clin Radiol 39:534–536

52. Bhargava DK, Tandon HD, Chawla TC (1985) Diagnosis of ileocaecal and colonic tuberculosis by colonoscopy. Gastrointest Endosc 31:68–70

53. De Silva R, Stoopack PM, Raufman J-P (1990) Esophageal fistulas associated with mycobacterial infection in patients at high risk for AIDS. Radiology 175:449–453

54. Tromba JL, Inglese R, Rieders B, TodaroR (1991) Primary gastric tuberculosis presenting as pyloric outlet obstruction. Am J Gastroenterol 86:1820–1822

55. McNamara M, Williams CE, Brown TS, Gopichadran TD (1987) Tuberculosis affecting the oesophagus. Clin Radiol 38:419–422

56. Chase RA, Haber MH, Pottage JC, et al. (1986) Tuberculous esophagitis with erosion into aortic aneurysm. Arch Pathol Lab Med 110:965–966

57. Savage PE, Grundy A (1984) Oesophageal tuberculosis: an unusual cause of dysphagia. Br J Radiol 57:1153–1155

58. Young TH, Hsieh JP, Chao YC, et al. (1996) Esophageal tuberculosis with supraclavicular lymph node involvement demonstrated by Ga-67 imaging. Clin Nucl Med 21:344

59. Gordon A, Marshall JB (1990) Esophageal tuberculosis: definitive diagnosis by endoscopy. Am J Gastroenterol 85:174–177

60. Gupta SK, Jaain AK, Agrawal AK, Berry K (1988) Duodenal tuberculosis. Clin Radiol 39:159–161

61. Misra D, Rai RR, Nundy S, et al. (1988) Duodenal tuberculosis presenting as bleeding peptic ulcer. Am J Gastroenterol 83:203–204

62. Nair KV, Pai CG, Rajagopal KP, et al. (1991) Unusual prentations of duodenal tuberculosis. Am J Gastroenterol 86:756–760

63. Desmond JM, Evans SE, Couch A, et al. (1989) Pyeloduodenal fistula: a report of two cases and a review of the literature. Clin Radiol 40:267–270

64. Edie DGA, Pollack DS (1968) A complicated aorto-duodenal fistula. Br J Surg 53:314–317

65. Singh MK, Arunbh, Kapoor VK (1987) Tuberculosis of the appendix – a report of 17 cases and a suggested aetiopathological classification. Postgrad Med J 63:855–857

66. Snider DE, Roper WL (1992) The new tuberculosis. N Engl J Med 326:703–705

67. Levine C (1990) Primary macronodular hepatic tuberculosis. Gastrointest Radiol 15:307–309

68. Wilde CC, Kueh YK (1991) Tuberculous hepatic and splenic abcess. Clin Radiol 43:215–216

69. Brauner M, Buffard MD, Jeantils V, et al. (1989) Sonography and computed tomography of macroscopic tuberculosis of the liver. J Clin Ultrasound 17:563–568

70. Kapoor R, Jain AK, Chaturvedi U, Saha MM (1991) Case report: ultrasound detection of tuberculomas of the spleen. Clin Radiol 43:128–129
71. Argawala S, Bhatnagar V, Mitra DK, et al. (1992) Primary tubercular abscess of the spleen. J Pediatr Surg 27:1580–1581
72. Kawamori Y, Matsui O, Kitagawa K, et al. (1992) Macronodular tuberculoma of the liver: CT and MR findings. AJR Am J Roentgenol 158:311–313
73. Malde HM, Chadha D (1991) The "cluster" sign in macronodular hepatic tuberculosis: CT features. J Comput Assist Tomogr 17:159–161
74. Satti MB, Al Freihi H, Ibrahim H, et al. (1990) Hepatic granuloma in Saudi Arabia: a clinicopathological study of 59 cases. Am J Gastroenterol 85:669–674
75. Moscovic E (1990) Macronodular hepatic tuberculosis in a child: computed tomographic appearances. Br J Radiol 63:656–658
76. Jeffrey RB, Tolentino CS, Chang FC, Federle MP (1988) CT of small pyogenic hepatic abscesses: the cluster sign. AJR Am J Roentgenol 151:487–489
77. Hahn PF, Stark DD, Saini S, et al. (1990) The differential diagnosis of ringed hepatic lesions in MR imaging. AJR Am J Roentgenol 154:287–290
78. Mathieu D, Vasile N, Fagniez P-L, et al. (1985) Dynamic CT features of hepatic abscesses. Radiology 154:749–752
79. Vasquez T, Evans DG, Schiffman H, Ashburn WL (1987) Fungal splenic abscesses in the immunosuppressed patient correlation of imaging modalities. Clin Nucl Med 12:36–38
80. Lozano F, Gomez-Mateos J, Lopez-Cortes L, Garcia-Bragado F (1991) Tuberculous splenic abscesses in patients with the acquired immune deficiency syndrome. Tubercle 72:307–308
81. Wolff MJ, Bitran J, Northland RG, Levy IL (1991) Splenic abscesses due to M. Tuberculosis in patients with AIDS. Rev Inf Dis 13:373–375
82. Pedro-Botet J, Maristany MT, Miralles R (1991) Splenic tuberculosis in patients with AIDS. Rev Infect Dis 13:1069–1071
83. Ohta H, Fufuyama T, Sakamoto M, et al. (1996) Liver tuberculoma detected by Ga-67 imaging. Clin Nucl Med 21:575–576
84. Kao P-F, Tzen K-Y, Chou Y-H, et al. (1996) Accumulation of Ga-67 citrate in a tuberculous splenic abscess. Clin Nucl Med 21:49–52
85. Yang S-O, Lee YI, Chung DH, et al. (1992) Detection of extrapulmonary tuberculosis with gallium-67 scan and computed tomography. J Nucl Med 33:2118–2123
86. Cho KC, Lucak SL, Delany HM, et al. (1990) CT appearance intuberculous pancreatic abscess. J Comput Assist Tomogr 14:152–154
87. Stambler JB, Klibaner MI, Bliss CM, Lamont JT (1982) Tuberculous abscess of the pancreas. Gastroenterology 83:922–925
88. Radin DR (1991) Intra-abdominal Mycobacterium tuberculosis vs Mycobacterium avium-intracollulare infections in patients with AIDS. AJR Am J Roentgenol 156:487–491
89. Crowson MC, Perry M, Burden E (1984) Tuberculosis of the pancreas: a rare cause of obstructive jaundice. Br J Surg 71:239
90. de Miguel F, Beltran J, Sabas JA, et al. (1985) Tuberculous pancreatic abscess. Br J Surg 72:438
91. del Castillo CF, Gonzalez-Ojeda A, Reyes E, et al. (1990) Tuberculosis of the pancreas. Pancreas 5:693–696
92. Morris DL, Wilkinson LS, Al Mokhtar N (1993) Emphysematous tuberculous pancreatitis diagnosed by ultrasound and computed tomography. Clin Radiol 48:286–287
93. Lepke RA, Paganii JJ (1982) Pancraetic Castelman disease simulating pancreatic carcinoma on computed tomography. J Comput Assist Tomogr 6:1193–1195
94. Boudghene FP, Deslandes PM, LeBlanche AF, Bigot JMR (1994) US and CT imaging features of intrapancreatic metastases. J Comput Assist Tomogr 18:905–910
95. Jain R, Sawhney S, Bhargava D, Berry M (1995) Gallbladder tuberculosis: sonographic appearance. J Clin Ultrasound 23:327–329
96. Alvarez SZ, Sollano JD (1998) ERCP in hepatobiliary tuberculosis. Gastrointest Endosc 47:100–104
97. Mathieu D, Ladeb MF, Guigui B, et al. (1986) Periportal tuberculous adenitis: CT features. Radiology 161:713–715
98. Lee Y, Park KS, Chung SY (1994) Cervical tuberculous lymphadenitis: CT findings. J Comput Assist Tomogr 18:370–375
99. Reede DL, Bergeron RT (1985) Cervical tuberculous adenitis: CT manifestations. Radiology 154:701–704
100. Jeffrey RB, Nyberg DN, Bottlesn K (1986) Abdominal CT in acquired immunodeficiency syndrome. AJR Am J Roentgenol 146:7–13
101. Scatarige JC, Fishman EK, Kuhajda FP, et al. (1983) Low attenuation nodal metastases in testicular carcinoma. J Comput Assist Tomogr 7:682–687
102. Oliver TW, Bernardino ME, Sones PJ (1983) Monitoring the response of lymphoma patients to therapy. Correlation of abdominal CT findings with clinical course and histological cell type. Radiology 149:219–214
103. Deutch SJ, Sandler MA, Alpern MB (1987) Abdominal lymphadenopathy in benign disease: CT detection. Radiology 163:335–338
104. Ferreiros J, Gomez-Leon N, Mata MI, et al. (1989) Computed tomography in abdominal Castleman's disease. J Comput Assist Tomogr 13:433–436
105. Banerjee AK, Coltart DJ (1990) Abdominal tuberculosis mimicking lymphoma in a patient with sickle cell anaemia. Br J Clin Pract 44:660–661

CHAPTER 7

Tuberculosis of the Genito-Urinary Tract

■ Introduction

Apart from tuberculous infection of the pleura and of the lymphatic system, tuberculosis (TB) of the renal tract is the most common non-pulmonary type of infection [1, 2]. It is a disease of relatively young people; the age distribution, in most cases, lying between 20 years and 40 years. More males than females are affected [2–4].

Tuberculous infection of the renal tract is a chronic, insidious infection involving all the components of the urinary pathway. Commonly, the kidneys, ureters and bladder are affected and, less commonly, the urethra. Both male and female genital organs are often secondarily involved, either by downward extension or haematological spread of the disease.

As is the case in most mycobacterial infections, considerable pathological change has usually occurred before the infection is discovered. Minimal constitutional change is usually present, and symptoms of occasional abdominal pain, dysuria, nocturia and urgency, coupled with a laboratory finding of microscopic haematuria, are often discounted. Sterile acid pyuria is initially the only definite finding, though even this may be intermittent, and the whole clinical presentation is, unfortunately, often minimised by both patient and physician until irreversible pathological changes have taken place. Culture of the urine for acid-fast bacilli is very important, but even this is not a constant finding, as distal stenoses may prevent the infected urine from reaching the exterior. Because of this, repeated cultures may be necessary before a positive finding is made [2–4].

■ The Pathological Basis for Imaging Findings

Renal-tract TB arises secondarily from haematological spread. The primary focus, in most cases, is to be found in the lungs or in a lymph node. The initial lesions in the kidney are microscopic miliary granulomas affecting both kidneys and confined to the peri-glomerular regions. As in the case of Rich focuses elsewhere, the initial nidus is an aggregation of polymorphonuclear leucocytes surrounded by macrophages and fibroblasts. As the granuloma develops, the macrophages elongate to become epithelioid cells, the surrounding fibroblasts are joined by lymphocytes and central giant cells are seen, with central caseation. In most instances, however, the lesions resolve as cell-mediated immunity develops. Some lesions do not resolve completely but lie dormant, while still containing mycobacteria, and may reactivate many years later as the immune state of the patient alters.

During the reactivation stage, distal migration of the mycobacterium through the nephron to the tubules and papillae allows the characteristic lesion of the papillae to develop. These lesions are ulcerative–necrotising and cause cavities close to the pericalyceal region.

The images presented to the radiologist are of a broad range, depending on many factors. First, there are no detectable changes in at least 15% of patients. In those cases that do show changes, the first detectable signs include haziness of a calyx on urography. As ulceration develops, pericalyceal destruction leads to deformity of calyces and to the formation of small pericalyceal abscesses [1–5].

The filling of these abscess cavities is gravity dependent, as no excretion occurs directly into them. Later in the disease process, these cavities may be large and may be mistaken for hydronephrotic calyces [5, 6]. At any stage of development, they may be filled with fluid or caseous or calcifying material, each presenting differing radiological appearances. As fibrotic change due to partial healing occurs, overlying parenchymal scarring in the cortex and on the surface of the kidney may be visible on both intravenous urography (IVU) examination and ultrasound. However, this scarring cannot be differentiated from that seen in pyogenic infections of the kidney. The common early change in the urinary pathway, as opposed to in the renal parenchyma, is stenosis of the calyceal infundibulum. This, in turn, leads to failure of the affected calyx to fill, described at urographic examination as a "phantom calyx" [4]. Stenosis involving groups of calyces or of the renal pelvis results in caliectasis or general or local hydro-nephrosis.

Mucosal oedema in the distal ureter is a common early finding, and this can also lead to hydroureter or hydronephrosis. Until fibrotic healing is advanced, these pathological changes are reversible, but the usual progression is to chronic obstructive and functional changes. Two types of common change are seen in the renal pelvis. The first is ballooning of the pelvis, with a pelvi-ureteric obstruction. The second is the result of gradual fibrotic shrinkage of the renal pelvis while, proximally, dilatation of the calyces remains.

As the disease advances, granulomatous space occupation develops in the renal pyramids and, as these lesions caseate, calcifications develop. Quite large mass lesions may develop, and the calcification may be stippled, crescentic or more extensive and lobular. The end product of this is often total calcification of the involved organ.

Fibrosis also develops when healing results from anti-tuberculous chemotherapy, so treatment does not always end the pathological process. Stenotic lesions lead to functional impairment of the medulla and cortex, proximal to the obstruction. This, combined with cavitation, caseation and calcification, gives rise to a failing kidney. These lesions also affect the perfusion of the kidney, as stretching of vessels and arteritis lead to loss of renal cortex, scarring and diminution cortical of function. Over a period of months and years, the kidney fails, and so-called autonephrectomy occurs. The ability of these silent kidneys to act as a focus of infection for further haematological spread is a point of dispute. Perfusion is minimal, but some authorities still recommend nephrectomy. As fibrotic healing develops, the ureter undergoes shrinkage and rigidity to form a pipe-stem ureter. Later, ureteric calcification may occur. The lower ureteral orifice is often irregular and gaping, resulting in cysto-ureteric reflux [7].

Granulomatous disease in the mucosa of the bladder causes bladder-wall thickening, contraction and reduction of bladder volume, so dysuria and urinary frequency are common symptoms of the disease. Renal TB is usually unilateral, although low-grade changes in the contralateral kidney are often present, and full-scale contralateral infection may develop at any time. The infection is usually confined within the renal tract, although cases of perinephric infection are rarely described. Communication of sinus tracts with the skin, colon and the duodenum and small bowel are also uncommon and seem to depend on the presence of proximal obstruction in a functioning, active kidney [8]. Reno-duodenal fistula usually involves the right kidney, where the bare area of the kidney is in contact with the third or fourth

parts of the duodenum. These fistulae may develop in reverse when duodenal TB perforates into a normal renal pelvis. Distal fistulas are uncommon, except in urethral TB, which in itself is rare. Multiple perineal fistulas have been described, but most cases were reported before the advent of chemotherapy.

■ Imaging Methods

In renal TB, the plain radiograph is still of great importance in diagnosis. The excretory urogram is also a major method of examination. Both ultrasonography and computed tomography (CT) scanning are of value, but ultrasound has proved disappointing in its failure to define some of the early changes visible on the other modalities of investigation.

Plain Radiography

Various types of calcification may be seen. The calcification of stone disease is unusual in TB. Papillary calcification is often stippled, as is that in developing caseation (Fig. 7.1). In more advanced cases, extensive areas of calcification, of a lobular or arcuate–crescentic pattern, are observed. The kidney size is unhelpful apart from suggesting renal disease, as both small and large kidneys may be seen. Calcification in other areas of the system, such as the ureters, seminal vesicles or prostate, is usually only seen in advanced cases [1–4, 6–8].

Excretory Urography

It must be emphasised that, in up to 15% of patients at the time of presentation, there are no visible changes on urography. The initial lesion in the calyceal wall is a result of granulomatous infiltration and oedema. This produces minor deformity of the calyx and may lead to calyceal cut-off or failure to fill. In the next phase, focal necrosis in the pericalyceal region results in cavitation (Fig. 7.2). These cavities may be seen as small, contrast-filled abscesses. Infundibular stenosis may the reason for failure of a calyx to fill or, in the early phases, for caliectasis of an affected calyx. Later, the subsegment of cortex servicing the calyx may develop atrophy and surface scarring. As the disease progresses, the underlying pathology produces two distinct areas of urographic change. In the substance of the kidney mass lesions resulting from granuloma formation, and in the collecting systems, fluid-filled lesions are due to cavitation and the development of distal obstructions. The calyceal patterns are changed by displacement and stretching

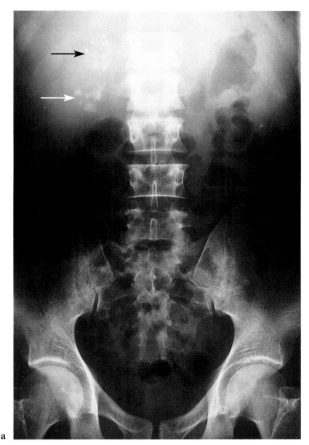

a

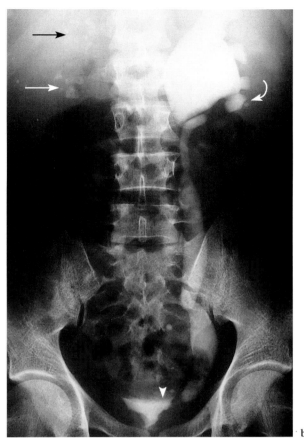

b

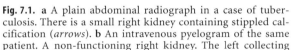

Fig. 7.1. a A plain abdominal radiograph in a case of tuberculosis. There is a small right kidney containing stippled calcification (*arrows*). **b** An intravenous pyelogram of the same patient. A non-functioning right kidney. The left collecting system is enlarged with pyelocaliectasis. On the *right*, a small pericalyceal cavity is seen (*curved arrow*). The left ureter is wide and tortuous and leads to a small, contracted bladder (*arrowhead*)

(Fig. 7.3). Enlargement of a calyx may be the result of cavitation and not raised pressure. Fibrosis in the renal pelvis will diminish the volume of the pelvis, while focal stenosis produces hydronephrosis. Eventually, diminished renal function due to high pressure or to parenchymal change causes inability to visualise the affected kidney (Fig. 7.4).

In the renal pelvis and ureter, both stenotic lesions and kinking are common (Kerr's kinks). Calcification of the ureter is a late-change manifestation [1, 7].

As dysuria is the common presentation of the disease, the pathological changes in the bladder are usually advanced by the time of diagnosis and, on urography, the bladder is seen as thick walled and small in volume (Figs. 7.5). The changes in the lower ureters are related to the bladder-wall infection. Gaping, deformed ureteric orifices, often with reflux, characterise the disease in this sector.

Calcification in the bony pelvis is more likely to be in the seminal vesicles or in the female adnexa than in the bladder wall. TB of the prostrate gland may produce extensive calcification on the plain radiograph in a very small number of cases (Fig. 7.7).

Ultrasound Examination

Early TB of the renal system is seldom diagnosed and, in most instances, clear pathological change is visible in the kidneys, ureters and bladder when the first sonogram, urograph or CT is carried out [6]. The role of ultrasound in the diagnosis of these cases has not yet been defined. So far, it is unclear if the early ulcero-necrotic lesions of the renal papillae would be recognised by standard ultrasound examination. In theory, the dilation of a single calyx should be visible on ultrasound, and all of the later changes, such as hydrocalyx, hydronephrosis, mass lesions and pelvic obstruction, are all common conditions demonstrated by ultrasound. One change that is suggestive of

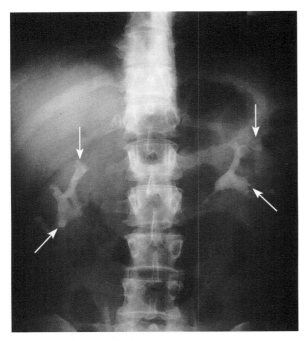

Fig. 7.2. Renal tuberculosis. An intravenous urogram showing small pericalyceal abscesses (*arrows*)

TB, but which is not a specific finding, is due to fibrotic changes in the renal pelvis. The diminution in size of the renal pelvis, accompanied by dilatation of the calyces, is highly suggestive of TB. Varying degrees of papillary and parenchymal calcification may be less readily defined by ultrasound than by plain radiography or CT scanning (Fig. 7.8).

It seems clear that, if tuberculous urinary-tract infection is suspected, then ultrasound investigation should be linked with some other investigation (for instance, excretory pyelography), as a normal ultrasound examination does not exclude renal-tract TB. In the later stages, high echogenicity is seen in the renal papillae, the renal medulla and the renal sinus, as well as the renal pelvic region. Echographically, the dilation of obstructed calyces must be differentiated from the hypoechoic cavities seen in the medulla and renal parenchyma in advanced cases. These are usually present in non-functioning kidneys, and a disadvantage of ultrasound is that it gives no information about renal function. Careful examination of the contralateral kidney may show early evidence of bilateral disease [5].

In the lower renal tract, ultrasound is of considerable value. The thickness and irregularity of the

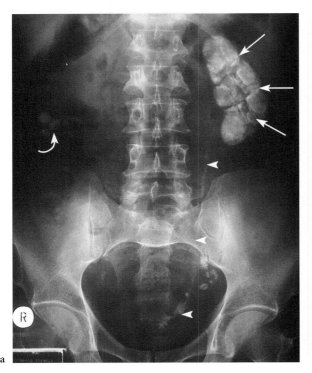

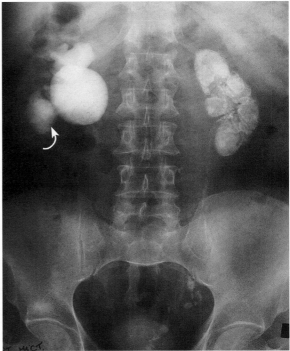

a   b

Fig. 7.3. a A plain abdominal radiograph. There is lobular calcification throughout the left kidney (*arrows*), in the left ureter (*arrowheads*) and in the right lower pole (*curved arrow*). **b** An intravenous pyelogram. The calcified left kidney does not function. The collecting system on the right is dilated, with the appearances of pelvi-ureteric stenosis. The right lower-pole calcification lies in a cavity (*curved arrow*)

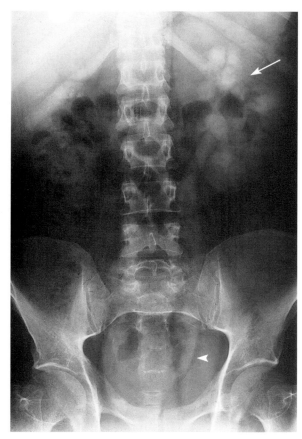

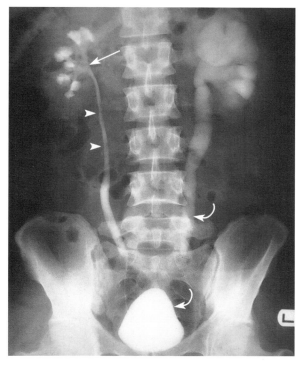

Fig. 7.5. Renal tuberculosis. Bilateral disease. There is a contracted collecting system on the right, and the renal pelvis is small (*arrow*). The right ureter is straightened (*arrowheads*). There is dilatation of the left collecting system, with a dilated ureter and a contracted bladder (*curved arrows*)

Fig. 7.4. An intravenous pyelogram in a case of tuberculosis. The right kidney is small. The concentration of the contrast is poor on both sides. On the left, there is hydronephrosis (*arrow*) and hydroureter (*arrowhead*)

bladder wall and mucosa is easily confirmed, as are changes in the calibre of the lower and intramural portion of the ureter. Measurements of the bladder capacity are also possible; this is usually much reduced by the time of presentation.

Computed Tomography

In established renal-tract TB, all of the morphological changes of the disease are visible on axial scanning. Some indication of the state of function may also be gathered from CT examination; the degree of cortical enhancement and transfer to the renal pelvis mirrors function to a certain point and may be compared with the normal contralateral side. Focal lack of perfusion of the cortex, may be seen in the wedge area beyond affected calyces. The disease may be segmental or polar, and this is readily demonstrated on axial scanning. All the changes in the collecting system seen on IVU are demonstrable

on CT scanning. Distortion of the calyces, ulcerative deformity of the papillae and caliceal distension are visible.

The presence of a small or apparently absent renal pelvis (the result of fibrosis) combined with caliectasis is suggestive of TB. On axial scanning, the calyceal pattern and absent renal pelvis produces an appearance similar to a flower and is called a "daisy pattern". Calcification is more easily visible on CT than on urography. The different types of calcification – solid, stipples or the characteristic "putty-like" calcification, which probably represents calcifying caseation – are all clearly visible (Fig. 7.9) [6, 7].

Mass lesions due to inflammatory granulomatous tissue that enhances, and necrotic caseating material, which does not enhance, may be difficult to differentiate from tumours or other granulomas. The recent trend of older patients developing TB causes overlap of the age groups for TB and renal transitional cell carcinoma. Xanthogranulomatous lesions, although demonstrating similar CT patterns, will probably also show long-standing stone disease [3, 6, 9, 10]. CT also differentiates between the radiographic density of the various collections of fluid in the diseased kidney. Dilated calyces and a hydronephrotic renal

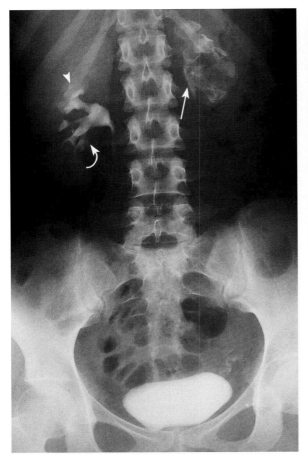

Fig. 7.6. Renal tuberculosis. Intravenous contrast study demonstrates autonephrectomy of the left kidney, with lobular calcification and calcification of the contracted renal pelvis (*arrow*). On the *right*, there is deformity of the upper-pole calyx (*arrowhead*) and a phantom lower-pole calyx (*curved arrow*)

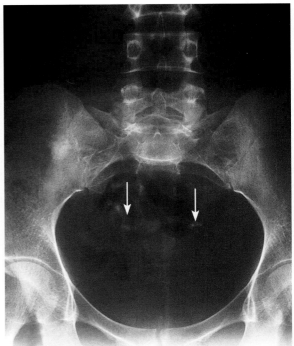

Fig. 7.7. Bilateral calcification of the fallopian tubes in tuberculosis (*arrows*)

pelvis contain urine in the early stage, with a density of 0–10 Hounsfield units (HU). As the disease develops, debris and necrotic material increase the density. Caseating or necrotic material measures 10–30 HU. As calcification occurs, the densities slowly move higher, 50–120 HU, until the dense calcification of autonephrectomy develops, above 120 HU [2, 9].

Perinephric abscesses and sinus formation are rare but are more liable to be diagnosed on CT and ultrasound than on urography. Ureteral calcification will be seen on pre-contrast plain scans, and the changes in the lower ureter are visible and defined by intravenous contrast as long as the kidney remains functioning [1, 2]. The bladder-wall pathology is also discernable and may affect both ureteric orifices, whether the contralateral kidney is infected or not. The incidence of cysto-ureteric reflux in ureters affected by TB is, so far, not well documented.

Although not a specific sign, there may be calcified mesenteric lymph nodes, the result of previous lymphoid TB. These will be seen both on CT examination and on plain-film radiography.

Magnetic Resonance Imaging

The presence of calcification in tuberculous lesions is such an important and often subtle sign of the infection that magnetic resonance (MR) is at a disadvantage compared with IVU and CT examination. The low-intensity signal of calcification is difficult to interpret on MR, and this, combined with the necessity for cardiac and respiratory gating and the long scanning times, diminishes the value of examination of the renal tract. One area in which it is of value is in the differentiation of macronodular, tuberculous lesions from other mass lesions. Mass lesions of the kidney tend to be hypodense on T1 and of high signal on T2 and T1-gadolinium (Gd) images. In tuberculous lesions, the presence of caseation, calcification and free radicals results in hypodense or isodense images on T2 acquirements, and caseating tissue fails to enhance. These appearances are similar to those seen on MR examination in other areas of the body [11].

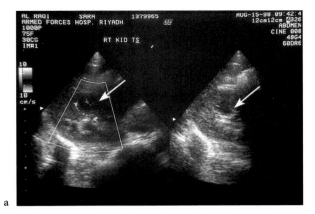

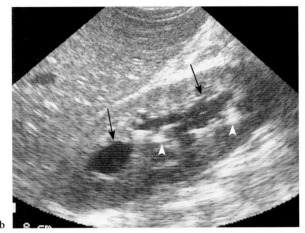

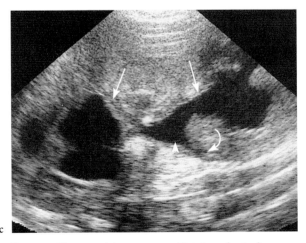

Fig. 7.8. a Ultrasound demonstrates dilatation of a single upper-pole calyx in early tuberculosis. There was acid pyuria, and alcohol acid-fast bacilli were cultured from the urine (*arrows*). **b** Ultrasound demonstrates irregular caliectasis in childhood tuberculosis (*arrows*); the caliectasis is linked with echogenic foci in the parenchyma (*arrowheads*). **c** Irregular cavitation (*arrows*), a small renal pelvis (*arrowhead*) and dilatation of the upper ureter with uro-epithelial thickening (*curved arrows*). Images **b** and **c** by courtesy of Dr. B.J. Cremin, Red Cross Hospital, Cape Town

■ Seminal Vesicles and the Prostate Gland

TB of these structures may be silent or accompanied by mild dysuria. Symptoms are more likely if the infection is secondary to downward spread from TB of the renal tract than if the pathway of infection is haematogenous from a distant focus. In both organs, abscesses may develop, causing constitutional symptoms. Infertility is a common later development and, as healing occurs, calcification may develop in the glands themselves and in the vas deferens. This calcification cannot be distinguished from that commonly seen in diabetes or, in endemic areas, the calcification of schistosomiasis [2, 12 – 15].

Calcification will be evident on plain radiographs, IVU and CT, but CT will be necessary to delineate soft-tissue mass lesions in the seminal vesicles. Transrectal ultrasound demonstrates patchy, hypodense lesions in the tuberculous prostate gland, but these are non-specific findings, and the differential diagnosis includes prostatic carcinoma. However, the younger age group involved in tuberculous infections is a helpful pointer in differentiating this. Aspiration biopsy should always include specimens sent for bacteriological study [13].

Tuberculous stricture of the male urethra is rare but may be a complication of long-standing infection of the urinary tract. On urethrography, the lesion will be indistinguishable from stricture due to other causes. It is usually in the membranous segment and may be associated with multiple cutaneous fistulae. This condition is called "watering-can perineum". Penile tuberculous ulcer is even more rare, but does occur. The chancre-like lesion is important, as it may lead to or result from sexually transmitted TB.

■ Pelvic TB in Females

TB of the female internal genitalia is haematogenous in origin and, in endemic regions, is a common cause of secondary infertility. Tuberculous salpingitis and salpingitic abscesses are common [1, 2]. In the case of females, the communication of the salpinx with the peritoneal cavity can lead to tuberculous peritonitis. Careful gynaecological assessment is, therefore, essential in all female patients with abdominal TB (Fig. 7.10).

■ TB of the Scrotal Contents

A small number of patients with TB of the renal tract develop tuberculous epididymitis or orchitis [2, 12, 15]. Estimates of the numbers vary between 1% and 23% of those with upper-renal-tract infection.

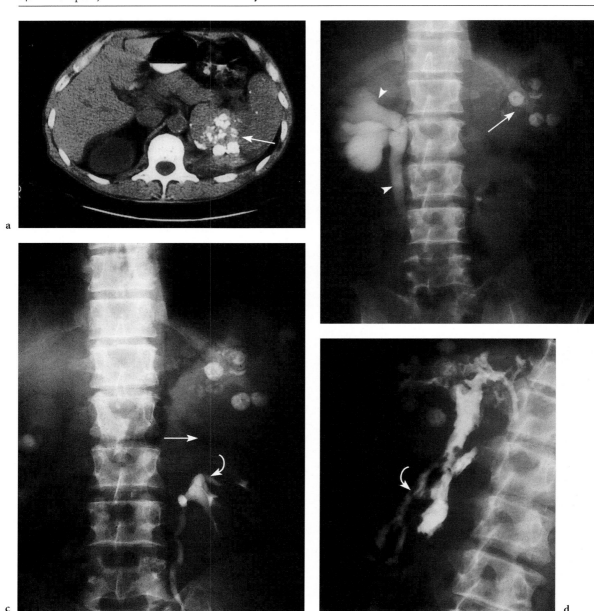

Fig. 7.9 a – d. A 40-year-old man with a discharging tuberculous sinus in the left flank. **a** Non-contrast computed tomography demonstrates numerous calcified granulomas in the spleen (*arrow*). **b** Intravenous pyelography shows right hydronephrosis, deformity of the renal pelvis and hydroureter (*arrowheads*). The splenic calcification is seen (*arrowhead*), but no apparent left-sided renal function. **c** A delayed image. The left kidney functions and shows a drooping-flower appearance in the collecting system (*curved arrow*). The kidney is displaced downwards by the enlarged spleen (*arrow*). **d** A sinogram reveals perisplenic infection. The contrast enters the left renal collecting system (*curved arrow*)

Primary epididymo-orchitis without urinary tract infection is thought to be of haematogenous origin and is even rarer than infection due to downward spread.

In previous decades, the number of cases was in decline. The incidence in south-east England between 1978 and 1988 roughly halved [15]. However, in the literature, there have been a number of recent papers, mainly from endemic areas. These probably reflect the more advanced methods of imaging now available rather than an increase in the number of patients. The clinical presentation is of painful scrotal swelling, testicular enlargement, a palpable irregular and hard epididymus and, in long-standing cases, cutaneous sinuses may be present. Sterile pyuria is found in up to 75% of cases. Recognisable changes of renal TB on IVU are absent in up to 25% of cases. Kim

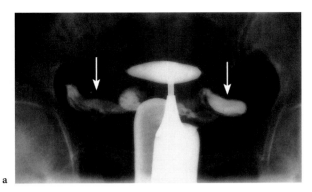

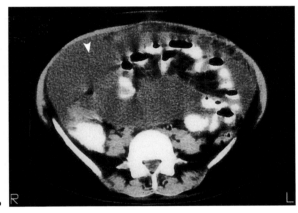

Fig. 7.10. a A hysterosalpingography showing bilateral pyosalpinx (*arrows*). **b** Computed tomography in the same young woman demonstrates high-density ascites in the pelvis (*arrowhead*). The aspirate cultured positive for alcohol acid-fact bacilli

of increased echogenicity. Diffuse enlargement of the epididymus develops, but the tail of the structure appears to be more markedly affected in tuberculous infection than in non-tuberculous epididymitis. In the later stages, calcification is revealed as high focal echoes with acoustic shadowing. Limited hydrocoele may also be a feature [15, 16].

The echographic appearances of tuberculous orchitis are impossible to differentiate from those of neoplasm. Focal hypoechoic tissue often confined to a testicular pole is present and may develop into echolucent tissue with posterior acoustic enhancement indicating fluid contents. Caseating material will be echogenic, giving rise to inhomogeneity [17]. Doppler study of the inflamed testis will demonstrate an increased blood flow when compared with the normal testis. This is not in any way specific, as some testicular tumours, particularly metastasis, may be highly vascular [18].

Surgical exploration of the scrotum may reveal para-epididymal masses of granuloma tissue, abscess formation, testicular granulomatous masses, necrosis or pus [15, 16]. Sometimes, frozen sections and auramine-stained bacteriological slides fail to demonstrate TB, and orchidectomy is resorted to. In one case reviewed by Koyama, the mass had reached a considerable size (6 × 5 × 4 cm), and the urine was constantly negative for alcohol acid-fast bacilli. At operation, it proved impossible to visually exclude neoplasm, the pus was bacteriologically negative and the diagnosis was only made from post-operative histological and bacteriological examination [19].

In other cases, alcohol acid-fast bacilli were isolated from the intra-scrotal contents, and the condition was cured with anti-tuberculous chemotherapy. Using MR imaging (MRI), Hamrick-Turner et al. have demonstrated, with perfect anatomical detail, a case of intra-scrotal TB. In their case, sonography suggested both epididymitis and orchitis, but MRI demonstrated a markedly enlarged epididymus indenting the testis. In this case, granulomatous prostatitis was also present. Culture of the urine and of a number of cutaneous ulcers confirmed the diagnosis of disseminated TB [20].

et al. describe a case where, although the IVU seemed normal, cystoscopy revealed tuberculous changes in the bladder wall. Those cases with renal-tract TB may have accompanying symptoms, such as dysuria, urgency or frequency, if the bladder is involved but, in most cases, the presenting illness will be confined to the scrotal contents. In these cases, in addition to urinalysis, IVU should be carried out to exclude early tuberculous renal infection. Infection is usually by peripheral spread from the seminal vesicles or prostate through the vas deferens. Epididymitis is the result. Orchitis appears to be the result of direct spread from the infected epididymus and is a late-stage development. Scrotal or testicular abscess formation may lead to scrotal sinus formation. Plain radiographs may show calcifications suggestive of TB, and both IVU and scrotal ultrasound examinations are of great value.

Epididymal and testicular tuberculous disease is usually unilateral. The epididymal appearances on ultrasound are dependent upon the duration of the infection. Early homogeneous hypoechogenicity gives way to inhomogeneous changes with mixed areas

Fine-Needle Aspiration Biopsy: Histological Diagnosis and Bacterial Culture in Renal TB

The constitutional symptoms of renal-tract TB can be limited and can lead to the infection being overlooked. Sterile pyuria may be the only pointer to the diagnosis. In 15% of the cases, there are no identifiable changes on IVU, so urine cultures may be negative. Repeated cultures are recommended.

The mycobacterium may be absent from the distal renal tract or only intermittently present for physical reasons. The kidney may be non-functional. Hydronephrosis or ureteral stenosis may be present, or an isolated calyceal or papillary lesion not communicating distally can be the cause. In these circumstances, sonographic or CT-guided trans-lumbar fine-needle aspiration can clinch the diagnosis. The aspirate is often comprised of necrotic material containing epithelioid cells and Langerhans' cells. The residue in the needle should be washed out and cultured using an accelerated culture method [21]. Das et al. suggest staining the material for direct bacteriological study [21], but Baniel et al. [22] point out that non-tuberculous mycobacteria may be present, leading to false-positive diagnosis. Haematoma is a possible complication of the procedure. Trans-abdominal puncture should be avoided in view of the theoretical spread of the infection to the peritoneum. In theory, miliary dissemination is also possible, and early institution of chemotherapy as soon after diagnosis as possible is advised.

■ Renal-Tract TB after Bacille Calmette-Guerin Therapy

Instillation of bacille Calmette-Guerin (BCG) (a live, attenuated form of *M. bovis*) into the bladder, as a means of treatment of superficial transitional cell carcinoma of the bladder, is a widely accepted method of treatment. The development of extra-vesicular granulomatous disease has been described in a small number of cases as a complication of this treatment. Granulomas have been observed in the liver, lungs, lymph nodes, spleen and bone marrow. Infection in the vertebral column and in long bones has been referred to in earlier chapters. In the renal tract, prostatic and epididymal lesions are described, as are renal granulomas. Lesions in the kidney, in these cases, result from cysto-ureteric reflux, a common feature after trans-urethral resection of bladder tumour. It is also likely if a double-J stent is in place [23]. The dissemination of tuberculous infections from these granulomas has led to some fatalities and should be treated by anti-tuberculous therapy as soon as suspected. The bacillus is seldom retrieved from the lesions or urine, so clinical suspicion is of great importance.

■ TB of the Adrenal Glands

When Addison described his eponymous disease in 1853, TB was the most common infectious cause of death. Six of his nine cases were the result of TB.

Addison described the syndrome of chronic adrenal insufficiency but, because of the decline in numbers of cases of TB, the most common cause of adrenal insufficiency today is idiopathic adrenal atrophy based on autoimmune disease [24]. Granulomatous infection counts for only a small proportion of cases at the moment, but the recent association of acquired immunodeficiency syndrome (AIDS)-related TB and Addison's disease should alert physicians to a change in the pattern in the future. In AIDS cases, the pathological organism may be an atypical mycobacterium [25]. The common cause of adrenal enlargement, replacement by metastatic tissue in cases of carcinoma of the lung and the breast, is rarely associated with gland hypofunction [25, 26]. This is because 90% of adrenal tissue must be replaced before the advent of adrenal insufficiency. Tubercular infection of the adrenal glands is a subacute or chronic state. In the first years of granulomatous disease, the adrenals increase in size and, as caseation and caseating necrosis develops, punctate calcification is present. This is sometimes visible on plain radiographs but is more likely to be seen on CT images.

The enlarged adrenal glands can reach a considerable size. Wilms et al. [24] report an adrenal mass 10×15 cm in size, but this is unusual. The disease is invariably bilateral and, as central caseating necrosis occurs, the periphery of the gland enhances on computer-enhanced CT. If calcification is absent, the appearances may be difficult to differentiate from those of bilateral metastases. In both conditions, enlarged regional lymph nodes may be present, which also show peripheral enhancement but, in the case of TB, hypofunction of the adrenal glands is more likely to be present. In cases of adrenal TB of more than 2 years duration, patterns of change include total atrophy of the glands or, more commonly, nodular calcification or enlargement of the glands, with caseating necrosis.

Although, in Europe, Asia, Africa and most of the Americas, TB is the common cause of granulomatous adrenal disease, there are areas in the south-east and south-central areas of the USA, where disseminated histoplasmosis leads to a similar condition. The CT and MRI appearances are similar to those of tuberculous infection, with enlargement of the adrenals and calcification. The disseminated infection is unusual and is seen in patients who already have a debilitating disease, those with a compromised immune system and patients on steroid therapy. Fine-needle biopsy is the diagnostic method of choice since, in addition to tuberculous disease, other fungi, lymphoma, metastases and bilateral haemorrhages may produce similar appearances [27].

Other, less common diseases, such as adrenal adenoma and primary carcinoma, are usually unilateral. The rare lipid-storage condition, Wolman's disease, gives rise to hepatomegaly and mild adrenal insufficiency with visible adrenal calcification. So far, no MRI studies of this condition have been published. In theory, the increase in cellular lipids would lead to an increased MRI signal. The calcification will, of course, give rise to signal voids.

Imaging Methods

Plain Radiographs

Calcification of the adrenal glands must be distinguished from calcification in healed or healing psoas abscesses. In the latter, there will usually be an accompanying deformity of the nearby vertebral bodies (Fig. 7.11). Adrenal calcification is much less commonly seen than it was during the period 1930–1950, when 70% of cases of Addison's disease were caused by TB (Fig. 7.12). In infants, adrenal calcification is usually due to neuroblastoma.

Sonography

Increase in the size of the adrenals with or without calcification may be visible just above the renal pole. On the left side, the gland may be difficult to demonstrate due to the higher position of the left kidney.

Follow-up examinations after anti-tuberculous therapy are useful, and the lack of ionising radiation is an advantage. Calcification usually remains visible. Healing of the TB by no means guarantees the return of normal adrenal function.

CT Examination

This is the examination of choice. Axial views define the size and shape of the adrenals (or their absence, if atrophy has occurred). In the early stages of the disease, the glands tend to retain their shape but, as the disease progresses, a rounder silhouette is seen. In some cases, the changes are symmetrical; in others, there may be a size discrepancy between the two glands. Calcification is readily visible and may be punctate or nodular. CT-guided aspiration biopsy is facilitated, although the proximity of major blood vessels must be appreciated. Pseudo-tumour appearances are also described in the kidney, the liver, the colon and the inferior vena cava, so careful pre-biopsy assessment is essential [25, 26, 28, 29].

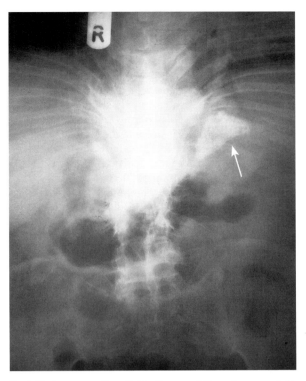

Fig. 7.11. Long-standing Pott's disease of the spine, with left-sided adrenal calcification (*arrow*)

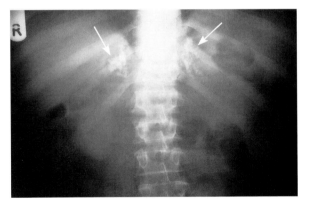

Fig. 7.12. Bilateral adrenal calcification in proven pulmonary tuberculosis (*arrows*)

Magnetic Resonance Imaging

The high-intensity signal of the peri-renal fat provides contrast and allows measurement of adrenal size and analysis of the morphology. T1-Gd enhancement defines central caseation necrosis and peripheral uptake of the contrast. Plain T1 images are either isodense or hypodense to muscle, and T2 images are slightly hyperdense. Calcification leads to signal voids.

The onset of the symptoms of subacute adrenal insufficiency, lethargy, weakness, cutaneous pigmentation and weight loss, together with hypotension in a patient with TB, should alert the physician to the possibility of Addison's disease. Up to 70 % of cases have an extra-adrenal focus of TB. In all cases of subacute insufficiency, the adrenals should be scanned to differentiate between atrophy and enlargement of the glands. If atrophy is present, the chance that TB is the cause is relatively low. If calcification is present, then idiopathic adrenal calcification has to be excluded by aspiration biopsy. Of the remaining cases with enlargement of the glands and calcification, a high proportion will be the result of granulomatous adrenal disease, either tubercular or fungal.

■ References

1. Elkin M (1990) Urogenital tuberculosis. In: Pollack HM (ed) Clinical urology. Saunders, Philadelphia, pp 1020–1052
2. Leder RA, Low VHS (1995) Tuberculosis of the abdomen. Radiol Clin North Am 33:691–698
3. Cohen MS (1986) Granulomatous nephritis. Urol Clin North Am 13:647–657
4. Kenney PJ (1990) Imaging of chronic renal infections. AJR Am J Roentgenol 155:485–494
5. Cremin BJ (1987) Radiological imaging of urogenital tuberculosis in children with emphasis on ultrasound. Pediatr Radiol 17:34–38
6. Premkumar A, Lattimer J, Newhouse JH (1987) CT and sonography of advanced urinary tract tuberculosis. AJR Am J Roentgenol 148:65–69
7. Birnbaum BA, Friedman JP, Lubat E, et al. (1990) Extrarenal genitourinary tuberculosis: CT appearance of calcified pipe-stem ureter and seminal vesicle abscess. J Comput Assist Tomogr 14:653–655
8. Desmond JM, Evans SE, Couch A, Morewood DJW (1989) Pyeloduodenal fistulae. A report of two cases and a review of the literature. Clin Radiol 40:267–270
9. Goldman SM, Fishman EK, Hartman DS, et al. (1985) Computed tomography of renal tuberculosis and its pathological correlates. J Comput Assist Tomogr 9:771–776
10. Feeney D, Quesada ET, Sirbasku DM, Kadmon D (1994) Transitional cell carcinoma in a tuberculous kidney: case report and review of the literature. J Urol 151:989–991
11. Murata Y, Yamada I, Sumiya Y, et al. (1996) Abdominal macronodular tuberculomas: MR findings. J Comput Assist Tomogr 20:643–646
12. Premkumar A, Newhouse JH (1988) Seminal vesicle tuberculosis: CT appearance. J Comput Assist Tomogr 12:676–677
13. Wang J-H, Chang T (1991) Tuberculosis of the prostate: CT appearance. J Comput Assist Tomogr 15:269–270
14. Kumar A, Srivastava A, Mishra VK, et al. (1994) Tubercular cavity behind the prostate and bladder: an unusual presentation of genito-urinary tuberculosis. J Urol 151:1351–1352
15. Heaton ND, Hogan B, Michell M, et al. (1989) Tuberculous epididymo-orchitis: clinical and ultrasound observations. Br J Urol 64:305–309
16. Kim S, Pollack M, Cho KS, et al. (1993) Tuberculous epididymitis and epididymo-orchitis: sonographic findings. J Urol 150:81–84
17. Chung T, Harris RD (1991) Tuberculous epididymo-orchitis: sonographic findings. J Clin Ultrasound 19:367–369
18. Tessler FN, Tublin ME, Rifkin MD (1998) US case of the day. Radiographics 18:251–253
19. Koyama Y, Iigaya T, Saito S (1988) Tuberculous epididymo-orchitis. Urology 31:419–421
20. Hamrick-Turner J, Abbitt PL, Ros PR (1992) Tuberculosis of the lower genitourinary tract: findings on sonography and MR. AJR Am J Roentgenol 158:919
21. Das KM, Vaidyanathan S, Rajwanshi A, et al. (1992) Renal tuberculosis: diagnosis with sonographically guided aspiration cytology. AJR Am J Roentgenol 158:571–573
22. Baniel J, Manning A, Leiman G (1991) Fine needle cytodiagnosis of renal tuberculosis. J Urol 146:689–691
23. Goh PYT, Htoo MM, Yeong KY (1996) Case report: renal granuloma following intra-vesicle Bacillus-Calmette-Geurin. Clin Radiol 51:69–71
24. Wilms GE, Baert AL, Kint EJ, et al. (1983) Computed tomographic findings in bilateral adrenal tuberculosis. Radiology 146:729–730
25. Doppman JL (1990) Diseases of the adrenal cortex. In: Pollack HM (ed) Clinical urology. Saunders, Philadelphia, pp 2338–2343
26. Dunnick NR (1990) Hanson lecture. Adrenal imaging: current status. AJR Am J Roentgenol 154:927–936
27. Wilson DA, Muchmore HG, Tisdal RG, et al. (1984) Histoplasmosis of the adrenal glands studied by CT. Radiology 150:779–783
28. Villabona CM, Sahun M, Ricart W, et al. (1993) Tuberculous Addison's disease. Utility of CT in diagnosis and follow up. Eur J Radiol 17:210–213
29. Jagannath A, Brill PW, Winchester P (1986) Addison's disease due to tuberculosis in a 13-year old girl. Pediatr Radiol 16:522–524

CHAPTER 8

Extrapulmonary Tuberculosis in Acquired Immunodeficiency Syndrome

■ Introduction

Limitation of the cell-mediated response in acquired immunodeficiency syndrome (AIDS) patients, due to the reduction of T-helper lymphocyte levels, removes the main defence against *Mycobacterium tuberculosis* [1, 2]. The resulting co-infection of AIDS and tuberculosis (TB) has become so commonplace in the USA that, in 1987, the Centers for Disease Control (CDC) expanded its AIDS surveillance case definition, to include human immunodeficiency virus (HIV)-positive patients with extrapulmonary TB and, in 1993, to include HIV-positive patients with pulmonary TB or clinically suspected pulmonary TB.

The changes in immune response in the co-infection have led to a different pattern of disease, and this has had an impact on the clinical and imaging characteristics of TB in these cases. In the lungs, cavitating upper-lobe disease is replaced by a wider pattern of non-cavitating pulmonary infiltration associated with lymphadenopathy. In other parts of the body, pericardial, peritoneal, gastrointestinal, meningeal and miliary disease become common complications although, in intravenous (IV)-drug abusers with AIDS, bone and joint infection remains an important feature.

It is apparent that both the HIV-positive state and AIDS accelerate the progress of TB, and TB is often the primary indication of impending AIDS in HIV-positive patients. Villoria et al demonstrate a number of cases of AIDS where tuberculous meningitis was the presenting disorder, and the prodromal signs of listlessness, headache, fever and altered consciousness were the first indication of meningitis linked to AIDS [3]. The role played by the radiologist in recognising these new patterns and in helping to confirm the diagnosis cannot be overemphasised.

Beginning in the 1950s, there was a continuous, and initially rapid, decline in the number of cases of TB reported annually in the USA [4, 5]. Between 1977 and 1985, the decline was 5% annually. This was not the case with extrapulmonary TB, where the percentage rose from 14% to 17% as the numbers remained relatively constant during the same period [5–7].

After 1985, the annual number of cases began to rise and, by 1991, the CDC estimated that 39,000 more cases than expected had been noted [5]. This rising curve continues today. Many authors have linked the rise to the increase in HIV-positive cases, and this is indeed one of the factors. However, socio-economic conditions, immigration, widespread drug abuse, non-compliant patients and the emergence of drug-resistant strains of TB are also important reasons for the rise in case numbers.

The dramatic rise is not nationwide, but in the north-east coastal urban areas and in Florida there is a very high proportion of TB amongst AIDS patients [7]. In areas such as Tennessee, where AIDS is less of a problem even in urban areas, the number of TB cases has remained almost constant, and extrapulmonary cases have, in fact, fallen due to an unexplained fall in genito-urinary TB [6]

In patients attending TB centres and hospitals in the USA, roughly 3.4% are positive for HIV. However, the rate varies widely, from as high as 46% in New York City to less than 1% in Honolulu [7]. Pulmonary TB was the most common form but, in HIV-positive patients, 19% had extrapulmonary TB, compared with 10% of sero-negative patients [7]. In patients with AIDS, between 70% and 89% have extrapulmonary manifestations [4]. In San Francisco, Theurs found 28% sero-positive in a group of 60 non-Asian, tuberculous patients [2]. In general, the co-infection affects the sexually active age groups, and TB is uncommon in AIDS patients below the age of 10 years [8]. It is, then, of vital importance to test tuberculous patients for HIV, and HIV patients for TB.

In Africa, the same pattern of "new tuberculosis" is emerging. As sputum culture is often relied upon to make the diagnosis and, in Africa, other methods of diagnosis may be lacking, the new form of pulmonary TB is diagnosed with difficulty [9].

The co-infection is also seen in increasing numbers. The recently quoted numbers of HIV-positive patients in groups of tuberculous patients were 110/188 (59%) in Zambia, in Uganda 58%, 137/403 (34%) in Zimbabwe and 105/656 (16%) in Nairobi [10].

In Latin America, Haitians show a high sero-positive prevalence amongst TB patients. In Brazil, 21% of 5219 HIV cases had TB and, in Spain, the association reaches 67% among AIDS patients who are also IV-drug abusers [3, 5, 10, 11]. In theory, TB in these groups should be curable if the organism is sensitive to chemotherapy. However, in AIDS patients where the CD4 cell count is less than 200/mm^3, there is a high mortality, often due to associated opportunistic infections.

Mortalities are 36% for patients with a CD4 cell count under 200/mm^3, 8% if the cell count is between 200/mm^3 and 500/mm^3 and 2% if it is above 500/mm^3. If, however, there is multi-drug resistance, then mortality is extremely high, and death is rapid. A common mortality rate is 72–89%, with death within 4–16 weeks [1]. Early diagnosis and appropriate treatment are of vital importance. Rapid methods of bacteriological examination are of great help here, and the anergic response of many AIDS patients must be borne in mind if tuberculin testing is undertaken. Chest radiography is of value, as up to 80% of these cases have evidence of pulmonary TB.

Central Nervous System TB in Patients with AIDS

In HIV-positive and AIDS patients, all areas of the central nervous system (CNS) may be affected by TB. The infection may be due to reactivation of a pre-existing focus or rapid spread from a newly acquired infection.

In the brain, both meningitis and parenchymal TB occur and, in the spinal-cord, arachnoiditis, radiculomyelitis, myelitis, oedema, infarction and mass lesions are seen. These lesions may be tuberculous or due to other common conditions in AIDS, such as virus infections, HIV myelitis, cytomegalic inclusion virus or progressive multifocal leukoencephalopathy. These, as well as fungal disease and neoplasms, must all be considered in addition to the less common involvement by TB.

The infection is often seen in the early stages of the immunosuppressed state; it is emphasised that the infection is sometimes a precursor, the HIV-positive state being confirmed after the onset of TB [5, 12]. There is a more rapid progression of the illness in those patients with very low CD4 lymphocyte counts, and there are differences between the manifestations of the neurological infection in HIV/AIDS patients and in immunocompetent patients.

The rate of CNS infection of 10% is much higher than the 2% recorded in tuberculous cases in the general population. Also, the presence of co-infections and malignancies of the nervous system lead to clinical states differing from those in immunocompetent patients [5, 13]. Up to 65% of cases have evidence of tuberculous infection in other parts of the body, usually in the lungs. In cases with meningitis, study of the cerebrospinal fluid (CSF) is atypical for TB meningitis in that, in almost 50% of cases, the protein levels are not raised.

The rate of positive CSF cultures for *M. tuberculosis* is high, with 16 of 24 patients positive in Whiteman's study [12]. Assessment of the CSF adenosine deaminase estimation is a helpful test. In some centres, direct CSF smears have been positive for alcohol acid-fact bacilli.

In patients already diagnosed as having AIDS, the development of CNS symptoms may be slow, with headache and changes in mentation at the forefront. Similar symptoms arise due to the many other opportunistic conditions that affect this group of patients, making diagnosis difficult.

Localised CNS signs are uncommon, and seizures are rare. Tuberculous meningitis (TBM) has developed during anti-tuberculous therapy, and it is postulated that this was due to paradoxical expansion of an already-present cerebral focus [13, 14].

Imaging

Tuberculous Meningitis

The classical triad of basal meningeal enhancement, hydrocephalus and basal ganglia infarction is present in roughly 33% of cases. The intense basal-meningeal enhancement usually present on computed tomography (CT) and magnetic resonance imaging (MRI) images after IV contrast medium injection is not seen in the more common cryptococcal meningitis of AIDS. Metastatic meningeal lymphoma, however, enhances intensely, and CSF examination, both bacteriological and histological, is helpful in differentiating TBM from lymphoma. Biopsy at lymph-node sites in other areas of the body may also be helpful.

The enhancement of the surface of peripheral nerve roots in the lumbar regions due to metastatic carcinoma and lymphoma, called "sugar coating" or "frosting", is also seen in tuberculous radiculomyelitis [15]. Enhancing ependymal lesions confined to the ventricles are seen in cytomegalic inclusion virus (CMV) infections. Ependymitis in TBM is usually only seen in the terminally ill and is always accompanied by extensive meningeal enhancement, which is absent in CMV.

Tuberculous Parenchymal Lesions

In the AIDS-infected population, tuberculous mass lesions in the parenchyma are less common than TBM and, when they occur, they usually do so in combination with TBM [5]. In up to 20% of cases with neurological TB and AIDS, true TB abscesses are seen; this compares with 4–8% of sero-negative patients [12].

The pattern of the distribution of parenchymal lesions is similar in both groups of patients. The cortico-medullary junction predominates, but periventricular and pericisternal lesions are described. In both populations, supra-and infra-tentorial parenchymal lesions are seen, but the latter are much less frequent. The size of the granulomata is generally smaller in AIDS patients, usually less than 1 cm in diameter and causing little surrounding oedema or displacement [3, 5, 12].

Cryptococcus is a more common infection in AIDS patients than TB. It is usually meningeal but, when parenchymal lesions occur, they usually cannot be differentiated from tuberculoma by axial imaging. Cryptococcal lesions that do not enhance on T1-gadolinium (Gd) contrast images have been described, and it is postulated that these represent dilated Virchow-Robin spaces in and around the midbrain. In another pattern, small multiple calcifications are present in the brain parenchyma and the leptomeninges. Hydrocephalus is uncommon in cryptococcal infection, probably due to the low grade of the associated inflammatory reaction, which causes negligible interference to the flow of CSF. This type of pattern has not been described in TB. MRI is more sensitive in demonstrating these different lesions than CT [16].

Toxoplasma gondii is the most common organism affecting the brain in AIDS patients. Toxoplasmic granulomata are usually periventricular, in the basal ganglia or in the midbrain. Although they may be solid or ring-like and enhancing, their distribution differs from the common cortico-medullary pattern of tubercular parenchymal lesions. However, by imaging alone, they are difficult to differentiate from TB granulomas. A rising titre of serum-specific antibody for toxoplasmosis is taken as evidence of infection. Both diseases may be present at the same time [17].

Both primary and metastatic lymphoma of the CNS may mimic tubercular lesions. Primary lymphoma is present in 2–6% of AIDS patients with neurological symptoms, and metastatic lymphoma in 1–5%. Primary lymphoma in AIDS patients is often multi-centric and similar in appearance to multiple tuberculomas, which in AIDS may be represented by a mix of solid and centrally caseating lesions. Single primary lymphoma is often a deep lesion in the region of the thalamus and may cross the midline. Tuberculomas do not grow across the midline, though they may displace midline structures.

Metastatic lymphoma is often meningeal. It enhances and can be confused with tuberculous, gyral cerebritis or with tuberculoma en plaque. Both types of lymphoma take up the radioactive tracer thallium-201. This isotope may be utilised with single-photon emission computed tomography images to outline lymphoma tissue in the brain. Tuberculomas do not concentrate the isotope [18].

Central necrosis in tuberculomas must be differentiated from true tuberculous abscess. In AIDS patients, true abscesses tend to be larger than tuberculomas, often reaching 3 cm in diameter. They are often single, unlike the multiple tuberculomata found in AIDS. The clinical pattern of focal cerebritis and space occupation develops rapidly. Peripheral enhancement is similar to that in pyogenic cerebral abscess, which is rare in AIDS but is the alternative diagnosis, especially in IV-drug users. Drainage will be necessary and reveals large numbers of tubercle bacilli.

Both CT and MRI images are of value in investigating these cases. Villoria found MRI T1-Gd images more sensitive in demonstrating meningeal enhancement than computer-enhanced CT. Also, cerebritis, juxta-pial lesions and small infarctions are readily seen on MRI, whereas CT beam-hardening artefacts and infra-tentorial limitations are well known.

TB of the Gastrointestinal Tract and Abdominal Organs in Patients with AIDS

A wide spectrum of infections and malignant conditions affect those with AIDS, and both clinical findings and imaging patterns overlap the characteristic lesions of abdominal TB. AIDS itself produces malaise and weight loss. Any opportunistic infection of the gastrointestinal tract adds abdominal pain and diarrhoea to the pattern of symptoms. *Candida*, *Cryptosporidium*, CMV infection, herpes simplex and *Mycobacterium avium intracellulare* (MAI), all result in clinical states with high morbidities and similarities to infection by *M. tuberculosis*.

AIDS-related lymphoma (ARL) and Kaposi sarcoma (KS) are the common malignancies occurring in AIDS and cause widespread nodal disease similar to TB. Early diagnosis of TB and treatment leads to cure of the infection, but MAI infection is highly resistant to anti-mycobacterial drugs and, as it is usually found in patients with low CD4-lymphocyte levels, it is a common cause of death.

Tuberculous infection of the lymph nodes is usually associated with solid-organ or gastrointestinal TB infection. Both mesenteric and retroperitoneal groups are involved. On CT examination, central hypodensity (due to caseation) with rim enhancement is seen after contrast injection. Biopsy with culture is necessary to make the diagnosis.

In both KS and MAI, lymph-node groups in the abdomen and in the inguinal regions are common. In disseminated KS, the nodes are often uniformly hyper-attenuating after contrast injection, without central hypodensity [19].

The most common causes of abdominal lymphadenopathy in AIDS patients, according to Jeffrey et al., were ARL, KS and MAI [20]. There may, however, be geographical differences, as Radin suggests TB to be the most common cause in his group of 259 patients, with MAI second, ARL third and KS next [21]. Sansom [22] suggests that this may be due to a higher incidence of TB among the AIDS population of southern California, because, in England, in a group of 156 patients, MAI was first, ARL second KS third and TB fourth. In a further group of 29 autopsies on AIDS patients with a confirmed diagnosis of TB, the most commonly affected organs were lymph nodes (59%), lungs (56%), spleen (53%), liver (45%) and kidneys (37%) [23–25].

MAI is difficult to differentiate from infection due to *M. tuberculosis*. Both infections involve the solid organs, gastrointestinal tract and lymph nodes. MAI has been labelled the Whipple's disease of AIDS, as it characteristically affects the jejunum and the mesenteric nodes.

Extensive, diffuse wall thickening in the small bowel is seen, accompanied by diarrhoea. Lymph nodes are enlarged between 1.5 cm and 3 cm and are described as bulky by Nyberg et al. [26]. Radin emphasises that the lymph nodes are often homogeneous and of soft-tissue density, which is similar to the density of muscle [27]. Marked hepato-splenomegaly is also more often seen in MAI than in TB. Fine-needle biopsy is, however, necessary to make a certain diagnosis.

Although common in the distal gastrointestinal tract and abdominal lymph nodes in the general population, tuberculosis of the oesophagus and stomach are uncommon. In the oesophagus, it is postulated that both the pH and constant passage of saliva preclude the deposition of mycobacteria in the mucosa. In patients with AIDS, oesophageal tuberculosis is reported more often. This may be the result of co-existing opportunistic infections, *Candida*, herpes, CMV and breach of the defence mechanisms of the mucosa by *Cryptosporidium*, allowing oesophagitis to develop.

In the general sero-negative population, the usual initially infected focus is in a mediastinal lymph node, and the oesophagus is secondarily affected, often with fistula formation between the mediastinum, or a bronchus and the oesophagus [28]. In AIDS patients, both this mechanism and true oesophagitis occur, and de Silva et al. reported six patients encountered over a 7-month period. One case had MAI, the others TB. In all cases, there was fistula development [29].

True mucosal oesophagitis is rare, and transmural lesions with fistula formation are more usual. Goodman describes a case with both fistula formation and mucosal ulceration, characteristically longitudinal in direction (Fig. 8.1) [30]. In immunocompetent patients, TB infection of the stomach usually infects the pyloric segment and leads to stricture, stenosis and gastric retention. In AIDS patients, strictures have been described in another opportunistic infection, *Cryptosporidium*. This has to be differentiated from TB and MAI by biopsy and culture.

In the case described by Brody, the tuberculous lesion is, unusually, at the gastric fundus. There was also an associated soft-tissue mass in the lesser sac, as demonstrated on CT scanning. Endoscopically, the intraluminal lesion appeared malignant. Later histological examination revealed necrotising granulomas, and TB was cultured from a mesenteric lymph node [31].

Beyond the pylorus, tuberculous infection of the intestines is relatively common and, as in sero-negative patients, in TB with AIDS the ileocaecal region is the favoured site. This is in contradistinction to MAI infection, where segmental, small-bowel lesions combined with hepato-splenomegaly are usual, as is a more florid type of lymphadenopathy that often affects the glands of the inguinal region in addition to mesenteric and retroperitoneal lymph nodes.

Bargallo et al. report that, in Spain, the incidence of TB in AIDS patients is 30%, rising to 67% in IV-drug abusers and recidivists. Four of six patients that she describes demonstrated pulmonary as well as gastrointestinal lesions (Fig. 8.2) [11]. Although the imaging findings in this group of AIDS patients were generally similar to those seen in sero-negative patients with intestinal tuberculosis, the degree of bowel-wall thickening and the extent of adenopathy was greater in the sero-positive group.

CT examination has the advantage of demonstrating the bowel-wall changes, solid-organ lesions, lymphadenopathy and high-density ascites. Barium studies afford a more detailed view of the changes in the intestinal mucosa. In Bargallo's study, a duodenal fistula was demonstrated by both CT and barium studies.

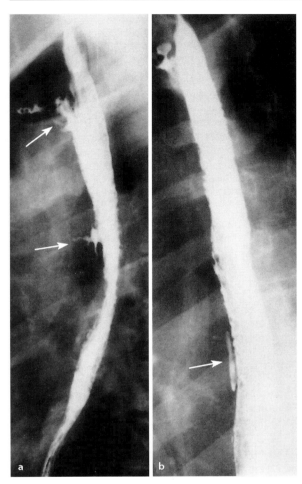

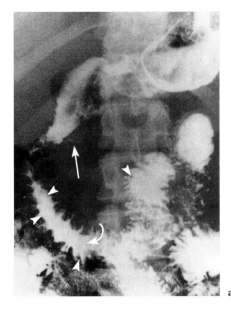

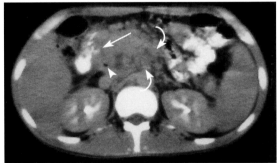

Fig. 8.1. a Barium swallow shows characteristic sinus tracts arising from ulcers on the anterior wall of the oesophagus and passing into the mediastinum (*arrows*). **b** Shallow, longitudinal ulceration is demonstrated (*arrow*). Abundant mycobacteria were obtained at oesophagoscopy. Pulmonary tuberculosis was also present. Images by courtesy of Dr. P. Goodman, University of Texas Medical School, Houston

Fig. 8.2. a Duodenal tuberculosis in a case of acquired immunodeficiency syndrome presented with widening of the duodenal loop (*arrowheads*), with thickening of the mucosal folds (*curved arrow*), and a fistulous tract (*arrow*). **b** Computed tomography study at the level of the duodenum reveals the fistula (*arrow*) together with a hypodense mass of lymph nodes (*curved arrow*). There is also extra-luminal gas present (*arrowhead*). Images by courtesy of Dr. Nuria Bargallo. Hospital Clinic i Provincial, Barcelona, Spain

Ultrasound is also of great value in demonstrating bowel-wall thickening in the area of the ileocaecal valve, peritoneal changes in associated TB peritonitis and focal lesions in the liver and spleen. As in non-AIDS TB, the pre-pancreatic group of lymph nodes is often markedly enlarged and must be differentiated from a pancreatic mass.

Tuberculosis of Solid Abdominal Organs in AIDS Patients

Splenic Tuberculosis

As is the case with CNS TB, splenic tuberculosis may be the initial sign of conversion from the HIV-positive state to AIDS [32]. Recent publications suggest that multiple splenic lesions are more frequent in AIDS cases than was previously thought. This may be an expression of disseminated tuberculosis as, in most reported cases, chest radiographs demonstrate lymphadenopathy with or without pulmonary parenchymal disease.

Lesions discovered at splenectomy are multiple, round, soft, caseating masses that contain many TB organisms. Biopsy of the lesions produces tissue showing caseating necrosis but with poorly formed granulomas. This is to be expected, in view of the lowered inflammatory responses of AIDS patients. Hepatomegaly may also be present [30–32].

Imaging, by ultrasound, of multiple hypoechoic splenic lesions is the norm, as is hepatomegaly with a homogeneous structure. CT study points to hypodense splenic lesions but, in the cases published so far, there is no mention of the response to IV contrast agents. In non-sero-positive patients with splenic TB, the lesions may enhance solidly or show ring enhancement, and it is to be expected that similar findings will be present in AIDS patients. Most authors confirmed the diagnosis by image-guided splenic aspiration biopsy and recorded no complications; however, a case of hepatosplenic tuberculosis with hypersplenism has been reported, so careful haematological assessment is necessary before biopsy [33]. Treatment with a standard four-drug regime produced a good response in most recorded cases.

Hepatic TB in AIDS is suspected in the differential diagnosis of those patients with abnormal liver enzymes. Macronodular tuberculous liver disease in AIDS has not yet been reported in the literature, and widespread microscopic involvement with diffuse hepatomegaly is more usual.

In a series of ten patients with AIDS and abnormal liver enzymes, hepatic granulomas were observed on blind liver biopsy in all ten patients [34]. Only one case had TB, and five had MAI. Three others showed granulomas, but no mycobacteria were found, and one case was of cryptococcal infection. Imaging methods and liver size were not recorded but, from the experience of these authors, hepatic TB and MAI infection may be much more widespread than has so far been appreciated.

In a female drug abuser known to be HIV positive, presenting with a history of fever, pulmonary miliary disease was seen on chest radiography with hilar lymphadenopathy. Abdominal ultrasound revealed a 7-cm-diameter true abscess in the liver, which required percutaneous drainage and contained large numbers of tubercle bacilli. After drainage, the patient responded well to anti-tuberculous chemotherapy. In a second case, a young male drug abuser was found to have a tuberculous abscess of the prostate gland. In both of these cases, a diagnosis of pyogenic abscess would be expected in view of the IV-drug abuse [35].

Physicians should no longer be surprised by the unexpected discovery of tuberculous infection, especially among AIDS patients; nor should it be surprising, when an unusual extra-pulmonary expression of TB is found, that the patient proves to be HIV positive.

Bone and Joint Tuberculosis in AIDS Patients

In addition to the usual spectrum of musculoskeletal tuberculosis, there are sites of infection in AIDS patients suggestive of the syndrome. Destructive lesions of the ribs, with an associated cold abscess, are relatively common while, because of the relatively high proportion of IV-drug abusers, tuberculous infection of the costo-chondral junctions and the sterno-clavicular joints is common. Pulmonary changes are present in up to 73 % of these cases, and sputum specimens often show *M. tuberculosis*. Biopsy may nevertheless be necessary to exclude concomitant fungal or pyogenic disease [36].

References

1. Cohn DL (1994) Treatment and prevention of tuberculosis in HIV-infected persons. Infect Dis Clin North Am 8:399–412
2. Theuer CP, Hopewell PC, Elias D, et al. (1990) Human immunodeficiency virus infection in tuberculous patients. J Infect Dis 162:8–12
3. Villoria MF, de la Torre J, Fortea F, et al. (1992) Intracranial tuberculosis in AIDS: CT and MRI findings. Neuroradiology 34:11–14
4. Buckner CB, Leithiser RE, Walker CW, et al. (1991) The changing epidemiology of tuberculosis and other mycobacterial infections in the USA: implications for the radiologist. Am J Roentgenol 156:255–264
5. Villoria MF, Fortea F, Moreno S, et al. (1995) MR imaging and CT of central nervous system tuberculosis in patients with AIDS. Radiol Clin North Am 33:805–820
6. Mehta JB, Dutt A, Harvill L, et al. (1991) Epidemiology of extrapulmonary tuberculosis. Chest 99:1134–1138
7. Onorato IM, McCray E (1992) Prevalence of human immunodeficiency virus infection among patients attending tuberculosis clinics in the USA. J Infect Dis 165:87–92
8. Braun MM, Byers RH, Heyward WL, et al. (1990) Acquired immunodeficiency syndrome and extrapulmonary tuberculosis in the USA. Arch Intern Med 150:1913–1916
9. Harries AD (1990) Tuberculosis and human immunodeficiency virus infection in developing countries. Lancet 335:387–390
10. Pitchenik AE (1990) Tuberculosis control and the AIDS epidemic in developing countries. Ann Intern Med 113:89–91
11. Bargallo N, Nicolau C, Luburich P, et al. (1992) Intestinal tuberculosis in AIDS. Gastrointest Radiol 17:115–118
12. Whiteman M, Espinoza L, Post MJ, et al. (1995) Central nervous system tuberculosis in HIV-infected patients: clinical and radiographic findings. Am J Neuroradiol 16:1319–1327
13. Berenguer J, Moreno S, Laguna F, et al. (1992) Tuberculous meningitis in patients infected with the human immunodeficiency virus. N Engl J Med 326:668–672
14. Teoh R, Humphries MJ, O'Mahoney G (1987) Symptomatic tuberculoma developing during treatment of tuberculosis: a report of 10 patients and a review of the literature. QJM 63:449–460
15. Holz AJ (1998) The sugarcoating sign. Radiology 208:143–144
16. Tien RD, Chu PK, Hesselink JR, et al. (1991) Intracranial cryptococcosis in immunocompromised patients. Am J Neuroradiol 12:283–289
17. Ramsey RG, Geremia GK (1988) CNS complications of AIDS: CT and MR findings. Am J Roentgenol 151:449–454

18. Ruiz A, Ganz WI, Post MJ, et al. (1994) Use of thalium-201 brain SPECT to differentiate cerebral lymphoma from toxoplasma encephalitis in AIDS patients. Am J Neuroradiol 15:1885–1894

19. Herts BR, Megibow AJ, Birnbaum BA, et al. (1992) High-attenuation lymphadenopathy in AIDS patients: significance of findings at CT. Radiology 185:777–781

20. Jeffrey RB, Nyberg DA, Bottles K, et al. (1986) Abdominal CT in acquired immunodeficiency syndrome. Am J Roentgenol 146:7–13

21. Radin R (1995) HIV infection: analysis in 259 consecutive patients with abnormal abdominal CT findings. Radiology 197:712–722

22. Sansom H, Seddon B, Padley SGP (1997) Clinical utility of abdominal CT scanning in patients with HIV disease. Clin Radiol 52:698–703

23. Abdel-Dayem HM, Naddaf S, Aziz M, et al. (1997) Sites of tuberculous involvement in patients with AIDS. Clin Nucl Med 22:310–314

24. Nyberg DA, Federle MP, Jeffrey RB (1985) Abdominal CT findings of disseminated mycobacterium avium-intracellulare in AIDS. Am J Roentgenol 145:297–299

25. Radin DR (1991) Intraabdominal mycobacterium tuberculosis vs mycobacterium avium-intracellulare infections in patients with AIDS. Am J Roentgenol 156:487–491

26. Ramakantan R, Shah P (1990) Tuberculous fistulas of the pharynx and esophagus. Gastrointest Radiol 15:145–147

27. de Silva R, Stoopack PM, Raufman J-P (1990) Esophageal fistulas associated with mycobacterial infection in patients at risk for AIDS. Radiology 175:449–453

28. Goodman P, Pinero SS, Rance RM, et al. (1989) Mycobacterial esophagitis in AIDS. Gastrointest Radiol 14:103–105

29. Brody JM, Miller DK, Zeman RK, et al. (1986) Gastric tuberculosis: a manifestation of acquired immunodeficiency syndrome. Radiology 159:347–348

30. Wolff MJ, Bitran J, Northland RG, et al. (1991) Splenic abscesses due to mycobacterium tuberculosis in patients with AIDS. Rev Infect Dis 13:373–375

31. Lozano F, Gomez-Mateos J, Lopez-Cortes L, et al. (1991) Tuberculous splenic abscesses in patients with aquired immune deficiency syndrome. Tubercle 72:307–308

32. Pedro-Botet J, Maristany MT, Miralles R, et al. (1991) Splenic tuberculosis in patients with AIDS. Rev Infect Dis 13:1069–1071

33. Choi BI, Im J-G, Han MC, et al. (1989) Hepatosplenic tuberculosis with hypersplenism: CT evaluation. Gastrointest Radiol 14:265–267

34. Orenstein M.S, Tavitian A, Yonk B. et al. (1985) Granulomatous involvement of the liver in patients with AIDS. Gut 26:1229–1225

35. Moreno S, Pacho E, Lopez-Herce JA, et al. (1988) Mycobacterium tuberculosis visceral abscesses in the acquired immunodeficiency syndrome. Ann Intern Med 109:437

36. Goodman PC (1995) Tuberculosis and AIDS. Radiol Clin North Am 33:707–717

CHAPTER 9

Tuberculous Disease in the Paediatric Age Group

■ Introduction

Tuberculosis (TB) of infants and children is a serious infection, often leading to death or major incapacity. The underlying process of primary TB varies in intensity from a silent event to a rampant infectious condition. Delay in diagnosis is one of the major factors leading to complications. This delay is often the result of the varied clinical presentation of the patient, which suggests other common conditions; the delay is also a result of the inexperience of doctors in the West, who are often being confronted by the condition for the first time [1, 2].

Infants are particularly vulnerable to the infection, which in the very young almost invariably has a pulmonary presence but is rapidly disseminated through the lymph nodes, central nervous system and abdominal organs. There is a high death rate and morbidity, showing a relationship to the delay before the instigation of anti-tuberculous drugs [2, 3].

In America, until 1984, childhood TB was in decline but, since that time, there has been an annual increase in case numbers, parallel to the changes seen among adults [4]. In Africa and the Far East, there have always been high levels of TB among the young and, due to the turbulent conditions in many areas in the last few years, there is anecdotal evidence of a general increase in childhood disease. However, the collection of data has ceased in many areas where wars have occurred.

Every new childhood case indicates transfer of the infection from a contagious source in the community, as reactivation TB does not occur in childhood. The source is invariably a family member or close social contact [5, 6].

In Africa, poor housing conditions and overcrowding allow the spread of the bacillus by airborne droplet infection. Malnourished and underweight children are a target group for the infection. In the West, however, both Strouse and Hooijboer describe childhood TB in immunocompetent children living under Western social conditions [2, 7].

In children, 30 % of TB cases are extra-pulmonary, but it is impossible to separate these cases from those with pulmonary disease, as 90 % of all cases have pulmonary manifestations. The pulmonary primary complex spreads to the hilar or mediastinal lymph nodes. Compression of the major airways is the common result and, in the infant, gives rise to a clinical picture of stridor and tachypnoea. Erosion of a venule or arteriole allows the dissemination of the disease as miliary infection. Evidence of meningeal or abdominal infection may predominate, but it is difficult, on clinical grounds, to differentiate between TB and pyogenic disease. Hepato-splenomegaly, with or without jaundice, is a common presentation and, in the very young, may be the only sign of the infection [3].

Infants with meningeal disease often show few signs of meningism, and there may be an indolent onset, with lethargy, floppiness and gaze disturbances linked with fever. Careful retinal examination reveals choroidal tubercles [1]. Even in the very young, the imaging triad of basal meningeal enhancement, hydrocephalus and cerebral infarction is often established at the time of presentation. The cerebrospinal fluid (CSF) changes of lymphocytic pleomorphism, increase in protein and low sugar content are important in differentiating these cases from pyogenic meningitis. Smear examination of the CSF, rapid methods of bacterial culture and CSF adenosine deaminase levels are helpful. Dystrophic calcification in the meninges and gyri has been seen at an early stage in children [8, 9].

■ Congenital TB

There has been a ninefold increase in TB among pregnant women in New York City in recent times. An increase in the number of cases of congenital TB can be expected as long as the present epidemic of the disease continues. One of the difficulties in making the diagnosis is that the site of infection in the mother is often extra-pulmonary. Unsuspected genital TB is commonly the source [10].

Congenital TB is a relatively rare condition, as *Mycobacterium tuberculosis* does not normally cross the placental barrier. If miliary disease occurs in the mother, tubercle formation in the placenta leads to rupture of granulomas either into the foetal circulation or the amniotic fluid [10, 11]. The bacillus then either passes through the umbilical veins to form a primary complex in the liver or is ingested by the foetus from the amniotic fluid. Rare cases of middle-ear TB have arisen from exposure of the external auditory canal or the Eustachian tube to infected amniotic fluid [12].

Infected babies rarely reach term and are usually born prematurely in the last trimester. At delivery, tubercles are visible on the surface of the placenta and, in cases where a mother has been febrile during the pregnancy, placental material should be saved and submitted for histology and culture.

Before the availability of isoniazid (INH), there was a 100% mortality rate but, since the introduction of effective chemotherapy, this has been reduced to 50%. However, the characteristic miliary, pulmonary, hepatic and bone-marrow spread can lead to irreversible complications and multi-organ failure. Serious haematological complications develop, disseminated intravascular coagulopathy (DIC) may be found and bone-marrow study demonstrates haemophagocytic syndrome in some cases.

Neonatal fever, jaundice and hepato-splenomegaly are usually present with miliary changes and mediastinal lymph-node enlargement on chest radiography. Choroidal tubercles are often seen on fundal examination. Ultrasound demonstrates the hepatic and splenic enlargement, but there are usually no focal solid-organ lesions. However, abdominal lymphadenopathy is present, and hepatic or lymph-node biopsy confirms the diagnosis.

The protein purified derivative (PPD) test is often negative, as the immune status of these often pre-mature infants is immature. In those babies that present later in the neonatal period, it is important to screen the family and contacts as well as the mother to confirm that the infection is congenital and to discover any other source [11].

■ Abdominal TB in Infants and Children

Only 1–5% of cases of childhood pulmonary TB develop extension of the disease to the abdominal organs [13]. These cases may be subdivided into gastrointestinal TB, peritoneal TB and solid-organ TB. Extensive lymph-node disease may be present with any of these forms. With the exception of renal TB, solid-organ TB is very rare in childhood. Peritonitis is also uncommon. Nagi describes 5 cases of peritonitis among 38 examples of abdominal TB [14].

The age group most affected is from 2 years to 15 years of age, and the swallowing of infected sputum in children with pulmonary TB plays a role in the pathogenesis of the disease [9]. Haematogenous spread also occurs but, in endemic areas, the ingestion of non-pasteurised milk is still an important method of infection.

As in other forms of childhood tuberculous infection, those under 5 years of age are particularly vulnerable to the disease and, unless an early diagnosis is made, there is a 50% mortality rate [15]. After multiplication of the organism in the abundant lymphatic tissue of the sub-mucosa of the intestine, extension of the enteric lesion occurs followed by spread of the infection to the regional and central abdominal lymph nodes (Fig. 9.1).

The common presentation as in adults is as an ileocaecal lesion, often accompanied by a lymphoid

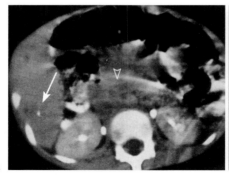
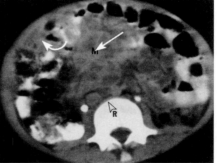

a   b

Fig. 9.1 a, b. Abdominal computed tomography (CT) scan of a 2-year-old African boy who had been suffering weight loss and abdominal pain for 3 months. **a** Both low-density and calcified granulomas are present in the liver (*arrow*) and a midline mass of lymph nodes (*open arrow*). **b** At a lower level, there is

a large midline mass of lymph nodes demonstrating ring enhancement (*M*). There are also retroperitoneal lymph nodes (*open arrow*) and a low-density mass in the omentum (*curved arrow*). Images by courtesy of Dr. F. M. Denath, Baragwanath Hospital, Johannesburg

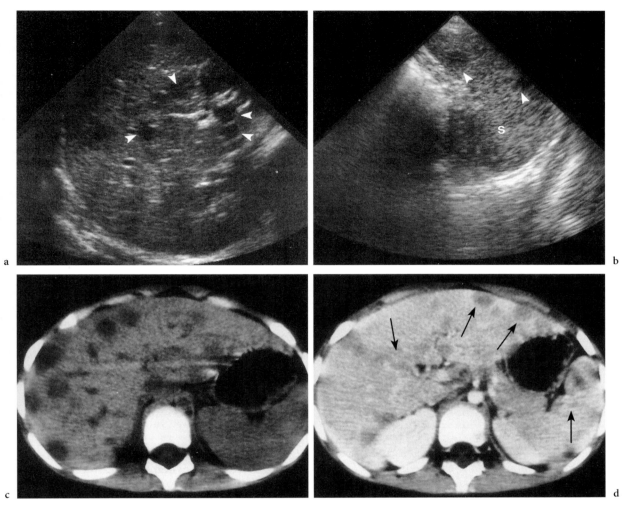

Fig. 9.2 a – d. A febrile 5-year-old Caucasian boy. Open biopsy of the liver revealed caseating granulomas with a few alcohol acid-fact bacilli. Ultrasound of the liver (**a**) and spleen (**b**) revealed multiple, rounded hypo-echoic and anechoic granulomas (*arrowheads*). **c, d** Pre- and post-contrast computed tomography at the level of the liver and spleen shows multiple, rounded, hypo-dense granulomas scattered through the liver. The post-contrast study (**d**) demonstrated rim enhancement in both the liver and spleen granulomas (*arrows*). Images by courtesy of Dr. C. Levine, Missouri School of Medicine, USA

mass. In children, the onset is insidious, and there may be considerable debilitation and wasting before help is sought. Abdominal pain and distension are usually present.

If tuberculous peritonitis is present, then findings similar to those in adults occur, with wet, dry and plastic types being portrayed. Plain radiographs, ultrasound and computed tomography (CT) scanning are all of value, and classical barium studies are usually necessary to show the full extent of mucosal enteric disease, although CT is of considerable help in pin-pointing affected areas (Fig. 9.2).

Calcification in the lymph nodes and, less commonly, in the liver or spleen is more often seen as an end result of childhood than of adult disease and is demonstrated both on radiographs and on CT examination (Fig. 9.1). High-density ascitic fluid can be documented on CT as can solid-organ and lymph-node lesions [9, 13, 15, 16]. Ultrasound is of great value in these children, with bowel mesenteric, lymphatic and solid-organ abnormalities being visualised (Fig. 9.3) [9, 13].

Acute presentation is often due to arising complications, and these are similar to those of the adult disease. Intestinal obstruction, perforation and acute appendicitis are all common, and TB as an underlying cause must be considered so that the necessary bacteriological specimens are submitted for study at the time of surgery. If surgery is not essential, then medical treatment should be initiated. Surgery, while

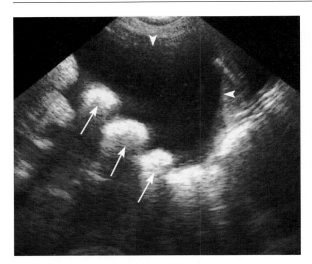

Fig. 9.3. Tuberculous peritonitis in a child shows matted loops of echogenic bowel (*arrows*) contrasting with anechoic ascites (*arrowheads*). Courtesy of Dr. B. J. Cremin, Red Cross Hospital, Cape Town

essential in some cases, has been shown to have a high morbidity [17].

In the liver and spleen, the origin of the lesion is by haematogenous spread, either systemically from a distant focus, or through the portal venous system from the bowel. In theory, lymphatic spread to the liver is also possible. Splenic lesions are rare and, in a series of 362 splenic abscesses, Chun and Nelken noted only a single tuberculous lesion [18]. However, in acquired immunodeficiency syndrome (AIDS) cases, tuberculous splenic abscesses are becoming more numerous than in the pre-AIDS period and, in

endemic areas of the co-infection, abdominal TB in children occurs [13].

The images seen are in no way specific and are more likely to be initially interpreted as the result of malignancy. Macro-nodular hepatic lesions (either single or multiple) and abdominal lymphoid masses are more often due to lymphoma than to an infection. Careful analysis of bodily fluids with rapid culture methods is essential, but the gold standard is the discovery of *M. tuberculosis* on aspiration biopsy or from other tissues (Fig. 9.4).

■ Renal TB

The pathogenesis of renal TB is such that overt infection in childhood is uncommon. The initial, bilateral haematological spread of infection initially heals. Unilateral reactivation is the pattern of development. This mostly occurs in the young adult. When it occurs in childhood, the usual age range is 8–15 years.

All of the imaging presentations seen in adult patients are also described in children. One important feature is apparently the result of the slow, sub-clinical progress of the disease in symptomless children. Considerable permanent destructive change has often occurred before presentation of the patient, and the infection has often destroyed the affected kidney to such an extent that no excretion is visible on urography [9, 19].

Ultrasound examination of these non-functioning kidneys reveals destruction of pericalyceal tissues to produce cavitation. This may simulate the appearance of hydronephrosis [19]. The widened or fibrotic ureter is also visible on ultrasound. The changes in the bladder – general contraction, wall thickening and golf-hole ureteric orifices – are important supportive evidence for the diagnosis, which is confirmed by culture of the urine. Fine-needle aspiration

Fig. 9.4 a, b. Tuberculous hepatic granulomas. **a** Rounded hypo-echoic lesions. **b** Hypo-echoic granuloma showing an echogenic centre (*arrow*). Courtesy of Dr. B. J. Cremin, Red Cross Hospital, Cape Town

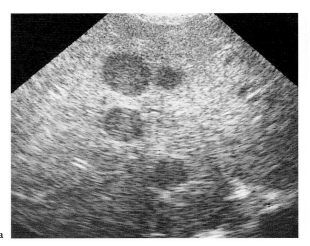

a

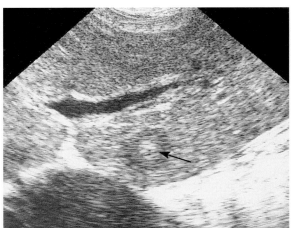

b

biopsy of granulomatous masses in the kidney may be necessary if the lower urinary tract is obstructed on the infected side, as the bacterium is unable to reach the urine [20].

Central nervous System TB in Children

Tuberculous meningitis (TBM) has a predilection for infants and young children. Untreated, it is a fatal disease, and the outcome after treatment is directly proportional to the stage at which the patient presents. Delay in initiation of anti-tubercular chemotherapy leads to a high proportion of neurological sequelae [2]. In the West, the highest proportion of patients is among immigrant populations, but it is essential to bear the diagnosis in mind when confronted by non-immigrant children with symptoms of meningitis. The disease is slow in development, with headache, irritability and lethargy being early symptoms and vomiting occurring as raised intracranial pressure develops. Unfortunately, most patients have reached an advanced stage by the time they or their parents seek help [2, 8].

Once ventriculomegaly has developed, the outlook for complete recovery is diminished. Infarction leads to focal neurological signs and such developments as mono- or hemiplegias; in addition, the level of consciousness is affected. Basal exudates that cause the arterial changes leading to infarction also result in cranial nerve deficits in up to 30 % of children with TBM [8, 21].

The diagnosis may be accelerated by correlating the chest radiographs, CSF analysis, PPD results and computer-enhanced CT (CECT) findings. Only 30 % or less of cases show signs of pulmonary TB and, apart from anergic cases, a high proportion of these children show positive PPD reactions. The CECT changes are non-specific, and similar appearances have been described in bacterial and fungal meningitis. The extent and intensity of the changes is usually lower in these other conditions.

Tuberculomata

In many areas where TB is endemic, parenchymal tuberculomas are the most common intracranial space-occupying lesions. This is particularly the case in children. The prodromal symptoms are quite different from those of TBM. Headache, lack of concentration and other mentation deficits, focal fits and focal neurological signs are indications of the underlying condition. In children, infra-tentorial tuberculomata are more usual than the supra-tentorial preference noted in adults. This, is of course, the case

in sporadic tuberculoma as, in the parenchymal tuberculomata complicating TBM, a supra-tentorial or combined distribution is more common [4, 21].

Cremin points out that the common form of tuberculoma has a gummatous histological structure, where the granulomatous tissue necroses. A less common form contains many cellular elements, and the necrosis of these often leads to true abscess formation [9]. When this type of abscess develops, it cannot be distinguished from a pyogenic abscess by imaging techniques. These abscesses also contain large numbers of *M. tuberculosis*, and the chance of seeding along the needle track is high when aspiration is undertaken [20]. Abscess development is less likely in children than in young adults.

The treatment of tuberculoma is often rewarded by complete recovery, although the duration of chemotherapy is long. The degree of post-contrast enhancement of the lesion on CECT and T1-weighted, gadolinium-contrast magnetic resonance imaging (MRI) is taken as an indication of activity. Calcification may develop in the lesion in the healing period, and the calcification process takes years rather than months. Encephalomyelopathy of the overlying brain tissue may also be a long-term development, and this may lead to permanent neurological deficits, depending on the site of the lesion.

In children, spinal-cord changes are almost invariably the result of tuberculous spondylitis (TS). Granulomatous disease of the cord or arachnoid is very rare. The introduction of MRI studies on a wider scale may lead to the discovery of more cases [9]. Studies using contrast-enhancing techniques demonstrate granulomatous deposits in the arachnoid and the nerve roots. Non-enhancing lesions may be due to infarction or oedema. Syrinx may also be associated with intra-medullary granulomas. In the late stages of both cranial and spinal meningitis, there is conversion of granulomatous arachnoid tissue into fibrous tissue, which is avascular and does not enhance [22].

Tuberculous Disease of the Spine in Children

TS is, in most geographical areas, a disease of young adults. In Africa, India and the Far East, it is also a disease of childhood and creates an abundance of paraplegic young children. Cremin reviewed 30 patients with an average age of 5 – 6 years whereas, in the West, the average age is more usually in the late 30 s [23].

At its onset, the disease is painless until stress resulting from mechanical factors or neurological complications supervene. In the uncommon cervical region lesions, the condition is painful from the out-

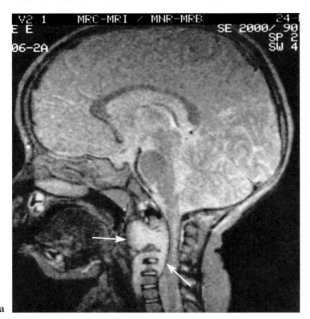
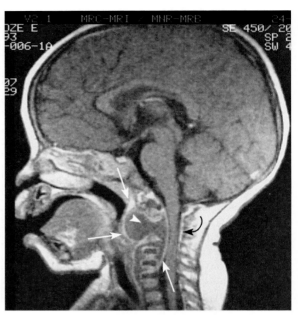

a   b

Fig. 9.5. a T2-weighted magnetic resonance image of a destructive lesion of the upper cervical spine from C2 to C4. Anterior and posterior tuberculous abscess are present (*arrows*). **b** T1-weighted post-gadolinium scan. The peripheries of the abscesses enhance (*arrows*), but the central caseous material does not (*arrowhead*). Note the spinal-cord compression (*curved arrow*). Courtesy of Dr. B. J. Cremin, Red Cross Hospital, Cape Town

set due to muscle spasm and torticollis (Fig. 9.5) [9]. In children, an initial lytic lesion close to the end plate is seen in the vertebral body. Narrowing of the disc space occurs at an earlier stage than in adults as a result of the more extensive vascularity of the paediatric annulus fibrosus. Implosion of the vertebral body is seen at an early stage, leading to fragmentation of the vertebral-body structure [23].

Although most of these changes are visible on plain radiographs and plain lateral tomography, analysis of CT or MRI will be necessary to assess posterior-element disease. The presence or absence of this will dictate the approach in any surgical intervention.

In children, the advance of the disease to affect the disc space and two or more contiguous vertebral bodies is rapid, and kyphosis is also seen at an early stage. In young groups of patients, paravertebral abscess formation is often extensive and may lead to erosion of the anterior margins of a number of vertebral bodies, of a type more often seen in aortic aneurysm in older individuals. Ultrasound examination of the loin is of value in children in mapping paravertebral collections and the extent of any psoas-sheath abscess.

The differential diagnosis in children is similar to that in adults, except that both pyogenic spondylitis and histiocytosis are relatively common in children. In pyogenic disease, the disc is destroyed at an earlier

stage, due to the presence of proteolytic enzymes, which are not produced by mycobacteria.

Histiocytosis leads to early vertebral-body collapse, often to vertebra plana. The disc space is preserved, and the characteristic well-circumscribed lesions of the condition are almost invariably seen in other bones, particularly the skull.

Cervical spine TB is not only painful but, in children, is much more extensive than in adults. Hsu, in a series of 1100 patients seen over a period of 30 years, described 46 patients with cervical TS. In children under the age of 10 years, the number of vertebrae involved was greater than in the adult patients, and the extent of abscess formation was much wider. In infants, nocturnal crying attacks due to muscle spasm and painful torticollis were a feature and, in three infants, stridor due to a large anterior collection compressing the airway occurred. Despite the extent of the anterior cervical abscess in this group of children, the posterior extent was limited, and fewer children developed spinal compression than adults [24].

In Hsu's cases, 42% of those with TS between C2 and C7 developed significant spinal compression syndromes. In children, 50–60% of the intra-spinal area must be compromised before spinal compression occurs. Kyphosis worsens the situation, as the canal contents are stretched over the angulation as well as over the anterior extra-dural abscess

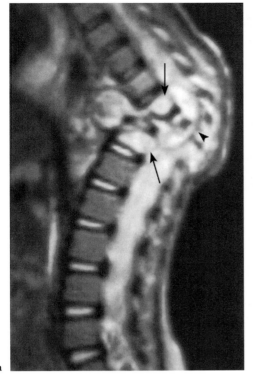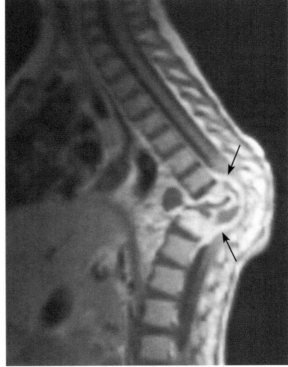

Fig. 9.6. Classic Pott's disease in a child. **a** On sagittal T2-weighted images, the bodies of T9 and T12 show a high-intensity signal (*arrows*). The intervening T10 and T11 bodies have been destroyed. There is an acute kyphosis, and the cord is compressed (*arrowhead*). **b** The post-gadolinium T1 image shows the extent of the abscess (*arrow*), and the low intensities signal necrotic contents. Courtesy of Dr. B. J. Cremin, Red Cross Hospital, Cape Town

(Fig. 9.6). Assessment of the lesion is difficult without access to CT or MRI [9]. Myelography, if available, will demonstrate the lower end of the spinal block but gives no information on the condition of the pedicles. Cremin suggests six aims for the radiologist, in cases of TS:

1. Demonstrate the number of vertebrae involved.
2. Assess the severity of bone destruction.
3. Demonstrate the site of involvement within the vertebrae.
4. Assess the angle of kyphosis.
5. Demonstrate the extent of soft-tissue involvement.
6. Demonstrate the extent of cord compression.

For those with access to axial scanning, all six aims are achievable but, for those without CT, plain-film radiography and tomography bring four of the aims within reach.

■ Osteoarticular Tuberculous Lesions in Children

As in adults, arthritic disease is more common than pure osteitis, and the main weight-bearing joints – the hip and the knee – are the usual sites. Mono-articular disease predominates and, as this begins as an effusion, it may be difficult to differentiate from mono-articular rheumatism in the early stages. Early aspiration and culture before irreversible changes have occurred in the joint are important in these cases. Aspiration is recommended in all persistent arthritides in children and, if culture reveals no organism, then needle biopsy of the synovium should be carried out [25]. The absence of pain is an important feature in tuberculous arthritis. Also, while in adults erosions at the margin of the joints are common, Cremin has not noted them in children [9]. As in adults, hyperaemic osteopenia occurs but, in children, this leads to enlargement of the epiphyses of the infected joint. The gradual development of joint-space loss, articular-surface destruction, sub-chondral cystic bone destruction and bone fragmentation as a result of caseation are paralleled by similar changes seen in the adult patient. As in all tuberculous joints, the infection characteristically crosses the epiphyseal line [26].

■ Osteitis

In general, the distribution and imaging features are similar to those in adults, but there are some features that are predominately seen in children. In the long bones, symmetrical lesions in both limbs are an example, and there is also a predilection for cystic lesions in flat bones (such as the scapula), which is less common in adults (Fig. 9.7).

Spina ventosa is much more common in children than in adults, as are lesions of the calvarium. Calvarial lesions may be isolated or part of a multi-centric osteitis. Tsui et al., reported of a 13-year-old Chinese girl presenting with pleurisy and multiple lesions of the flat bones and vertebrae. Even after 1 month of chemotherapy, further lesions developed in the vault of the skull and in vertebrae at other levels. The lesions slowly improved but, after 1 year, supra-clavicular lymphadenopathy was seen, together with a number of destructive calvarial osteitic lesions in the frontal and parietal regions. These skull lesions had sequestrated and had to be excised before further chemotherapy led to healing almost 3 years after the initial pleuritic lesion [27].

In infants, lesions of the ends of long bones may exhibit exuberant periosteal reaction, an effect commonly seen in primary bone neoplasm. In infants inoculated with Bacille Calmette-Guerin, osteitic lesions may develop as late as 2–5 years after vaccination. Although rare, if undiagnosed, this leads to the development of a lytic lesion in bone. Usually, a long bone is affected, but vertebral and flat-bone lesions have been reported. The osteitis invariably develops on the same side of the body as the inocultion. The lesions are diagnosed by the histological appearance and bacteriological study of biopsy tissue [28].

■ References

1. Kibel M (1996) Clinical spectrum and diagnosis in childhood tuberculosis. In: Cremin BJ, Jamieson DH (eds) Childhood tuberculosis: modern imaging and clinical concepts. Springer, Berlin Heidelberg NewYork, pp 107–113
2. Hooijboer PJA, van der Vliet AM, Sinnige LGF (1996) Tuberculous meningitis in native Dutch children: report of four cases. Pediatr Radiol 26:542–546
3. Schaaf HS, Gie RP, Beyers N, et al. (1993) Tuberculosis in infants less than 3 months of age. Arch Dis Child 69:371–174
4. Vallejo JG, Ong LT, Starke JR (1994) Clinical features, diagnosis and treatment of tuberculosis in infants. Pediatrics 94:1–7
5. Snider DE, Rieder HL, Combs D, et al. (1988) Tuberculosis in children. Pediatr Infect Dis J 7:271–278
6. Starke JR, Jacobs RF, Jereb J (1992) Resurgence of tuberculosis in children. J Pediatr 120:839–854
7. Strouse PJ, Dressner DA, Watson WJ, et al. (1996) Mycobacterium tuberculosis infection in immunocompetent children. Pediatr Radiol 26:134–140
8. Wallace RC, Burton EM, Barrett FF, et al. (1991) Intracranial tuberculosis in children: CT appearance and clinical outcome. Pediatr Radiol 21:241–246
9. Cremin BJ, Jamieson DH (1996) In: Cremin BJ, Jamieson DH (eds) Childhood tuberculosis: modern imaging and clinical concepts. Springer, Berlin Heidelberg NewYork, pp 51–67
10. Abughali N, van der Kuyp F, Annable W, et al. (1994) Congenital tuberculosis. Pediatr Infect Dis J 13:738–741
11. Foo AL, Tan KK, Chay OM (1993) Congenital tuberculosis. Tuber Lung Dis 74:59–61
12. Naranbhal RC, Mathiassen W, Malan AF (1989) Congenital tuberculosis localised to the ear. Arch Dis Child 64:738–740
13. Ablin DS, Jain KA, Azour EM (1994) Abdominal tuberculosis in children. Pediatr Radiol 24:473–477
14. Nagi B, Duggal R, Gupta R, et al. (1987) Tuberculous peritonitis in children. Pediatr Radiol 17:282–284
15. Denath FM (1990) Abdominal tuberculosis in children: CT findings. Gastrointest Radiol 15:303–306
16. Moskovic E (1990) Macronodular hepatic tuberculosis in a child: computed tomographic appearances. Br J Radiol 63:656–658
17. Bhansali SK (1977) Abdominal tuberculosis. Am J Gastroenterol 67:324–337
18. Argarwala S, Bhatnagar V, Mitra DK, et al. (1992) Primary tubercular abscess of the spleen. J Pediatr Surg 27:1580–1581

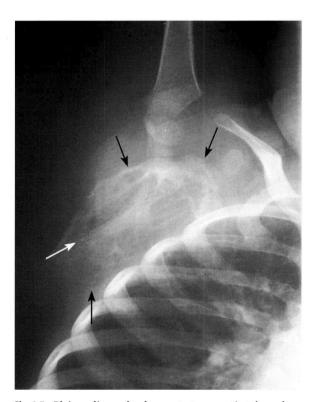

Fig. 9.7. Plain radiography demonstrates a cystic tuberculous lesion of the scapula, with marked bone expansion (*arrows*). Courtesy of Dr. B.J. Cremin, Red Cross Hospital, Cape Town

19. Cremin BJ (1987) Radiological imaging of urogenital tuberculosis in children with emphasis on ultrasound. Pediatr Radiol 17:34–38
20. Baniel J, Manning A, Leiman G (1991) Fine needle cytodiagnosis of renal tuberculosis. J Urol 146:689–691
21. de Castro CC, de Barros NG, Campos ZM, et al. (1995) CT scans of cranial tuberculosis. Radiol Clin North Am 33:753–769
22. Jinkins JR, Gupta R, Chang KH, et al. (1995) MR imaging of central nervous system tuberculosis. Radiol Clin North Am 33:771–786
23. Cremin BJ (1994) CT in tuberculous spondylitis. Clin Radiol 49:433–434
24. Hsu LCS, Leong JCY (1984) Tuberculosis in the lower cervical spine (C2–C7). J Bone Joint Surg Br 66:1–5
25. Jacobs JC, Li SC, Ruzal-Shapiro C, et al. (1994) Tuberculous arthritis in children: diagnosis by needle biopsy of the synovium. Clin Pediatr (Phila) 33:344–348
26. Haygood TM, Williamson SL (1994) Radiographic findings of extremity tuberculosis in childhood: back to the future. Radiographics 14:561–570
27. Ip M, Tsui I, Wong KL, Jones B, et al. (1993) Disseminated skeletal tuberculosis with skull involvement. Tuber Lung Dis 74:211–214
28. Arias FG, Rodriguez M, Hernandez JG, et al. (1987) Osteomyelitis deriving from BCG vaccination. Pediatr Radiol 17:166–167

CHAPTER 10

Less Common Forms of Extra-Pulmonary Tuberculosis

■ Tuberculosis of the Ear, Nose and Throat

Tuberculosis of the Larynx and Pharynx

In the pre-chemotherapy era, the larynx and pharynx were common sites of secondary tuberculous infection, and infections at these sites occurred in patients with long-term, sputum-positive disease; these patients were usually undergoing sanatorium treatment for cavitatory pulmonary tuberculosis (TB). During that period, up to 30% of patients developed laryngeal disease [1].

Since the introduction of chemotherapy, occurrence of infection at this site has become uncommon, occurring in 1% of patients. Furthermore, the disease itself seems to be changing. The age group has shifted from the young and middle aged to an older group of patients and is seen in those with moderate infiltrative pulmonary disease as well as cavitatory disease.

The area of the larynx infected has also altered in comparison with earlier cases. The anterior structures and the epiglottis are now the prime targets. This has raised the conjecture that the pathway of spread may now be haematogenous or via the lymphatics, as opposed to via airborne infection. The disease is highly contagious, and it is essential to make an early diagnosis to prevent spread to family members or health-care workers.

In the older age group, laryngeal carcinoma is the usual provisional diagnosis at patient presentation. Amongst the symptoms common to both conditions, hoarseness, dysphagia, weight loss and a fairly rapid clinical course predominate. Direct laryngoscopy reveals anterior disease, with oedema, tissue thickening and, occasionally, ulceration of the vocal cords, false cords, aryepiglottic folds and epiglottis. There may be extension of the changes to surrounding tissues, and the inflammatory lesions are usually bilateral. The sub-glottic region is rarely involved, and there is an absence of cartilage or vocal-cord destruction. Cord mobility is usually unimpaired.

Computed tomography (CT) scanning confirms the findings. Thickening of the vocal cords and false cords is seen, as well as epiglottic thickening and small mass lesions, some of which may be hypodense. Small regional lymph nodes may show enlargement, with low-density centres and rim enhancement after intravenous contrast injection. The internal jugular group are the glands usually enlarged. On their chest radiograph, 70% of patients will show changes of TB, which may only be infiltrative, and only 25% of these have cavitating TB.

Carcinoma is the main differential diagnosis. In TB, the bilaterality and lack of destruction of the cartilage are a pointer to the diagnosis, and sub-glottic spread is unusual. The lymph-node enhancement of carcinoma is often solid enhancement. However, the appearances are not specific and, in addition to carcinoma, other granulomatous lesions must be excluded. These include sarcoidosis, syphilis, leprosy, fungal diseases and lethal midline granuloma. Biopsy and smears produce a high proportion of positive results, either immediate recognition of alcohol acid-fast bacilli (AAFB) or positive cultures [1].

Swallow et al. [2] describe a patient presenting with a mass lesion thought to be a squamous cell carcinoma of the larynx. Laryngoscopy confirmed the presence of the lesion, and CT demonstrated a mass lesion involving the anterior portion of the larynx, both lateral hypo-pharyngeal walls, the aryepiglottic folds and the false and true cords.

Contrast-enhanced CT demonstrated the laryngeal mass and thickening of the supra-glottic and infra-glottic folds. There was narrowing of the supra-glottic larynx and poor definition of the peri-glottic fat planes. CT of the lungs demonstrated extensive upper-lobe tuberculous pneumonia bilaterally, with cavitation on the right. The right hilar lymph nodes were also enlarged.

Laryngoscopic biopsy produced positive samples for both direct smear and for culture. Having been exposed to the patient, 100 hospital staff underwent screening and, of these, four developed new positive skin reactions to protein purified derivative. They were treated with prophylactic chemotherapy [2].

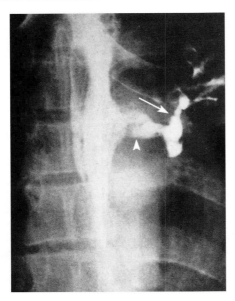

Fig. 10.1. Oesophagogram in a 35-year-old male presenting with a cough with expectoration and left-sided chest pain. Contrast leakage through an oesophageal fistula (*arrowhead*), passing into the left main bronchus (*arrow*). Image by courtesy of Dr. Ravi Ramakatan, King Edward Memorial Hospital, Mumbai, India

Pharyngeal TB

Rare in the West, pharyngeal TB has been described in endemic areas and is usually associated with sinus formation. Ramakantan describes a case presenting as a left supra-clavicular sinus track, developing silently without symptoms. Treatment with antibiotics was of no avail, so the sinus was biopsied, and granulomatous lesions were seen. Because of this, a barium swallow was carried out as most tuberculous lesions commence in the pharynx or in the oesophagus. A track was demonstrated arising from the left pyriform fossa and passing downwards. This responded well to anti-tuberculous therapy [3] (Fig. 10.1).

Tuberculous Otitis Media and Mastoiditis

In the pre-chemotherapy era, tuberculosis otitis media was a common disease. In 1915, Turner and Fraser commented that 50 % of otitis media in infants was tuberculous, the percentage falling to 2 % in adolescents. After the introduction of effective anti-tuberculous treatment in the 1950 s, Jeanes and Friedman found only 12 cases among 23,000 instances of otitis media. By 1980, the disease was found in 14 of 4000 biopsies from the middle ear [4].

Today, in the West, it is a rare disease, although sporadic cases occur in Caucasians. Many of the recent cases in the West have been in immigrant patients. In South Africa, the infection is common among the socially deprived. In Natal, it is a common cause of facial palsy in childhood. In Singh's 43 patients, 17 developed lower motor-neuron seventh-nerve palsy [5]. Although rare, if not diagnosed, it remains a chronic, disagreeable condition that leads to deafness in the affected ear. Complications such as bony sequestration, sinus formation and intracranial infection may arise. In some cases, profuse otorrhoea continues for many years, and the condition is normally painless. The source, in most cases, is haematogenous from a distant active or reactivated source although, in theory, infection via the Eustachian tube can occur.

In young African patients, pulmonary TB is present in 50 % of cases, and otitis media may be part of a more widespread disease with central nervous system, hepatic, renal or spinal disease. Often, the infection is bilateral. In the West, isolated otitis media is more common. Target groups with immune problems are infected, and one of Lee and Drysdale's patients had been treated with steroids for rheumatoid arthritis [6].

The pathological process may affect any part of the aural anatomy but commonly affects the middle ear and mastoid. Vestibulitis is sometimes reported [6]. The eardrum is slowly destroyed, as are the ossicles, and the middle-ear chamber fills with caseous material. Rarely, the cochlea is destroyed. The mastoid is not always affected. Occasional postmastoid cutaneous sinuses develop. Lymphadenitis occurs around the ear and in the neck.

The clinical presentation is of painless, profuse otorrhoea linked with hearing loss. In young children, facial nerve palsy is common and is sometimes seen in adults. There is severe or total hearing loss. Physical examination reveals perforation or partial or total destruction of the drum. Early descriptions were of multiple perforations but, more recently, single perforation has been described [4]. Visually, the drum and mucosa are pale, and pale granulations are present. These do not glisten like the tissue of cholesteatoma, and their appearance has been described as being like "cottage cheese" [4]. Biopsy of the granulations reveals caseating granulomas, and immediate screening may discover AAFB. It is essential to send materials for tuberculous culture, as secondary infection with pyogenic organisms will invariably be present and is misleading.

Imaging Methods

Imaging by plain radiographs may show clouding of the mastoid cells and destruction of bone, in some cases. Plain tomography will demonstrate destructive changes in the middle ear.

Axial scanning is, of course. much superior to conventional radiography, and standard middle-ear protocols are of great help. Bone destruction, soft-tissue masses and destruction of the ossicles can be documented (Fig. 10.2).

Magnetic resonance imaging (MRI) T1-gadolinium (Gd) images demonstrate the extent of the inflammatory change. Granulomatous tissue enhancing and caseation remain isodense [7]. MRI imaging is also useful in demonstrating intracranial spread.

The usual complications that arise are tuberculous meningitis (TBM), tuberculomata and inflammatory changes and neural deficits in nearby cranial nerves (VI, VII, XI and XII; Fig. 10.3) [5]. Differentiation from other chronic conditions depends on biopsy and culture. Otomastoid cholesteatoma, fungal granulomatous diseases, Wegener's granulomatosis, histiocytosis X, rhabdomyosarcoma and recurrent bacterial infections can all produce similar pictures [8].

■ TB of the Parotid Gland

Parotid-gland TB is an uncommon cause of parotid swelling [9]. In a study in Leicester in England, it was noted in a small group of Asian immigrants. During a 5-year period, 177 parotid masses in native English patients were diagnosed histologically as adenoma

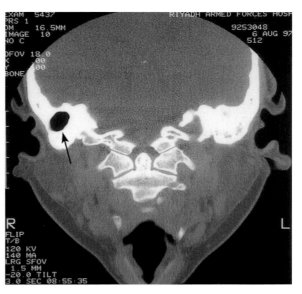

Fig. 10.2. Computed tomography scan shows a large, bony defect in the right temporal bone (*arrow*). The patient had a long history of discharge from the right ear. Auroscopy revealed pale granulation tissue, and alcohol acid-fast bacilli were cultured from the discharge

and lymphadenoma. There were no cases of TB. During that same period, there were 14 cases of parotid-gland masses in Asians, and four of these were tuberculous. AAFB was found on biopsy in two instances and on partial parotidectomy in the other

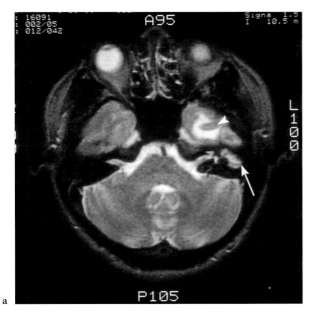

a

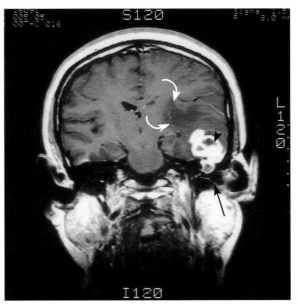

b

Fig. 10.3. a Post-gadolinium T1 image demonstrating enhancement of a left-sided tuberculous infection of the middle ear (*arrow*). There is infection in the temporal lobe (*arrowhead*). **b** A coronal image confirms the middle-ear infection (*arrow*)

and the associated temporal-lobe tuberculoma. Central areas of caseation are seen (*arrowhead*), as is a surrounding zone of oedema (*curved arrows*). **c** *on p. 172*

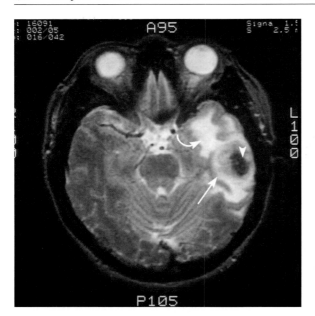

Fig. 10.3 (*continued*). **c** T2-weighted axial image of the same tuberculoma (*arrow*), central necrosis (*arrowhead*) and surrounding oedema (*curved arrow*)

two cases [10]. Tumour and TB are indistinguishable clinically, and aspiration biopsy and culture are the advised methods of investigation to avoid unnecessary parotidectomy.

■ TB of the Breast

The breast appears resistant to many systemic diseases and infections. Local infection is almost invariably the result of breast feeding. TB depends on the disruption of cell-mediated immunity. This is diminished in pregnancy and in the post-partum state, so it is no surprise that, in the developing world, young women during the childbearing period are a group in which breast TB occurs.

In developed countries, it is a rare disease but has already been seen in the early phases of acquired immunodeficiency syndrome [11]. More commonly in the West, it is reported as a secondary condition, an extension of intra-thoracic infection passing through the chest wall to affect the overlying breast. These cases are usually reported in elderly patients, while those from Asia and Africa are of childbearing age.

The morphology of the pathological process in primary breast TB has been divided into three groups: nodular, diffuse and fibrotic or sclerotic. These are not radiological classifications. The nodular form must be differentiated from benign or malignant lesions, diffuse changes must be differentiated from inflammatory disease and inflammatory cancer, and fibrotic changes must be differentiated from sclerosing types of neoplasm. The formation of abscesses is not considered in this classification, a modification of Morgen (1931) [12]. In both primary and secondary tuberculous mastitis, focal necrosis of granulation tissue is common, and the ensuing abscess is readily defined by sonography and CT. Sinus formation is also a frequent complication in the primary form, and a sinus passing from the thorax to the breast lesion is present, by definition, in the secondary form.

Sinus formation is often the initial complaint in the developing countries, as the mammary mass lesion is usually painless and non-tender on palpation. Patients are then often symptomless, and the mass may have been present for 1–2 years before presentation to the doctor. There are no systemic symptoms in the primary type unless TB is present at another site. Nipple retraction may be noticed and, in the pre-sinus phase, a cutaneous swelling is sometimes visible. Although the chest radiograph is usually normal, a history of TB in the past has been described, as has contact with tubercular family members.

The affected breast may appear smaller, and palpation reveals a non-tender mobile mass. In the secondary form, the mass will be fixed to the chest wall. Axillary lymph nodes are often present, and the common clinical diagnosis is of malignancy [13].

Imaging Methods

Mammography

There is often a generalised coarse reticular texture. The focal lesion is commonly in the upper outer quadrant, and the appearance is of diffuse increase in density, with ill-defined margins (Fig. 10.4). There is no micro-calcification. Alternative appearances are of nodular lesions with irregular margins similar to fibroadenomas or carcinomas but lacking in any radiating tissue. Overlying skin thickening is present, and there may be a skin bulge. Axillary lymph nodes are often demonstrated. A sinus track may be seen (Fig. 10.5) [13].

Ultrasound

Ultrasound reveals a general increase in the echogenicity of the breast stroma. The area of focal granulomatous infection is often hypo-echoic, showing

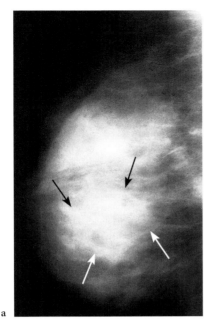

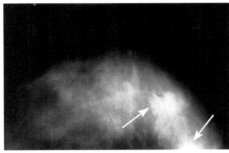

Fig. 10.4. a Mammography in a young Arabic woman reveals a rounded irregular inhomogeneous mass lesion in the lower part of the breast (*arrows*). Fine-needle aspiration (FNA) revealed tuberculosis. **b** A second case, with an irregular peripheral lesion passing deep to the retromammary area (*arrows*). FNA confirmed tuberculosis

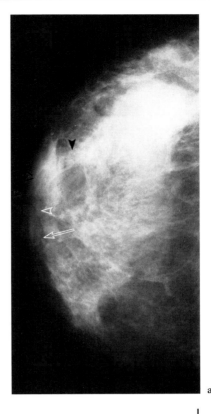

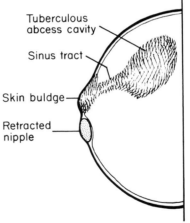

Fig. 10.5. a Breast tuberculosis. Cranio-caudal mammography. There is an ill-defined density in the upper outer quadrant connected by a dense linear tract (*black arrowhead*) to a localised area of skin thickening (*open arrow*) and a skin bulge (*arrowhead*). **b** A diagrammatic representation of the case. Courtesy of Dr. Dorothy Makanjuola, King Khalid University Hospital, Riyadh, Saudi Arabia

central fluid characteristics. This may contain necrotic debris. The contents may vary from fluid to caseous, so the transmission of echoes through the lesion varies from case to case. Granulomas in the walls of the lesion are seen as echogenic nodules (Fig. 10.6) [13].

Computed Tomography

CT is of major help in secondary tuberculous mastitis, detailing the intra-thoracic lesion, pleural changes and chest-wall lesions. Destruction of ribs is seen, as are abscesses penetrating the chest wall and sinus tracks, and retro-mammary and intra-mammary abscesses. These collections exhibit rim enhancement on contrast-enhanced CT. In primary cases, ultrasound and mammography are of much more value in defining the extent of the disease [14].

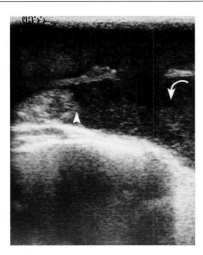

Fig. 10.6. Ultrasound of the breast in another case presenting with an ill-defined mass and a retracted nipple. The sonogram shows a septated fluid collection (*curved arrow*) with solid tissue in it (*arrowhead*). Courtesy of Dr. Dorothy Makanjuola, King Khalid University Hospital, Riyadh, Saudi Arabia

Isotope Examination

Technetium-99m sestamibi has been shown to be taken up by breast neoplasms and has a high diagnostic sensitivity [15]. Ohta et al. describe a case where there was intense uptake of the tracer in a painful breast mass due to tuberculous mastitis. If this isotope is used to differentiate between benign and malignant mass lesions, the examination of biopsy specimens should include culture for *Mycobacterium tuberculosis* [16].

Although most authors describe painless, non-tender mass lesions, two recent publications deal with painful swellings [13, 16]. Makanjuola also points out that, while the mammographic appearances show a non-specific a pattern, the presence of a cloudy density with a tract extending towards a skin bulge, combined with contraction of the breast, is highly suggestive of tuberculous breast abscess [13].

Other mass lesions must be excluded (for instance, pyogenic abscess), particularly in the lactating breast. Carcinoma is many times more common, with 180,000 cases per year in the USA, and is the cause of breast masses in up to 10% of European women. Diffuse inflammatory carcinoma may be particularly difficult to differentiate from tubercular mastitis.

At the turn of the century, TB and lymphoma commonly co-existed, both diseases depending on impaired cell-mediated immunity. Ewing remarked that "tuberculosis follows Hodgkin's disease (HD) like a shadow". Graeme-Cooke et al. describe a case where the reverse happened. A tuberculous breast mass was followed, after treatment, first by systemic HD and then by a discrete HD mass in the contralateral breast [11]. Other granulomas of the breast are rare, but syphilitic gummata and fungal-disease masses must also be considered.

■ Arterial Disease in TB

True tuberculous arteritis is rare except in TBM, where brain infarctions are the result of occlusion of the medium-sized arteries and the arterioles. These vessels are affected as they pass through the granulomatous basal exudates on their way to supply the brain parenchyma. Multiple, intramural, granulomatous lesions develop, and endarteritis obliterans results in distal closure of the smaller vessels.

Lehrer described the angiographic pattern of these changes as revealing widespread irregularity of calibre, early venous drainage and a stretched or hydrocephalic pattern due to the associated increase in size of the cerebral ventricular system.

Today, these changes can be demonstrated by magnetic resonance angiography [17, 18]. The areas usually involved are the basal ganglia, due to the granulomatous arteritis affecting the perforating branches of the posterior cerebral and posterior communicating arteries. In other arterial systems, two types of compromise occur: true arteritis and, much more commonly, localised inflammatory change in an arterial wall, due to the presence of adjacent granulomatous tissue or granulomatous lymph nodes. The arterial wall is then weakened, and pseudo-aneurysms may develop. This is similar to the development of Rasmussen aneurysms in cavitating TB. These are usually found in the branches of the bronchial artery system and may be large enough to be visible within a cavity on plain radiographs of the lung [19]. This type of arterial involvement may lead to life-threatening haemorrhages and, in patients with active TB, the development of aneurysm or pseudo-aneurysm must be borne in mind.

Cross et al. successfully treated a patient presenting with massive epistaxis associated with left-sided cranial neuropathies. This was the result of bleeding from a large pseudo-aneurysm of the petrous portion of the left carotid artery. The lesion was successfully occluded by placement of coils and a balloon. MRI of the lesion revealed miliary tuberculous granulomas of the cerebrum and cerebellum. The patient recovered after treatment with anti-tuberculous chemotherapy [20].

Arterial lesions may be multiple. In a 26-year-old Saudi Arabian woman, abdominal pain and low-grade fever were the presenting symptoms. The Mantoux reaction was strongly positive. Physical examination revealed an abdominal mass and hyper-

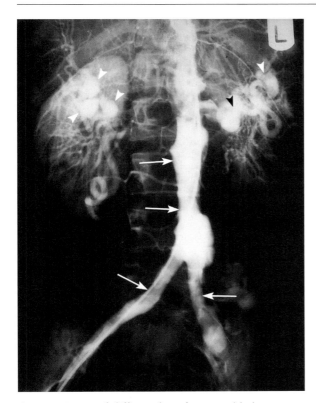

Fig. 10.7. A case of diffuse tuberculous arteritis in a young female. There is extensive irregularity of the aortic wall and its branches (*arrows*). There are multiple aneurysms of the hepatic, splenic and renal arteries (*arrowheads*). The superior mesenteric artery was occluded. Image by courtesy of Dr. Mona Al Shahed, Riyadh Military Hospital, Saudi Arabia

tension, which led to abdominal angiography. A large, abdominal aortic aneurysm, together with aneurysms of the right hepatic, left renal, inferior mesenteric and both iliac arteries were present (Fig. 10.7). At operation, very extensive peri-aortic, granulomatous inflammatory tissue was seen. The aortic aneurysm was treated with a Dacron graft. Other aneurysms were resected locally, where possible. The left kidney had to be sacrificed, as the renal artery aneurysm was deep in the renal hilum.

Histology of the aortic lesion revealed widespread, chronic inflammatory changes in the aortic wall, with numerous granulomas in the adventitia. These contained many histiocytes and multinucleated giant cells. No AAFB were seen or cultured, but the patient recovered after intense anti-tuberculous chemotherapy.

Pseudo-aneurysm of the hepatic artery is described in a single case by Husen et al. [21]. The diagnosis was made pre-operatively by means of Doppler ultrasound and confirmed by CT and angiography. The

aneurysm was successfully ligated [21, 22]. Kowole demonstrated that tuberculous lymph-node enlargement in the neck can result in carotid-artery occlusion while, in a second case, a massive pseudo-aneurysm of the abdominal aorta developed [23]. The thoracic aorta may become involved in the presence of tuberculous mediastinal lymphadenopathy. A case of tuberculous oesophagitis resulting in aorto-oeso-phageal fistula is also described [24, 25].

■ Tuberculous Pericarditis

Less common today than during the period before the introduction of effective chemotherapy, pericarditis leads, eventually, to the development of fibrotic tissue, which disturbs the cardiac function. Calcification of these tissues may be seen on plain radiographs and is often more readily visible on oblique views (Fig. 10.8). Axial scanning methods allow measurement of the pericardial thickening (Fig. 10.9) and, in the case of CT, the presence of calcification. Echocardiography allows measurement of the restrictive effect of these changes.

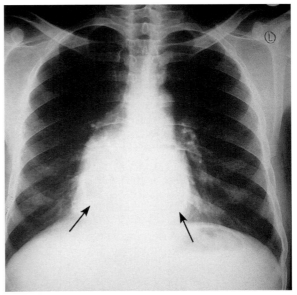

Fig. 10.8. Chest radiography demonstrates crescentic calcification of the pericardium (*arrows*) in a case of tuberculous constrictive pericarditis

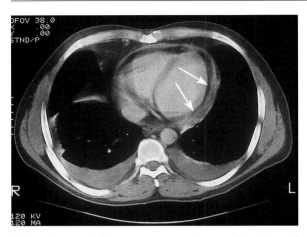

Fig. 10.9. Computed tomography scanning reveals pericardial thickening in a case of tuberculous pericarditis (*arrows*)

■ References

1. Moon WK, Han MH, Chang KH, et al. (1996) Laryngeal tuberculosis: CT findings. Am J Roentgenol 166:445–449
2. Swallow CE, McAdams HP, Colon E (1994) Tuberculosis manifested by a laryngeal mass on CT scans. Am J Roentgenol 163:179–180
3. Ramakantan R, Shah P (1990) Tuberculous fistulas of the pharynx and esophagus. Gastrointest Radiol 15:145–147
4. Buchanan G, Rainer EH (1988) Tuberculous mastoiditis. J Laryngol Otol 102:440–446
5. Singh B (1991) Role of surgery in tuberculous mastoiditis. J Laryngol Otol 105:907–915
6. Lee PYC, Drysdale AJ (1993) Tuberculous otitis media: a difficult diagnosis. J Laryngol Otol 107:339–341
7. Robertson K, Kumar A (1995) Atypical presentations of aural tuberculosis. Am J Otolarygol 16:294–302
8. Mumtaz MA, Schwartz RH, Grundfast KM, et al. (1983) Tuberculosis of the middle ear and mastoid. Pediatr Infect Dis 2:234–236
9. Adalla S, Garmole B (1996) Tuberculous parotitis: two cases in Libyan patients. Br J Clin Pract 50:62–63
10. Ubhi SS, Neoptolemos JP, Watkin DF (1988) Incidence and diagnosis of parotid gland tuberculosis in Asians in Leicester. Br J Surg 75:313
11. Graeme-Cook F, O'Briain DS, Daly PA (1988) Unusual breast masses: the sequential development of mammary tuberculosis and Hodgkin's disease in a young woman. Cancer 61:1457–1459
12. Chung SY, Yang I, Bae SH, et al. (1996) Tuberculous abscess in retromammary region: CT findings. J Comput Assist Tomogr 20:766–769
13. Makanjuola D, Murshid K, Al Sulaimani S, et al. (1996) Mammographic features of breast tuberculosis: the skin bulge and sinus tract sign. Clin Radiol 51:354–358
14. Schnarkowski P, Schmidt D, Kessler M, et al. (1994) Tuberculosis of the breast: US, mammographic and CT findings. J Comput Assist Tomogr 18:970–971
15. Khalkhali I, Cutrone J, Mena I, et al. (1995) Technetium-99m-sestamibi scintimammography of breast lesions: clinical and pathological follow-up. J Nucl Med 36:1784–1789
16. Ohta H, Ichii H, Arimoto A, et al. (1998) Tc-99m sestamibi uptake in tuberculosis of the breast. Clin Nucl Med 23:106–108
17. Lehrer H (1966) Angiographic tiad of tuberculous meningitis: a radiographic and clinico-pathological correlation. Radiology 87:829–835
18. Jinkins JR, Gupta R, Chang KH, et al. (1995) MRI imaging of central nervous system tuberculosis. Radiol Clin North Am 33:771–786
19. Santelli ED, Katz DS, Goldschmidt AM, et al. (1994) Embolisation of multiple Rasmussen aneurysms as a treatment of hemoptysis. Radiology 193:396–398
20. Cross DT, Moran CJ, Brown AP, et al. (1995) Endovascular treatment of epistaxis in a patient with tuberculosis and a giant petrous carotid pseudoaneurysm. Am J Neroradiol 16:1084–1086
21. Husen YA, Islam MU, Risvi IH (1997) Tuberculous hepatic artery aneurysm: multimodality imaging. Ann Saudi Med 17:354–356
22. Al-Hilli F (1998) The arteries in tuberculosis. Ann Saudi Med 18:191–192
23. Kolawole TM, Onadeko BO (1980) Vascular lesions in tuberculosis. Diagn Imaging 49:303–310
24. Catinella FP, Kittle CF (1988) Tuberculous esophagitis with aortic aneurysm fistula. Ann Thorac Surg 45:87–88
25. Chase RA, Haber MH, Pottage JC (1986) Tuberculous esophagitis with erosion into aortic aneurysm. Arch Pathol Lab Med 110:965–966

CHAPTER 11

Radionuclides in the Evaluation of Extra-Pulmonary Tuberculosis

D. Hamilton and J. Al Nabulsi

■ Introduction

It is widely acknowledged that nuclear medicine procedures are generally more sensitive than morphological imaging techniques for the localisation of sites of infection. With tuberculosis (TB), radionuclide imaging offers an indicator, of both the presence and the extent of active disease, which has been proven to be effective in the evaluation of suspected extra-pulmonary localisation, potentially revealing early abnormalities at unsuspected sites of sub-clinical disease [1–4]. It should be emphasised, however, that usually these techniques suffer a low specificity. In particular, multi-focal presentation can be confused with metastatic disease unless the scan appearances are interpreted in conjunction with a careful consideration of the clinical history.

■ Gallium-67 Citrate

The radiopharmaceutical most widely used currently in the evaluation of extra-pulmonary TB, and which has been labelled the best agent for imaging mycobacterial infections [5], is ^{67}Ga citrate. Compared with ^{99m}Tc, the main radionuclide used in routine clinical practice, ^{67}Ga has a relatively long half-life of 78 h. This allows for logistical considerations and facilitates protracted imaging protocols to accommodate slow accumulation in chronic and indolent infections, but limits the quantity that can be administered to a patient. This, together with the less-than-optimal imaging characteristics, means that the images are of poorer spatial resolution than would be obtained with ^{99m}Tc.

As with many radionuclide imaging procedures, one of the more important problems of the ^{67}Ga-citrate scan is its low specificity [4], and Yang et al. [2] counsel that correlation with computed tomography (CT) or ultrasound, and possibly biopsy or culture, is mandatory. Despite this, these authors recommend that, in patients with pyrexia of unknown origin (PUO) and no localising symptoms, inflammatory imaging methods such as this should be considered in the diagnostic work-up before the administration of drugs that may mask the site of infection.

In addition to its initial diagnostic capability, because abnormal ^{67}Ga-citrate accumulation is rare in inactive TB, the investigation is superior to radiography for assessing the response to chemotherapy or in establishing reactivation of the disease [1, 2, 6, 7]. The technique is recommended as a follow-up procedure in patients with documented extra-pulmonary TB [2, 8], because there are few other methods for determining disease activity [1, 2].

^{67}Ga: Mechanisms of Localisation

The exact mechanism of ^{67}Ga localisation in acute or chronic lesions of bacterial or non-bacterial origin is not clearly defined but probably involves a number of simultaneous processes. Ga is a group-III element and, in trace quantities, is handled biologically as a ferric iron analogue; the principle differences are that it has a lower affinity for most iron-binding molecules, such as a transferrin, and cannot be reduced in vivo, which prevents its incorporation into haem and several other biologically important proteins. After intravenous injection, it rapidly complexes with plasma proteins, especially transferrin but also at least two others, lactoferrin and ferritin; lactoferrin has a higher affinity than transferrin. Its subsequent distribution depends on its migration from plasma to tissue proteins and cells that have a stronger affinity for it. The increased blood supply and capillary hyper-permeability of the endothelium, characteristic of inflammation, allow ^{67}Ga bound to transferrin to enter the tissue non-specifically and increase its concentration in the extracellular fluid spaces of an inflammatory lesion. Intracellular localisation occurs in lysosomes or lysosome-like granules of cells, and it has also been found to bind to nuclear, mitochondrial and microsomal cell components of viable tissue.

Localisation may result from direct uptake by bacteria. At the site of bacterial infection, siderophores, which effectively bind and transport ferric iron, may be present and may play a role in the accumulation and retention of ^{67}Ga.

Neutrophils, lymphocytes and monocytes, but not red blood cells, accumulate Ga; neutrophils do so more than lymphocytes, in which ^{67}Ga binds to the surface of the lymphocyte plasma membrane. Thus, although leukocytes contribute to the accumulation and retention of ^{67}Ga, they are not essential for the uptake of the radionuclide in inflammatory lesions [9].

^{67}Ga: Normal Biodistribution

After intravenous administration, there is prominent accumulation of ^{67}Ga in the liver, with somewhat less uptake in the spleen. The concentration in the lungs at 48 h and beyond is normally low, making abnormal uptake easily recognisable, although faint bronchial activity may occasionally be seen in healthy individuals. There is some uptake in the bone and haematopoietic marrow in the bones of the cranium and jaw, within the normal rib cage and in the sternum, spine and the scapulae. In the extremities, the concentration is usually greatest in the epiphyseal region of the long bones and is prominent at the shoulders, elbows and knees. Additional sites of normal uptake include the lacrimal glands, where accumulation is variable, the nasopharynx, where activity is always present, and the saliva, which exhibits slight concentration.

During the first 24 h, ^{67}Ga is excreted primarily through the kidneys, and renal activity is, therefore, prominent; however, it is faint or absent afterwards, in the absence of renal disease. Thereafter, the major route of excretion is through the gastrointestinal tract, and activity is often present in the bowel, particularly in the ascending and transverse colon.

In most women, faint localisation of ^{67}Ga in breast tissue is seen and should usually be considered a normal variant that may change with variation in hormonal stimulation of mammary gland tissue (during menarche, with administration of cyclic oestrogen or progestational agents, in pregnancy and postpartum, when it can be particularly prominent). ^{67}Ga is excreted in human milk, and it is, therefore, necessary that breast feeding be replaced with formula feeding. Male patients normally have some uptake in the scrotum and testes.

In children, activity is seen in the epiphyseal regions and may be variably seen in normal thymus tissue. Surgical wounds usually remain positive for 1 week.

^{67}Ga: Imaging Considerations

Imaging protocols tend to be reasonably uniform. When no specific anatomical region is suspected, whole-body investigation is undertaken. When a specific region is of concern, tomographic images are often used as a means of improving the sensitivity. In a typical study, images are not acquired before 18–24 h, because high-background activity in the earlier images may mask lesions and produce false-negative results. This background activity generally diminishes to a visual optimum by 72–96 h. To overcome confusion presented by normal tracer accumulation in the bowel, it is common to acquire 48-h and possibly 72-h images, although early imaging has been advocated, for example, at 4 h to help identify patients with acquired immunodeficiency syndrome (AIDS)-related colitis [4]. Bowel preparations are often used but do not always eliminate intra-luminal activity. This will usually change position on delayed images except in cases of severe constipation or if the bowel is obstructed. If confusion persists, delayed images may be obtained for at least a week following administration.

Because the liver normally exhibits significant Ga uptake, hepatic abscesses may not accumulate ^{67}Ga citrate to higher concentrations than that of surrounding, uninvolved liver tissue. Therefore, if hepatic involvement is suspected, a colloid liver scan should be considered before ^{67}Ga citrate is administered. This will delineate any liver lesions as areas of decreased uptake. If any such area accumulates ^{67}Ga, even to a concentration less than in the surrounding liver tissue, it should be considered positive for ^{67}Ga abnormality.

^{67}Ga in Focal Disease

Twenty years ago, Sarkar et al. [6, 10] demonstrated that ^{67}Ga citrate could clearly delineate the spatial extent of active focal tubercular disease in the spine, kidney and peritoneum. They initially reported a study of five patients; positive scintigrams were obtained in three, and negative results were obtained in the two patients without extra-pulmonary involvement [10]. The following year, they reported a correct prediction of the presence or absence of active extra-pulmonary TB in all 11 patients studied [6].

It was only in the 1990s, however, that follow-up publications started to appear. The importance of the scan to the diagnostic process was established when it was reported to have shown extra-pulmonary foci in 8 of 16 patients with acute disseminated TB [3] and to have detected previously unrecognised foci without concomitant pulmonary disease, in 22% of 23 patients with known extra-pulmonary disease [2].

The primary aim of the latter study was to determine the sensitivity of the test. This was reported to be 83% and would have risen to 90% if two patients with small cervical lymphadenopathy were excluded [2]. The scan appearances were of focal or diffuse uptake at 48 h post-administration, persisting at 72 h. The authors state that the images obtained at 48 h were sufficient to localise the lesion in all cases except one, in which intestinal TB was detectable only on 72-h images.

Several case reports of particular localisations have been published. A splenic abscess appearing as three focal areas of increased ^{67}Ga accumulation in the left upper abdominal quadrant was shown by ^{99m}Tc sulphur colloid imaging to correspond to three photon-deficient areas in the spleen [11]. Two areas of increased ^{67}Ga accumulation in the liver were revealed to be tuberculoma by biopsy [12]. There have also been reports of oesophageal TB with supraclavicular lymph-node involvement [13], tuberculous enterocolitis [14] and a case in which the only site of extra-pulmonary disease identified was in a cervical lymph node [1].

Tuberculous spondylitis was studied in six patients by Lisbona et al. [8] who reported that all involved regions were detected on ^{67}Ga imaging. The scans also revealed: two additional skeletal foci, one in the sternum and the other in a sacroiliac joint, both of which were strikingly evident; paraspinal masses in two patients and two sites of soft-tissue involvement in different patients, one in the pre-auricular region and the other in the parainguinal area. The authors claim that the advantage of the scan is its ability to document the presence of para-spinal abscesses while highlighting distant foci in the soft tissues or skeleton, which could be more amenable to biopsy and/or culture than the spine itself (Fig. 11.1). They confirm the scan's relative sensitivity by reporting that radiographic studies, although abnormal in all patients, missed two of three sites of disease in a patient with multi-centric tuberculous spondylitis. They also confirm the lack of specificity, in that the scintigraphy was unable to differentiate between tuberculous and pyogenic spondylitis. They suggest an algorithm for the investigation of septic spondylitis, incorporating plain X-rays, ^{99m}Tc bone and ^{67}Ga citrate scintigraphy, CT, magnetic resonance (MR) and biopsy.

There has been some discussion as to whether scan appearances in recent cases of TB are consistent with the classically described pattern of the disease. Goldfarb et al. [15] performed whole-body scans on 22 patients and evaluated these for lung, intra-thoracic lymph-node and extra-pulmonary accumu-

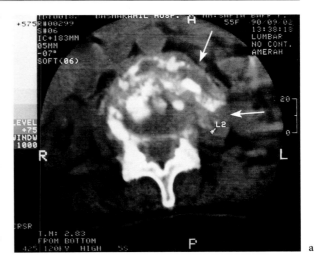

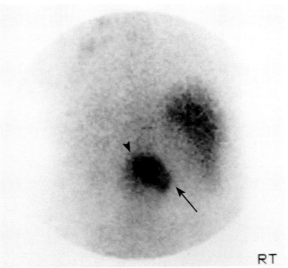

Fig. 11.1. **a** Computed tomography scan of the second lumbar vertebra in a case of multi-focal tuberculosis. The fragmented vertebral body is expanded, and the infection is apparent in the surrounding soft tissues (*arrows*). **b** A posterior ^{67}Ga-citrate scan of the same area indicates uptake in the soft tissues (*arrow*) and the vertebral body (*arrowhead*)

lation. Only five demonstrated unilateral or bilateral upper lobe uptake, which was the most frequent disease distribution in classical TB. In the others, uptake was diffuse in both lungs in five patients and variably affected one or both lower lobes or mid-lung zones in 12. Seven patients exhibited uptake in hilar or mediastinal nodes and six in cervical nodes. Extra-pulmonary lesions, mostly nodal, were present in five patients. The authors concluded that typical ^{67}Ga citrate patterns in recent cases of TB differed notably from the upper-lobe predilection of classical TB. Pulmonary parenchymal lesions are more heterogeneously distributed, and lymph-node involvement now occurs in the majority of cases.

⁶⁷Ga in Multi-Focal Disease

Although a multi-focal pattern has been described in lymphoma and solid tumours, TB must be considered when this pattern is observed [16] (Figs. 11.2, 11.3). An example of such a presentation shows intense accumulation at the left elbow, sternum, left anterior lower ribs and the lumbar and thoracic spine. The uptake was more intense than observed on previous ⁹⁹ᵐTc bone scintigraphy, which had revealed multiple foci of increased uptake in the left elbow, lumbar and thoracic spine, left shoulder, left maxilla and left temporo-mandibular joint, as well as faint sternal uptake. Coronal and sagittal slices of single-photon-emission CT studies showed a different pattern of increased activity with ⁶⁷Ga citrate than with bone scintigrams in that both sternal and vertebral accumulation extended beyond their anatomical borders. This was thought to be consistent with the soft-tissue component of the lesions.

⁶⁷Ga in TB Associated with AIDS

Lymph-node accumulation in patients with AIDS, in the presence or absence of parenchymal lung uptake, raises the possibility of TB, but the sensitivity of the test is reduced by anti-tuberculous treatment [4]. These authors studied 24 patients and regarded the scans as positive if accumulation was apparent in the lymph nodes, which transpired to be more common than parenchymal lung uptake. The sites noted were mediastinal, supra-clavicular, axillary, retro-peritoneal and inguinal. Sites of pulmonary uptake were only seen in five patients. There were 16 positive scans and, of these, only four patients were on anti-tuberculosis treatment. However, there were eight negative scans, and all these patients were on treatment.

In human immunodeficiency virus (HIV)-infected patients with unexplained fever, the scan is useful for the early diagnosis of TB [17]. The authors report a sensitivity of 85.7%, a specificity of 84.7%, a positive predictive value of 72.7% and a negative predictive value of 92.6% in 149 patients. The scan was considered positive if there was uptake in the hilar, mediastinal, axillary, supra-clavicular, sub-

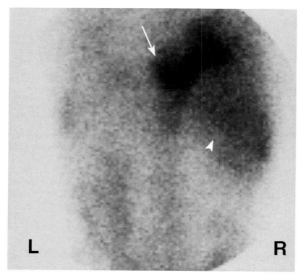

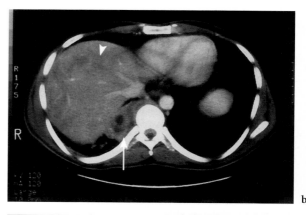

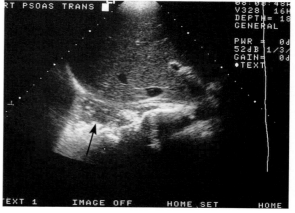

Fig. 11.2. a A posterior ⁶⁷Ga-citrate scan of a young man with hepatic, spinal and gastrointestinal tuberculosis. There is increased uptake of the tracer in the large liver (*arrowhead*) and in a para-spinal collection (*arrow*). **b** Computed tomography demonstrated patchy enhancement in the liver (*arrowhead*) and the para-spinal abscess (*arrow*). **c** The para-spinal collection was also visible on ultrasound examination (*arrow*)

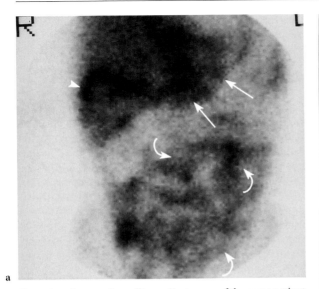

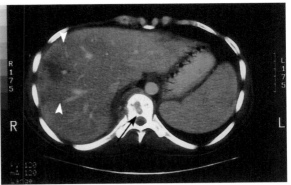

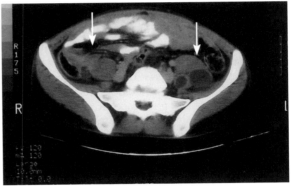

Fig. 11.3. a An anterior gallium-citrate scan of the same patient at 48 h demonstrates the large liver (*arrowhead*) and the para-spinal collection, which involves the body of L2 (*arrows*). The small bowel shows widespread uptake of the isotope (*curved arrows*). **b** The L2 lesion is outlined on the abdominal computed tomography (CT) study (*arrow*) as is inhomogeneous enhancement of the liver (*arrowheads*). **c** A lower CT image outlines matted loops of bowel due to enteric tuberculosis in both iliac fossae (*arrows*)

mandibular or cervical lymph nodes and negative if there was no uptake in the lymphoid regions. Positive results were obtained in intra-thoracic lymph nodes in 32.1% of scans, in peripheral lymph nodes in 25% of scans and in both sites in 28.6% of scans. Negative results were obtained in 14.3% of scans. The authors suggest that, while waiting for culture results, prompt empirical anti-tuberculous therapy can be initiated when a ⁶⁷Ga citrate scan of an HIV-infected patient in an area with a high prevalence of TB infection shows nodal uptake, because TB is unlikely when the scan does not show this appearance. They also suggest that the high sensitivity and specificity of the investigation may be of special relevance for those patients whose scans show only intra-thoracic uptake and from whom biopsy material is difficult to obtain, because these patients may benefit from early empirical administration of anti-tuberculous drugs.

⁶⁷Ga in Combination with Thallium-201 Chloride

A major problem with the use of ⁶⁷Ga citrate is its inability to differentiate mycobacterial infections from lymphoma, both of which commonly show fo-

cal uptake in the hila, mediastinum and lung parenchyma. In order to try to improve the specificity, Lee et al. [18] combined ⁶⁷Ga-citrate scans of the chest and abdomen with ²⁰¹Tl chloride in AIDS patients. Tl, in the form of the thallous ion, is a monovalent cation and an analogue of potassium, which shows high avidity for certain tumours, such as Kaposi sarcoma and lymphomas. The authors found local mismatches of ⁶⁷Ga and ²⁰¹Tl to be highly specific for mycobacterial infections.

Fourteen patients showed focal uptake of ⁶⁷Ga in hilar nodes and mediastinum, with no ²⁰¹Tl uptake. Of these, six were diagnosed with *Mycobacterium tuberculosis*, six with *M. avium-intracellulare* and one with cryptococcal infection; one diagnosis was not established. Seventeen patients demonstrated high ²⁰¹Tl uptake in lungs and mediastinum with ⁶⁷Ga absent or at different sites; of these, 14 had pulmonary Kaposi's sarcoma, and three diagnoses were not established. Eight patients had matched ⁶⁷Ga and ²⁰¹Tl uptake in the lungs and mediastinum; of these, seven had lymphoma, and one diagnosis was not established. Ten patients had both negative ⁶⁷Ga and ²⁰¹Tl scans, of which eight had no chest complications, and two diagnoses were not established.

■ Indium-111 Leukocytes

An alternative technique, widely used for the evaluation of infective foci, is the radiolabelled leukocyte scan. Compared with ^{67}Ga, however, this has
been reported to be less sensitive for the detection of
chronic and granulomatous lesions [19] and also to
be less sensitive for detecting TB in HIV-positive
patients [20]. Negative leukocyte scans can often
be observed, even in patients with extensive tuberculous lesions [5]. [67]Ga shows greater efficacy in
chronic, less pyogenic infections, probably because
of its multi-factorial mechanism of localisation not
matched by leukocytes, which localise mainly by
chemotaxis [14].

In extra-pulmonary TB, only leukocytes labelled
with ^{111}In have been used. This radionuclide has a
half-life (67 h) similar to that of ^{67}Ga but, because of
better physical characteristics, can produce superior
images. The alternative would be ^{99m}Tc, which with its
short 6-h half-life and physical characteristics almost
ideal for scintigraphy offers better image quality and
shorter acquisition times. However, its efficacy in
extra-pulmonary TB has not been assessed, possibly
because the half-life is considered too short to allow
acceptable accumulation in such an indolent infective process.

After intravenous injection, radiolabelled leukocytes rapidly distribute in the intravascular space.
Immediate scintigrams demonstrate activity in the
lungs, liver, spleen and blood pool, but images obtained at 24 h, the typical investigation time, show
activity only in the liver, spleen and bone marrow.
Useful scintigrams can be obtained at 4–6 h, or even
at 30 min, depending on the degree of inflammation.
However, image quality generally improves significantly as blood-pool activity decreases. Abnormalities most often present as areas of increased accumulation, but decreased uptake has been reported,
usually in areas rich in red marrow, where an abnormality will appear relatively less active than adjacent
areas of high activity.

A comparative study, using both ^{111}In leukocytes
and ^{67}Ga citrate in six patients with tuberculous
enteritis, revealed a slight but significant superiority
of [67]Ga [21]. When compared with endoscopy, the
sensitivity and specificity of ^{67}Ga citrate were 0.80
and 1.00, respectively, whereas those of ^{111}In leukocytes were 0.60 and 0.96. The authors stated that this
superiority is in agreement with the findings of
others that ^{67}Ga may be more reliable in the detection
of chronic inflammation, and that it does not rely on
vigorous leukocyte migration. However, it was also
observed that there was positive scintigraphy with
both radionuclides despite prolonged treatment,
indicating that leukocyte recruitment to areas of
tuberculous enteritis may continue for several weeks
despite optimum anti-tuberculous treatment.

■ [99m]Tc Bone Scan

Another technique that has been used extensively
for the assessment of extra-pulmonary TB is the bone
scan. First evaluated for this disease in 1974 using
radiolabelled stannous polyphosphate [22], it has
been investigated regularly ever since, unlike the
[67]Ga-citrate scan. In particular, more examples of
multi-focal presentation have been published. Introduced in 1975, methylene diphosphonate (MDP) is
now probably the most widely used label, although
the alternative, hydroxymethylene diphosphonate
(HMDP), is also popular. Both are attached to the
[99m]Tc radionuclide, which is used in over 80% of
radionuclide investigations and produces images
with excellent spatial resolution.

Like ^{67}Ga citrate, the ^{99m}Tc bone scan shows a remarkable sensitivity for the detection of active TB,
mainly in the skeleton in this case. It has been suggested that any confusing scan abnormality in a patient
from a population at risk may prove to be tuberculous [23]. It can, however, be insensitive to low-
grade, indolent or severely destructive osteomyelitis
[24], and a normal bone scan cannot exclude the
possibility of tuberculous bone infection [25]. Also, as
with ^{67}Ga citrate, abnormal appearances tend to be
non-specific.

Bone-phase scintigrams are acquired between 3 h
and 4 h post-administration. In the majority of instances, abnormalities will present as areas of increased accumulation, reflecting increased osteoblastic
activity and, to a lesser extent, increased vascularity.
Areas of decreased accumulation are less common
and are usually due to interference with the blood
supply by inflammatory products. Immediate vascular and blood-pool images are also used to evaluate
a possible infective process. These demonstrate the
degree of hyperaemia and, since osteomyelitis causes
increased blood flow, would be expected show increased accumulation in osseous TB.

Unlike the ^{67}Ga scan, which resolves within
months of initiation of anti-tuberculous chemotherapy, the ^{99m}Tc bone scan can remain abnormal
for a protracted period [6, 24] of up to 6 months
[22, 26, 27].

[99m]Tc Bone Scan in Focal Disease

Several publications have demonstrated the sensitivity of the scan in focal disease (Fig. 11.4). Even
using a rectilinear scanner rather than a gamma

camera, two cases of focal osseous TB in seven patients with bacteriologically proven tuberculosis were detected [22]. In one, the scan demonstrated increased uptake in the hand; this increase extended beyond the radiographic abnormality. In the other, the abnormality appeared in the sternum, and a repeat scan at 9 months indicated improvement, as did radiographs. The authors stated that, in tuberculous osteomyelitis, the scan abnormalities were, in their experience, unusually persistent compared with other, more acute osteomyelitic conditions, consistent with chronic infection.

A note of caution was introduced when two patients with spinal TB and normal scans were presented [24]. In one patient, three ^{99m}Tc bone scans over a 6-month period and ^{67}Ga-citrate imaging failed to detect any abnormality. However, radiographic changes over the same period were also too subtle for detection, not becoming positive until 6 months after the initial presentation. The authors postulated that these findings were likely to be due to the indolent nature of the infection. In the other patient, they reasoned that marked vertebral destruction with lack of bone reaction may have accounted for the normal scan. In these two patients, the normal images created more uncertainty and confusion rather than contributing towards the final diagnosis, and the authors emphasised that, if there is a strong clinical suspicion of skeletal TB, aspiration and biopsy of the tissue, with appropriate stains and culture, should be performed even if the nuclear-medicine studies are normal.

More optimistic reports appeared in the 1990s. An abscess presented as a well-delineated large area of increased uptake in extra-skeletal tissue and included an extremely avid upper portion conforming to the right gluteal region lateral to the iliac bone. The lower portion of the lesion spread down to the lower two-thirds of the right femur but maintained higher uptake than skeletal tissue [28].

An example of diffusely increased uptake at the hip joint was reported; it was more intense at the periphery and affected both the femoral head and acetabulum [29]. The authors stated that infectious processes in the hip show various presentations that depend on the extent of involvement in addition to the specific infectious organism. In tuberculous arthritis, large weight-bearing joints, such as the hip or knee, are most often affected, and mono-articular involvement is the rule. Plain-film radiography is usually sufficient to show the identifying features of tuberculous arthritis, although its early radiographic appearance is often indistinguishable from that of mono-articular rheumatoid arthritis. The radionuclide bone scan will show non-specific findings of increased uptake on both sides of the joint, which may also be seen in other conditions.

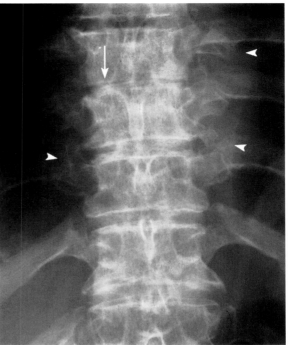

a

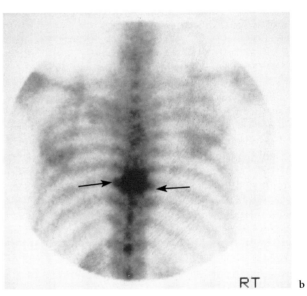

RT   b

Fig. 11.4. **a** A radiograph of early tuberculous spondylitis, with disc space narrowing and loss of the „white stripe" between T8 and T9 (*arrow*). There is a para-vertebral soft-tissue swelling (*arrowheads*). **b** A ^{99}Tc bone scan of the patient outlines increase in uptake of the tracer, confined to the two vertebral bodies and the associated costo-vertebral joints (*arrows*). There is little indication of para-vertebral disease

Two cases of increased uptake at the mid-tibial shaft and a destructive lesion of the superior ramus of the left pubic bone were presented [23]. Positive scans were reported in two patients with chronic tuberculous spondylitis. In both patients, the blood-pool phase and [99mTc] human immunoglobulin and [99mTc] monoclonal antibody investigations all gave false-negative results [30].

As with [67Ga] citrate, the specificity of the technique is poor. In comparison with plain radiography, CT and MR imaging, bone scintigraphy was found to be the least helpful in differentiating tuberculous from brucellar spondylitis [31]. However, in geographic areas where both infections are endemic, the authors suggest that bone scintigraphy is useful for screening patients suspected of having an infective spondylitis. They studied 13 patients and, using both anterior and posterior projections, they evaluated the scans for the presence or absence of increased uptake in the vertebral bodies. The ten patients with tuberculous spondylitis affecting the thoracic region had diffuse increased uptake at the affected sites; this uptake was indistinguishable from scintigraphic features of brucellar spondylitis. Vertebral architecture could not be seen on scintigrams in the three patients with lumbar spine involvement.

[99mTc] Bone Scan in Multi-Focal Disease

More examples of multi-focal scan abnormalities have been reported using the [99mTc] bone scan than using [67Ga] citrate. Such appearances would be regarded as unusual for pyogenic osteomyelitis, which usually presents as a single focal or regional lesion. Mycobacterium osteomyelitis is, however, a disseminated osseous process, and the [99mTc] bone scan accurately reflects this. Therefore, although multiple widespread lesions on a [99mTc] bone scan will usually represent metastatic disease, in the appropriate clinical setting, mycobacterium osteomyelitis should be considered [32]. Pulmonary involvement need not be present, and involvement may not be limited to the axial skeleton (Figs. 11.5, 11.6) [25].

An example of multi-focal abnormality included both shoulders and the mid-dorsal spine. After 2 months of treatment, there was radiographic evidence of healing, but the scan remained abnormal at many of the sites. After 6 months, the bone-scan appearances had improved but still remained abnormal [22].

A case in which most of the lesions were unsuspected clinically showed increased accumulation in the lumbar spine, ribs, thoracic spine and shoulder girdle [27]. A repeat scan undertaken 15 months later but 12 months after the patient had stopped taking

medication showed that, while most of the abnormalities were no longer apparent, some exhibited decreased accumulation. The authors state that, although the mechanism is unknown, a possible explanation would be fibrous replacement of the osteoid with healing, which would result in reduction of radiopharmaceutical uptake. A bone scan 7 months after restarting medication demonstrated a completely normal appearance.

The confusion that a multi-focal appearance can cause has been illustrated by a review of four cases, by Muraldi, in which the initial diagnosis was malignancy. Case 1 revealed increased uptake in the sternum, ribs (bilaterally), T11, T12, L1 and L2 and proximal diaphysis of the left tibia, right and left sacroiliac joints and right acetabulum. Case 2 showed increased uptake in the left fifth rib. Case 3 demonstrated increased uptake in the sternal area and the first lumbar vertebral body. Case 4 demonstrated increased uptake in the region of the left sacroiliac joint, with a limited scan of the pelvis, and a full scan revealed increased uptake in the left first and third ribs, the left medial clavicle and the left iliac crest. These cases were later shown to be due to TB [25].

[99mTc] Bone Scan in Conjunction with [111In] Bone-Marrow Scan

The multi-focal appearance of a [99mTc] bone scan can correspond with bone-marrow replacement by tuberculous inflammatory processes [26]. This postulate was developed from the results of complementary [111In] chloride bone-marrow scanning, which revealed that all of the numerous areas of increased accumulation in the ribs, spine and appendicular skeleton on the bone scan showed corresponding areas of decreased accumulation on the bone-marrow scan.

[99mTc] Diphosphonate Bone Scan Compared with [67Ga]

The [99mTc] bone scan is not as sensitive as [67Ga] citrate for the detection of extra-pulmonary TB. An example is a [67Ga] study that showed increased uptake in all the regions identified as abnormal on a bone scan, and also in both lungs, the posterior mediastinum and the left hilum [32]. Not only does [67Ga] show abnormalities at sites other than in the skeleton, it also reveals more abnormalities in bones.

In spinal TB, [67Ga] scanning has been shown to enhance the information that can be provided by bone scintigraphy [8]. In a study of six patients, these authors demonstrated that [67Ga] citrate not only

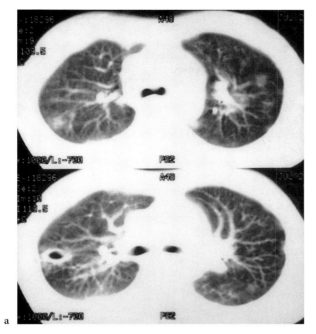

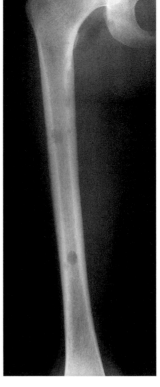

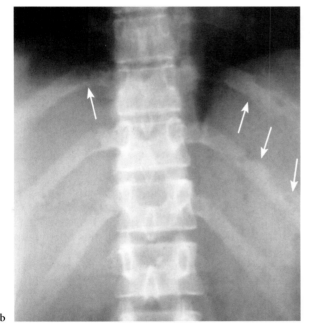

Fig. 11.5 a – c. A middle aged woman presented with a cough, expectoration, fever and widespread bone pain. **a** Computed tomography of the lungs confirmed that a right lower zone opacity contained a cavity. **b** Radiographs of the spine revealed multiple rib lesions similar to those seen in disseminated fungal disease in North America (*arrows*). **c** In the long bones, there were multiple, discrete, oval osteolytic lesions. There was no surrounding sclerosis, and the long axes were vertical, as is usually the case in tuberculous osteitis

detected spondylar lesions more vividly but also ascribed a septic origin to the less specifically increased vertebral uptake of the bone investigation. It also revealed the presence of para-spinal abscesses while highlighting distant septic foci in the soft tissues and skeleton; the authors comment that these foci could be more amenable to biopsy and/or culture than the spine itself. In their series of patients, the

bone scans were categorically abnormal at six sites, while the findings were more subtle at three remaining sites. Two additional skeletal foci of TB – one in the sternum and the other in a sacroiliac joint – were present. Both were strikingly evident on the 67Ga images, but the bone scans identified only the sternal focus of disease and failed to detect the tuberculous sacroiliitis.

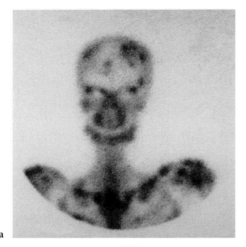

a

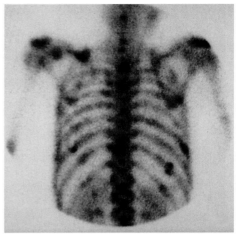

b

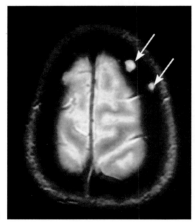

c

Fig. 11.6a – c. No alcohol acid-fast bacilli were present in the sputum. **a, b** Technetium bone scanning revealed multiple skeletal lesions. **c** Magnetic resonance imaging of the brain demonstrated no parenchymal lesions, but a number of high-signal foci in the dura of the skull vault were seen (*arrows*). Multiple metastases and multi-focal tuberculosis were considered as diagnoses. Biopsy of a superficial lesion grew cryptococcus. The patient was human immunodeficiency virus negative. Images by courtesy of Professor Price-Evans, Riyadh Military Hospital, Saudi Arabia

■ Other Radiopharmaceuticals

The efficacy of several miscellaneous radiopharmaceuticals has been investigated. Breast TB has, very recently, been successfully detected using ^{99m}Tc sestamibi [33]. For differentiating granulomatous inflammatory lesions from primary soft-tissue tumours, a combination of ^{99m}Tc(v) dimercaptosuccinic acid (DMSA) and ^{67}Ga citrate has been shown to be effective [34]. The authors state that, compared with DMSA, ^{67}Ga shows higher and more distinct uptake in most inflammatory lesions. DMSA shows the relatively hypervascular and hypermetabolic tissue surrounding an inflammatory lesion as a wider and less well-defined area of relatively lower uptake. ^{67}Ga shows fainter and less well-defined uptake in soft-tissue tumours. The example presented is a solitary muscular involvement by TB, which showed marked ^{67}Ga-citrate accumulation but ill-defined and faint DMSA uptake, implying the existence of a marked inflammatory reaction in the lesion.

A potential tracer for active TB has been described. This tracer is based on an effective anti-tuberculous agent that rapidly permeates the bacterial cell membrane and has been demonstrated to reach concentration levels, within the bacilli, 50 times greater than the surrounding environment [35, 36]. This is isonicotinic acid hydrazide (isoniazid) labelled with ^{123}I and ^{124}I. The normal biodistribution, in experimental animals, was shown to be greatest in the kidneys, heart and lungs, but human data has not been obtained.

■ Summary

It is widely acknowledged that nuclear-medicine procedures are generally more sensitive than morphological imaging techniques for the localisation of sites of infection. In TB, radionuclide imaging offers an indicator of both the presence and the extent of active disease. Such imaging has been proven to be effective in the evaluation of suspected extra-pulmonary localisation, potentially revealing early abnormalities at unsuspected sites of sub-clinical disease.

The radiopharmaceutical most widely used currently in the evaluation of extra-pulmonary TB is ^{67}Ga citrate. As with many radionuclide imaging procedures, one of the more important problems is its low specificity. Despite this, it is recommended that, in patients with PUO and no localising symptoms, such inflammatory imaging methods should be considered in the diagnostic work-up before the administration of drugs that may mask the site of infection.

Because abnormal ^{67}Ga-citrate accumulation is rare in inactive TB, the investigation is superior to radiography for assessing the response to chemotherapy or in establishing reactivation of the disease, in addition to its initial diagnostic capability. The technique is recommended as a follow-up procedure in patients with documented extra-pulmonary TB, because there are few other methods for determining disease activity. Although a multi-focal pattern is not characteristic only of TB – it has been described in lymphoma and solid tumours – TB must be considered when this pattern is observed. In patients with AIDS lymph-node accumulation in the presence or absence of parenchymal lung uptake, raises the possibility of TB but the sensitivity of the test is reduced by anti-tuberculous treatment. A major problem with the use of ^{67}Ga citrate is its inability to differentiate mycobacterial infections from lymphoma, both of which commonly show focal uptake in the hila, mediastinum and lung parenchyma. It has been found that local mismatches of ^{67}Ga and ^{201}Tl are highly specific for mycobacterial infections.

An alternative technique, widely used for the evaluation of infective foci, is the radiolabelled leukocyte scan. However, this has been reported to be less sensitive than ^{67}Ga, and negative leukocyte scans can often be observed, even in patients with extensive tuberculous lesions.

Another technique that has been used extensively in extra-pulmonary TB is the ^{99m}Tc bone scan. Like ^{67}Ga citrate, this shows a remarkable sensitivity for the detection of active TB (in this case, mainly in the skeleton). It has been suggested that any confusing scan abnormality in a patient from a population at risk may prove to be tuberculous. The scan can, however, be insensitive to low-grade, indolent or severely destructive osteomyelitis, and a normal bone scan cannot exclude the possibility of tuberculous bone infection. Also, as with ^{67}Ga citrate, abnormal appearances tend to be non-specific. More examples of multi-focal scan abnormalities have been reported using the ^{99m}Tc bone scan than using ^{67}Ga citrate. Although multiple, widespread lesions on a ^{99m}Tc bone scan will usually represent metastatic disease, in the appropriate clinical setting, mycobacterium osteomyelitis should be considered. Pulmonary involvement need not be present, and involvement may not be limited to the axial skeleton.

The multi-focal appearance of a ^{99m}Tc bone scan can correspond with bone-marrow replacement by tuberculous inflammatory processes. This postulate was developed from the results of complementary ^{111}In chloride bone-marrow scanning, which revealed that all of the numerous areas of increased accumulation in the ribs, spine and appendicular skeleton on the bone scan, showed corresponding areas of decreased accumulation on the bone-marrow scan.

The efficacy of several miscellaneous radiopharmaceuticals has been investigated. Breast TB has very recently been successfully detected with ^{99m}Tc sestamibi. A combination of ^{99m}Tc DMSA and ^{67}Ga citrate has been shown to be effective for differentiating granulomatous inflammatory lesions from primary soft-tissue tumours.

■ References

1. Moody EB, Glassmar SB, Hansen AV, Lawrence SK, Delbeke D (1992) Nuclear medicine case of the day. Case 1: miliary tuberculosis. Am J Roentgenol 158:1382–1386
2. Yang S-O, Lee YI, Chung DH, Lee MC, Koh C-S, Choi BI, Im J-G, Park JH, Han MC, Kim C-W (1992) Detection of extra-pulmonary tuberculosis with gallium-67 scan and computed tomography. J Nucl Med 33:2118–2123
3. Kao C-H, Wang S-J, Liao S-Q, Lin W-Y, Hsu C-Y (1993) Usefulness of gallium-67-citrate scans in patients with acute disseminated tuberculosis and comparison with chest X-rays. J Nucl Med 34:1918–1921
4. Abdel-Dayem HM, Naddaf S, Aziz M, Mina B, Turoglu T, Akisik MF, Omar WS, Di Fabrizio L, LaBombardi V, Kempf JS (1997) Sites of tuberculous involvement in patients with AIDS. Autopsy findings and evaluation of gallium imaging. Clin Nucl Med 22:310–314
5. McAfee JG (1996) Editorial comment. In: The year book of nuclear medicine. Mosby, London, pp 94–95
6. Sarkar SD, Ravikrishnan KP, Woodbury DH, Carson JJ, Daley K (1979) Gallium-67 citrate scanning – a new adjunct in the detection and follow-up of extrapulmonary tuberculosis: concise communication. J Nucl Med 20:833–836
7. Bekerman C, Bitran J (1988) Gallium-67 scanning in the clinical evaluation of human immunodeficiency virus infection: indications and limitations. Semin Nucl Med 18:273–286
8. Lisbona R, Derbekyan V, Novales-Diaz J, Veksler A (1993) Gallium-67 scintigraphy in tuberculous and non-tuberculous infectious spondylitis. J Nucl Med 34:853–859
9. Tsan M-F (1985) Mechanism of gallium-67 accumulation in inflammatory lesions. J Nucl Med 26:88–92
10. Sarkar SD, Ravikrishman KP (1978) Gallium-67 citrate scanning in extra-pulmonary tuberculosis. J Nucl Med 19:734
11. Kao P-F, Tzen K-Y, Chou Y-H, Lu S-Y, You D-L (1996) Accumulation of Ga-67 citrate in a tuberculous splenic abscess: report of a rare case. Clin Nucl Med 21:49–52
12. Ohta H, Fukuyama T, Sakamoto M, Kombuchi T, Shintaku M (1995) Liver tuberculoma detected by Ga-67 imaging. Clin Nucl Med 7:577

13. Young T-H, Hsieh J-P, Chao Y-C, Hsu C-T, Ho-Tom, Tang H-S (1996) Esophageal tuberculosis with supraclavicular lymph node involvement demonstrated by Ga-67 imaging. Clin Nucl Med 21:344

14. Brophey M, Lamki L, Barron B, Shah S (1995) Prominent small bowel Ga-67 uptake associated with yersinial and tuberculous enterocolitis. Clin Nucl Med 20:107–110

15. Goldfarb CR, Ongseng F, Finestone H, Colp C, Parmett SR (1995) Ga-67 scintigraphic appearances of tuberculosis in the "new" tuberculosis. J Nucl Med 36:23

16. Hardoff R, Efrat M, Gips A (1995) Multifocal osteoarticular tuberculosis resembling skeletal metastatic disease. Evaluation with Tc-99m MDP and Ga-67 citrate. Clin Nucl Med 20:279–281

17. Santin M, Podzamczer D, Ricart I, Mascaro J, Ramon JM, Dominguez A, Rufi G, Gudiol F (1995) Utility of the gallium-67 citrate scan for the early diagnosis of tuberculosis in patients infected with the human immunodeficiency virus. Clin Infect Dis 20:652–656

18. Lee VW, Cooley TP, Fuller JD, Ward RJ, Farher HW (1994) Pulmonary mycobacterial infections in AIDS: characteristic pattern of thallium and gallium scan mismatch. Radiology 193:389–392

19. Sfakianalkis GN, Al-Sheikh W, Head A (1982) Comparison of scintigraphy with In-111 leukocytes and Ga-67 in the diagnosis of occult sepsis. J Nucl Med 23:618

20. Palestro CJ, Swyer AJ, Kim CK, Goldsmith SJ (1991). Relative efficacy of In-111 leukocyte and Ga-67 imaging in HIV (+) patients. J Nucl Med 32:1003

21. Pettengell K, Garb M, Houlder A, Becker P, Simjee A (1990) Radionuclide scintigraphy in tuberculous enteritis. Gastrointest Radiol 15:148–150

22. Fanning A, Dierich H, Lentle B (1974) Bone scanning with ⁹⁹ᵐTc polyphosphate in tuberculous osteomyelitis. Tubercle 55:227–230

23. Abdelwahab IF, Kenan S, Hermann G, Lewis M, Klein M, Rabinowitz JG (1991) Atypical skeletal tuberculosis mimicking neoplasm. Br J Radiol 64:551–555

24. Pui MH, Chin-Sang HR, Rubenstein JD (1986) False-normal bone imaging in spinal tuberculosis. Clin Nucl Med 11:245–248

25. Muradali D, Gold WL, Vellend H, Becker E (1993) Multifocal osteoarticular tuberculosis: report of four cases and review of management. Clin Infect Dis 17:204–208

26. Nocera RM, Sayle B, Rogers C, Wilkey D (1983) Tc-99m MDP Indium-111 chloride scintigraphy in skeletal tuberculosis. Clin Nucl Med 8:418–420

27. Rust RJ, Park HM, Robb JA (1981) Skeletal scintigraphy in miliary tuberculosis: photopenia after treatment. Am J Radiol 137:877–879

28. Tamgac F, Baillet G, Alper E, Delporte MP, Moretti JL (1995) Extraskeletal accumulation of Tc-99m HMDP in a tuberculous cold abscess. Clin Nucl Med 20:1092

29. Greenspan A, Stadainik RC (1995) Increased uptake around the hip joint. Semin Nucl Med 25:283–286

30. Sciuk J, Brandau W, Vollet B, Stucker R, Erlemann R, Bartenstein P, Peters PE, Schober O (1991) Comparison of technetium-99m polyclonal human immunoglobulin and technetium 99m monoclonal antibodies for imaging chronic osteomyelitis. First clinical results. Eur J Nucl Med 18:401–407

31. Sharif HS, Aideyan OA, Clark DC, Madkour MM, Aabed MY, Mattsson TA, Al-Deeb SM, Moutaery KR (1989) Brucellar and tuberculous spondylitis: comparative imaging features. Radiology 171:419–425

32. Kimmel DJ, Klingensmith WC III (1980) Unusual scintigraphic appearance of osteomyelitis secondary to atypical myobacterium. Clin Nucl Med 5:189–190

33. Ohta H, Ichii H, Arimoto A, Ukikusa M, Awane H (1998) Tc-99m sestamibi uptake in tuberculosis of the breast. Clin Nucl Med 23:106–108

34. Kobayashi H, Kotoura Y, Hosono M, Tsuboyama T, Sakahara H, Konishi J (1995) Solitary muscular involvement by tuberculosis: CT, MRI and scintigraphic features. Comput Med Imaging Graph 19:237–240

35. Somawardhana CW, Lambrecht RM (1989) [Iodine-124]-2-iodoisonicotinic acid hydrazide: a potential radiotracer for tuberculoma. J Nucl Med 30:1756

36. Somawardhana CW, Sajjad M, Amartey JK, Lambrecht RM (1991) Synthesis of 2-[¹²³I and ¹²⁴I]-iodoisonicotinic acid hydrazide: potential radiotracers for tuberculosis. Appl Radiat Isot 42:215–220

Subject Index